New Perspectives in Rehabilitation after Traumatic Brain Injury

New Perspectives in Rehabilitation after Traumatic Brain Injury

Editors

Nada Andelic
Cecilie Røe
Eirik Helseth
Emilie Isager Howe
Marit Vindal Forslund
Torgeir Hellstrom

MDPI • Basel • Beijing • Wuhan • Barcelona • Belgrade • Manchester • Tokyo • Cluj • Tianjin

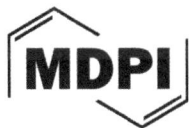

Editors

Nada Andelic
University of Oslo
Norway

Cecilie Røe
Oslo University Hospital
Norway

Eirik Helseth
Oslo University Hospital
Norway

Emilie Isager Howe
Oslo University Hospital
Norway

Marit Vindal Forslund
Oslo University Hospital
Norway

Torgeir Hellstrom
Oslo University Hospital
Norway

Editorial Office
MDPI
St. Alban-Anlage 66
4052 Basel, Switzerland

This is a reprint of articles from the Special Issue published online in the open access journal *Journal of Clinical Medicine* (ISSN 2077-0383) (available at: https://www.mdpi.com/journal/jcm/special_issues/Rehabilitation_Traumatic_Brain_Injury).

For citation purposes, cite each article independently as indicated on the article page online and as indicated below:

LastName, A.A.; LastName, B.B.; LastName, C.C. Article Title. *Journal Name* **Year**, *Volume Number*, Page Range.

ISBN 978-3-0365-5621-5 (Hbk)
ISBN 978-3-0365-5622-2 (PDF)

© 2022 by the authors. Articles in this book are Open Access and distributed under the Creative Commons Attribution (CC BY) license, which allows users to download, copy and build upon published articles, as long as the author and publisher are properly credited, which ensures maximum dissemination and a wider impact of our publications.

The book as a whole is distributed by MDPI under the terms and conditions of the Creative Commons license CC BY-NC-ND.

Contents

About the Editors vii

Preface to "New Perspectives in Rehabilitation after Traumatic Brain Injury" ix

Vanessa M. Young, Juan R. Hill, Michele Patrini, Stefano Negrini and Chiara Arienti
Overview of Cochrane Systematic Reviews of Rehabilitation Interventions for Persons with Traumatic Brain Injury: A Mapping Synthesis
Reprinted from: *J. Clin. Med.* **2022**, *11*, 2691, doi:10.3390/jcm11102691 1

Cathrine Tverdal, Nada Andelic, Eirik Helseth, Cathrine Brunborg, Pål Rønning, Torgeir Hellstrøm, Cecilie Røe and Mads Aarhus
In the Aftermath of Acute Hospitalization for Traumatic Brain Injury: Factors Associated with the Direct Pathway into Specialized Rehabilitation
Reprinted from: *J. Clin. Med.* **2021**, *10*, 3577, doi:10.3390/jcm10163577 19

Maud Stenberg, Britt-Marie Stålnacke and Britt-Inger Saveman
Health and Well-Being of Persons of Working Age up to Seven Years after Severe Traumatic Brain Injury in Northern Sweden: A Mixed Method Study
Reprinted from: *J. Clin. Med.* **2022**, *11*, 1306, doi:10.3390/jcm11051306 33

Daniel Løke, Nada Andelic, Eirik Helseth, Olav Vassend, Stein Andersson, Jennie L. Ponsford, Cathrine Tverdal, Cathrine Brunborg and Marianne Løvstad
Impact of Somatic Vulnerability, Psychosocial Robustness and Injury-Related Factors on Fatigue following Traumatic Brain Injury—A Cross-Sectional Study
Reprinted from: *J. Clin. Med.* **2022**, *11*, 1733, doi:10.3390/jcm11061733 51

Natascha Ekdahl, Alison K. Godbolt, Catharina Nygren Deboussard, Marianne Lannsjö, Britt-Marie Stålnacke, Maud Stenberg, Trandur Ulfarsson and Marika C. Möller
Cognitive Reserve, Early Cognitive Screening, and Relationship to Long-Term Outcome after Severe Traumatic Brain Injury
Reprinted from: *J. Clin. Med.* **2022**, *11*, 2046, doi:10.3390/jcm11072046 71

Laraine Winter, Janell L. Mensinger, Helene J. Moriarty, Keith M. Robinson, Michelle McKay and Benjamin E. Leiby
Age Moderates the Effect of Injury Severity on Functional Trajectories in Traumatic Brain Injury: A Study Using the NIDILRR Traumatic Brain Injury Model Systems National Dataset
Reprinted from: *J. Clin. Med.* **2022**, *11*, 2477, doi:10.3390/jcm11092477 83

Ida M. H. Borgen, Solveig L. Hauger, Marit V. Forslund, Ingerid Kleffelgård, Cathrine Brunborg, Nada Andelic, Unni Sveen, Helene L. Søberg, Solrun Sigurdardottir, Cecilie Røe and Marianne Løvstad
Goal Attainment in an Individually Tailored and Home-Based Intervention in the Chronic Phase after Traumatic Brain Injury
Reprinted from: *J. Clin. Med.* **2022**, *11*, 958, doi:10.3390/jcm11040958 93

Ingvil Laberg Holthe, Nina Rohrer-Baumgartner, Edel J. Svendsen, Solveig Lægreid Hauger, Marit Vindal Forslund, Ida M. H. Borgen, Hege Prag Øra, Ingerid Kleffelgård, Anine Pernille Strand-Saugnes, Jens Egeland, Cecilie Røe, Shari L. Wade and Marianne Løvstad
Feasibility and Acceptability of a Complex Telerehabilitation Intervention for Pediatric Acquired Brain Injury: The Child in Context Intervention (CICI)
Reprinted from: *J. Clin. Med.* **2022**, *11*, 2564, doi:10.3390/jcm11092564 111

Elinor E. Fraser, Marina G. Downing, Kerrie Haines, Linda Bennett, John Olver and Jennie Ponsford
Evaluating a Novel Treatment Adapting a Cognitive Behaviour Therapy Approach for Sexuality Problems after Traumatic Brain Injury: A Single Case Design with Nonconcurrent Multiple Baselines
Reprinted from: *J. Clin. Med.* 2022, 11, 3525, doi:10.3390/jcm11123525 135

Aleksi J. Sihvonen, Sini-Tuuli Siponkoski, Noelia Martínez-Molina, Sari Laitinen,
Milla Holma, Mirja Ahlfors, Linda Kuusela, Johanna Pekkola, Sanna Koskinen and
Teppo Särkämö
Neurological Music Therapy Rebuilds Structural Connectome after Traumatic Brain Injury: Secondary Analysis from a Randomized Controlled Trial
Reprinted from: *J. Clin. Med.* 2022, 11, 2184, doi:10.3390/jcm11082184 153

Francesco Latini, Markus Fahlström, Fredrik Vedung, Staffan Stensson, Elna-Marie Larsson,
Mark Lubberink, Yelverton Tegner, Sven Haller, Jakob Johansson, Anders Wall,
Gunnar Antoni and Niklas Marklund
Refined Analysis of Chronic White Matter Changes after Traumatic Brain Injury and Repeated Sports-Related Concussions: Of Use in Targeted Rehabilitative Approaches?
Reprinted from: *J. Clin. Med.* 2022, 11, 358, doi:10.3390/jcm11020358 165

Hui Xu, Xiuping Zhang and Guanghui Bai
Abnormal Dorsal Caudate Activation Mediated Impaired Cognitive Flexibility in Mild Traumatic Brain Injury
Reprinted from: *J. Clin. Med.* 2022, 11, 2484, doi:10.3390/jcm11092484 181

Qiang Xue, Linbo Wang, Yuanyu Zhao, Wusong Tong, Jiancun Wang, Gaoyi Li, Wei Cheng,
Liang Gao and Yan Dong
Cortical and Subcortical Alterations and Clinical Correlates after Traumatic Brain Injury
Reprinted from: *J. Clin. Med.* 2022, 11, 4421, doi:10.3390/jcm11154421 195

About the Editors

Nada Andelic

Nada Andelic (MD, PhD, Prof.) is a consultant physiatrist, Head of Research and Development, Dept of Physical Medicine and Rehabilitation, Oslo University Hospital, and Professor in Rehabilitation models and Services, Faculty of Medicine, University of Oslo. Her main research focus is on the outcomes of traumatic brain injury and multiple trauma, rehabilitation trajectories, rehabilitation- and health care needs and rehabilitation interventions.

Cecilie Røe

Cecilie Røe (MD, PhD, Prof.) is Head of the Dept. of Physical Medcine and Rehabilitation, Oslo University Hospital, Professor in Physical Medicine and Rehabilitation, Faculty of Medicine, University of Oslo and Head of the reasearch group painful conditions in the musculoskeletal system. She has an extensive research carereer, focused on the consequences of trauma, treatement and rehabilitation, as well as the underlying mechanisms, treatment and rehabiliation of long-term pain conditions.

Eirik Helseth

Eirik Helseth (MD, PhD, Prof.) is a consultant neurosurgeon at the Dept. of Neurosurgery, Oslo University Hospital, and Professor in Neurosurgery, Faculty of Medicine, University of Oslo. He has an extensive professional and research career focusing on the epidemiology of, risk factors for and outcomes after neurotrauma including traumatic brain injury.

Emilie Isager Howe

Emilie Isager Howe (Cand. Psych., PhD) is a clinical psychologist with a specialization in neuropsychology. She is employed at the Dept. of Physical Medicine and Rehabilitation, Oslo University Hospital and a member of the Rehabilitation after Trauma research group. She completed her PhD thesis on employment after traumatic brain injury, and has been involved in several national and international research projects.

Marit Vindal Forslund

Marit Vindal Forslund (MD, PhD) is a resident and postdoctoral fellow at the Dept. of Physical Medicine and Rehabilitation, Oslo University Hospital. Her main research focus is on outcomes, health care needs and rehabilitation interventions after traumatic brain injury.

Torgeir Hellstrom

Torgeir Hellstrom (MD, PhD) is a consultant physiatrist at the Dept. of Physical Medicine and Rehabilitation, Oslo University Hospital and a member of the Rehabilitation after Trauma research group. His main research focus is on outcomes after traumatic brain injuries and multiple trauma, rehabilitation interventions and imaging diagnostics.

Preface to "New Perspectives in Rehabilitation after Traumatic Brain Injury"

There has been increased focus on the evaluation of the scientific knowledge base within the field of traumatic brain injury (TBI) rehabilitation. TBI rehabilitation comprises several phases, from acute medical care to post-acute care in rehabilitation facilities and chronic care in the community. Rehabilitation is a multidisciplinary effort that covers the full spectrum of medical neuroscience, cognitive neuroscience, pharmacology, brain imaging, and assistive and smart technology. A future challenge is to integrate these areas to guide TBI rehabilitation into extensive research and clinical practice. Our goal is to provide a stronger base of scientific information on ongoing knowledge gaps and controversies, and focus on new perspectives regarding the rehabilitation and management of TBI.

Nada Andelic, Cecilie Røe, Eirik Helseth, Emilie Isager Howe, Marit Vindal Forslund and Torgeir Hellstrom

Editors

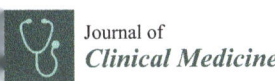

Review

Overview of Cochrane Systematic Reviews of Rehabilitation Interventions for Persons with Traumatic Brain Injury: A Mapping Synthesis

Vanessa M. Young [1], Juan R. Hill [2], Michele Patrini [3], Stefano Negrini [3,4,*] and Chiara Arienti [5]

[1] School of Social and Behavioral Sciences, Arizona State University, Phoenix, AZ 85051, USA; vmyoung1@asu.edu
[2] Independent Researcher, San Diego, CA 92108, USA; ricardo2hill@gmail.com
[3] Laboratory of Evidence-Based Rehabilitation, IRCCS Istituto Ortopedico Galeazzi, 20161 Milan, Italy; mikepatrini@gmail.com
[4] Department of Biomedical, Surgical and Dental Sciences, University La Statale, 20122 Milan, Italy
[5] IRCCS Fondazione Don Carlo Gnocchi, 20148 Milan, Italy; carienti@dongnocchi.it
* Correspondence: stefano.negrini@unimi.it

Abstract: Background: The World Health Organization has identified an unmet global need for rehabilitation interventions concerning 20 non-communicable diseases, traumatic brain injury included. This overview compiles and synthesizes the quality and quantity of available evidence on the effectiveness of rehabilitation interventions for traumatic brain injury from Cochrane systematic reviews (CSRs). The results will be used to develop the Package of Interventions for Rehabilitation. Methods: All CSRs on TBI tagged in the Cochrane Rehabilitation database published between August 2009 and September 2021 were included. Evidence mapping was implemented to extract study characteristics and evidence from the CSRs. Results: Six CSRs (42 studies; n = 3983) examined the effectiveness of either non-pharmacological or pharmacological interventions after TBI. Among 19 comparisons, 3% were rated as high in quality of evidence, 9% moderate, 54% low, and 34% very low. Non-pharmacological interventions with moderate quality, hospital-based cognitive rehabilitation and cognitive didactic therapy, likely produced minimal to no changes in the return-to-work rate. Anti-epileptic drugs and neuroprotective agents resulted in a minimal difference to the frequency of late seizure episodes in post-traumatic epilepsy. Conclusions: No prominent advances in treatment options were reported in any of the CSRs. The high rate of low and very low quality of evidence makes it difficult to ascertain the effectiveness of several recommended non-pharmacological interventions.

Keywords: brain injuries; traumatic; interventions; treatment outcome; rehabilitation; overview

1. Introduction

The World Health Organization (WHO) has described an unmet global need for the delivery of rehabilitation interventions in health systems, which is amplified in low- and middle-income countries with limited availability of resources [1–3]. The 'WHO Rehabilitation 2030 Call for Action' [2] was therefore launched. One of the main actions considered is the development of a Package of Interventions for Rehabilitation (PIR) [3,4]. The PIR aims at promoting favorable outcomes, accessibility, and the integration of multidisciplinary/interdisciplinary rehabilitation services into healthcare systems worldwide [3,4]. The WHO identified 20 major noncommunicable diseases to be investigated to develop the PIR; among these is traumatic brain injury (TBI) [4].

TBI is defined as 'any alteration in brain function or other evidence of brain pathology caused by an external force' [5] and it is estimated to affect 69,000 individuals worldwide annually [6]. Alterations in brain function may include any of the following: loss of (or decrease in) consciousness; loss of memory of events immediately preceding or following the injury; neurologic deficits (e.g., loss of balance or vision); or altered mental status, such as disorientation or confusion at the time of the injury [5]. TBI can be categorized into three possible diagnostic levels (mild, moderate, or severe), typically after evaluation using the Glasgow Outcome Scale or Glasgow Outcome Scale Extended [7,8] or by assessing structural imaging, loss of consciousness, altered consciousness, or post-traumatic amnesia.

Research has identified falls and road injuries as the two main causes of TBI worldwide [9,10], although causes of TBI have been found to differ across countries, depending on income, geographical region, and political circumstances [9,11]. Other common causes include sports-related concussions, assault, interpersonal violence, and blast injuries [12]. The direct consequences of a single TBI or repetitive insults include many possible long-term sequelae that vary according to age, sex, and the nature of the injury [13,14]. Common secondary pathophysiological conditions include seizures, sleep disorders, neurodegenerative diseases, neuroendocrine dysregulation, and psychiatric issues, each of which may persist throughout the long-term recovery process following moderate-to-severe TBI [15]. Due to these numerous clinical and demographic variables, TBI patients often experience nonlinear recovery trends, and those with moderate and severe cases are reported to show deteriorating Glasgow Outcome Scale Extended scores over time [16]. These unfavorable outcomes can hinder functioning, quality of life, and employment, and may worsen pre-existing conditions [17], further highlighting the chronic health issues associated with TBI as well as the need for complex rehabilitative programs and long-term services to support this group of patients [16].

A major step to the development of the PIR encompasses the "Best Evidence for Rehabilitation" (be4rehab) approach, which is applied to this work. Be4rehab supports the gathering of best evidence on the effectiveness and quality of pharmacological and non-pharmacological rehabilitation interventions for individuals with TBI and the delivery of this overview of Cochrane systematic reviews (CSRs) [4]. Overviews of systematics reviews are a methodological approach proposed by Cochrane to compile and synthesize data from multiple systematic reviews into one single, accessible document. All overviews requested by the WHO are restricted to CSRs to preserve the coherence and quality of the gathered evidence.

Supplemented by evidence mapping to aid in the synthesis of available evidence, this work aims at identifying the broad quality and the quantity of evidence, published in CSRs, on the effectiveness of rehabilitation interventions in person with TBI.

2. Materials and Methods

The WHO PIR adheres to methods designed from the collaborative efforts of the WHO Rehabilitation Programme and Cochrane Rehabilitation, and the directives from the WHO Guidelines Review Committee [4]. We used evidence mapping to synthesize and visualize study characteristics and evidence from CSRs on TBI. The overview was registered in Open Science Framework Registries (https://doi.org/0.17605/OSF.IO/M5XVG) and was reported following the Preferred Reporting Items for Systematic Reviews and Meta-analysis (PRISMA 2020 statement) [18].

2.1. Search Strategy

According to the methodology developed by the Cochrane Rehabilitation [19], CSRs relevant to rehabilitation are continuously tagged to maintain an up-to-date database (https://rehabilitation.cochrane.org/evidence, accessed on 1 September 2019). We initially searched all CSRs related to TBI published between August 2009 and August 2019 and reported the results to the WHO. We subsequently searched the Cochrane Library to August 2021 to preserve the timeliness of evidence. Eligible CSRs included those assessing interventions for persons with TBI provided or prescribed by rehabilitation professionals [19].

We included only tagged CSRs that examined rehabilitation interventions on individuals with TBI, of any age and gender. CSRs focused on persons with acquired brain injury or non-traumatic brain injury were excluded to ensure that the evidence synthesis is strictly applicable to persons who sustained a TBI.

2.2. Assessment of Methodological Quality of Included Studies

The methodological quality of each CSR was appraised by two assessors using the 16-item A Measurement Tool to Assess Systematic Reviews (AMSTAR) 2 tool. In this updated version, the 16 items are scored on a binary yes or no scale. AMSTAR-2 does not generate an 'overall score'; a high score may disguise weaknesses in 7 critical items [20]. The assessors adopted a process of 'considered judgment', which entails (1) interpreting weaknesses detected by the critical items and (2) reaching a consensus on the methodological quality of each CSR. Disagreements were resolved through discussion with a third assessor.

2.3. Data Extraction and Quality of Evidence Appraisal

The authors referred to the Table of Findings presented in each of the included CSRs; these contain the following data: type of outcome, outcome measure(s), number of primary studies, sample sizes, type of population, intervention, comparator(s), and effect (i.e., no effect, in favor of intervention, or in favor of comparator). Data were collected and entered into an Excel datasheet.

In addition, the quality of evidence for each outcome was extracted using the Grading of Recommendations Assessment, Development, and Evaluation (GRADE) rating system. For CSRs that did not include GRADE ratings, two members of the Cochrane Rehabilitation team independently appraised the quality of evidence for the primary outcomes only using the GRADE approach [21]. Any disagreement was resolved through consensus decision-making involving a third author [22]. The GRADE appraisal approach included two steps: (1) retrieval of the original primary studies included in each CSR; and (2) tabulation of the quality of evidence provided in Summary of Findings tables using GRADEPro software.

2.4. Summarizing the Data with an Evidence Map

Quality of evidence and effect data were transferred into evidence maps developed in Excel. The evidence map integrates the outcome and rehabilitation intervention values for each comparison. The magnitude of the effect (i.e., no effect, in favor of intervention, or in favor of comparator) and the quality of evidence (i.e., very low, low, moderate, or high) were presented laterally and color-coded for each outcome in order to generate a visual aid to facilitate the understanding of the overall judgement of the evidence.

Evidence mapping was employed as a complementary method to collating and appraising evidence from the CSRs, and subsequently used to summarize the results for the overview. The instrument collated outcomes and rehabilitation interventions and resulted in a comprehensive overview of the quality of evidence and effects. Because we did not consider other outcomes and interventions in addition to the those examined in the included CSRs, evidence mapping was not used to identify evidence gaps.

3. Results

The authors identified six tagged CSRs related to TBI: one published in 2013 [23], two in 2015 [24,25], and three in 2017 [26–28] (see Figure 1).

Three CSRs included only participants who sustained a TBI and excluded people with acquired brain injury and non-traumatic injury. Two CSRs included studies with a mixed population only when disaggregated data were reported to ensure that evidence was relevant to TBI. Finally, one CSR reported including studies where the etiology of the TBI is uncertain. The characteristics of the included systematic reviews are reported in Table 1.

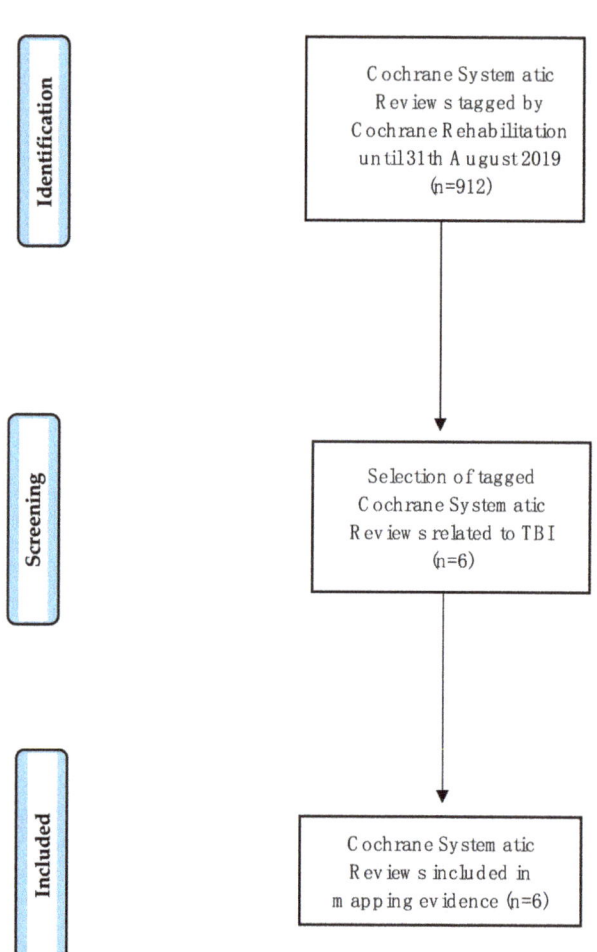

Figure 1. Flow chart displaying the tagging process of Cochrane systematic review.

Comprehensively, this mapping review encompasses 42 primary studies, 3983 participants, and 19 comparisons that examined the effectiveness and safety of either non-pharmacological or pharmacological interventions for individuals with TBI. Among non-pharmacological comparisons, four interventions (six outcomes) were categorized as very low quality of evidence, and eight interventions (16 outcomes) were deemed as low quality of evidence. Among the pharmacological comparisons, we found that four interventions (six outcomes) were rated very low and three interventions (three outcomes) were rated low in quality. The AMSTAR 2 assessment tool identified high methodological quality in the six CSRs; even when sources of funding were not reported. Results of the AMSTAR 2 assessment are displayed in Table 2.

Table 1. Characteristics of included systematic reviews.

Author (Year)	Population	Primary Outcome	Outcome Measure	Intervention	Comparator	Effect	Quality
Hassett et al., 2017 [26]	People with TBI; any age and sex	Cardiorespiratory fitness	Submaximal incremental cycle ergometer test	Exercise using large muscle	Usual care, a non-exercise intervention, or no intervention	Favor intervention	Low
Kumar (2017) [27]	Adults (≥16 years); any sex; any severity	Return to work	Attainment of work within 14 weeks (medium-term) of initiating intervention	Cognitive rehabilitation therapy	No treatment	None	Very low
		Community integration	Sydney Psychosocial Reintegration Scale (self-reported)	Cognitive rehabilitation therapy	No treatment	None	Low
		Return to work	Return to work status Follow-up: 6 months (medium-term)	Cognitive rehabilitation therapy	Conventional therapy	None	Low
		Independence in activities of daily living	Functional independence measure, with 18 items in basic and psychosocial functional activities	Cognitive rehabilitation therapy	Conventional therapy	None	Very low
		Community integration	Community integration questionnaire	Cognitive rehabilitation therapy	Conventional therapy	None	Low
		Return to work	Return to work status Follow-up: 24 months (long-term)	Hospital-based cognitive rehabilitation therapy	Home programme	None	Moderate
		Return to work	Return to work status follow-up: 1 year (medium-term)	Cognitive didactic therapy	Functional experiential therapy	None	Moderate
		Independence in activities of daily living	Structured interview follow-up: 1 year (medium-term)	Cognitive didactic therapy	Functional experiential therapy	None	Low
Synnot (2017) [28]	Children and adults who had skeletal muscle spasticity post injury. Any severity	Spasticity at up to 6 h after treatment	Ashworth Scale, 0–, with a higher score indicating greater spasticity	Intrathecal baclofen 50 µg (injected into the lumbar spine)	Saline placebo	Not reported	Very low
		Adverse events		Intrathecal baclofen 50 µg (injected into the lumbar spine)	Saline placebo	Not reported	Very low

Table 1. Cont.

Author (Year)	Population	Primary Outcome	Outcome Measure	Intervention	Comparator	Effect	Quality
		Spasticity at 4–12 weeks	Modified Ashworth scale, 0–5, at 12 weeks and Tardieu scale, 0–5, at 4 weeks	Botulinum toxin A × 1 dose (500/1000 U) or botulinum toxin A × 1 dose of 200 U + serial casting	Placebo (±casting)	Uncertain	Very low
		Adverse events		Botulinum toxin A × 1 dose (500/1000 U) or botulinum toxin A × 1 dose of 200 U + serial casting	Placebo (±casting)	Uncertain	Very low
		Spasticity at up to 6 h after treatment	Modified Ashworth scale, 0–4, with a higher score indicating greater spasticity	Repositioning splints equipped with participant-specific pseudoelastic hinges	Traditional splints with fixed angle braces	Uncertain	Very low
		Adverse events		Repositioning splints equipped with participant-specific pseudoelastic hinges	Traditional splints with fixed angle braces	Uncertain	Very low
Gertler (2015) [24]	Children and adults with depression after TBI; any severity	Depression	Beck depression inventory-II, Hamilton Rating Scale for Depression, and Hospital Anxiety and Depression Scale; higher score means more depressed	Cognitive behavioral therapy	Wait-list control	None	Very low
		Depression	Beck Depression Inventory; higher score means more depressed	Cognitive behavioral therapy	Supportive psychotherapy	None	Very Low
		Depression	Hamilton Rating Scale for Depression; higher score means more depressed	Repetitive transcranial magnetic stimulation	Repetitive transcranial magnetic stimulation plus tricyclic antidepressant	Favor control	Very low
		Depression	Beck Depression Inventory; higher score means more depression	Supervised exercises	Exercise as usual	None	Low

Table 1. *Cont.*

Author (Year)	Population	Primary Outcome	Outcome Measure	Intervention	Comparator	Effect	Quality
Thompson (2015) [25]	People with TBI who received prophylactic treatment with antiepileptic drugs or neuroprotective agents. Any age; any severity; acute	Early seizures Follow-up: 5–7 days	Count of Events	Antiepileptic drugs	Placebo or standard care	Favor intervention	Low
		Late seizures Follow-up: 3–24 months	Count of Events	Antiepileptic drugs	Placebo or standard care	None	Very low
		Early seizure Follow-up: 7 days	Count of Events	Neuroprotective agents	Placebo	None	Low
		Late seizure Follow-up: 6 months	Count of Events	Neuroprotective agents	Placebo	None	High
		Early seizure Follow-up: 7 days	Count of Events	Phenytoin	Other antiepileptic drugs	None	Low
		Late seizure Follow up: 6 months to 2 years	Count of Events	Phenytoin	Other antiepileptic drugs	None	Moderate
Wong (2013) [23]	People with TBI. Any age, sex, and severity	Post-treatment Modified Barthel Index-1 month post-treatment	Barthel index	Electro-acupuncture plus rehabilitation training	Rehabilitation training	Favor intervention	Low
		Post-treatment Modified Barthel Index-3 months post-treatment	Barthel index	Electro-acupuncture plus rehabilitation training	Rehabilitation training	Favor control	Low
		Post-treatment Fugl-Meyer assessment-1 month post-treatment	Fugl-Meyer Assessment	Electro-acupuncture plus rehabilitation training	Rehabilitation training	Favor intervention	Low
		Post-treatment Fugl-Meyer assessment-3 months post-treatment	Fugl-Meyer Assessment	Electro-acupuncture plus rehabilitation training	Rehabilitation training	Favor intervention	Low

Table 1. Cont.

Author (Year)	Population	Primary Outcome	Outcome Measure	Intervention	Comparator	Effect	Quality
		Post-treatment Glasgow Outcome score	Glasgow Outcome Scale	Needle acupuncture plus conventional medical intervention	Conventional medical intervention	Favor intervention	Low
		Post-treatment Glasgow Coma score	Glasgow Coma Scale	Needle acupuncture plus conventional medical intervention	Conventional medical intervention	Favor intervention	Low
		Frequency of normal post-treatment Glasgow Outcome score	Glasgow Outcome Scale	Electro-acupuncture plus conventional medical intervention	Conventional medical intervention	Favor intervention	Low
		Mortality		Electro-acupuncture plus conventional medical intervention	Conventional medical intervention	None	Low
		Frequency of post-treatment Barthel index above 60	Barthel index	Electro-acupuncture plus hyperbaric oxygen and rehabilitation training	Hyperbaric oxygen and rehabilitation training	Favor intervention	Low
		Frequency of post-treatment Barthel index above 40	Barthel index	Electro-acupuncture plus hyperbaric oxygen and rehabilitation training	Hyperbaric oxygen and rehabilitation training	None	Low

Abbreviation: TBI = traumatic brain injury.

Table 2. AMSTAR 2 Quality Assessment of Cochrane Systematic Reviews.

	Hassett 2017 [26]	Kumar 2017 [27]	Synnot 2017 [28]	Gertler 2015 [24]	Thompson 2015 [25]	Wong 2013 [23]
(1) Did the research questions and inclusion criteria for the review include the components of PICO?	Y	Y	Y	Y	Y	Y
(2) Did the report of the review contain an explicit statement that the review methods were established prior to the conduct of the review and did the report justify any significant deviations from the protocol?	Y	Y	Y	Y	Y	Y
(3) Did the review authors explain their selection of the study designs for inclusion in the review?	Y	Y	Y	Y	Y	Y
(4) Did the review authors use a comprehensive literature search strategy?	Y	Y	Y	Y	Y	Y
(5) Did the review authors perform study selection in duplicate?	Y	Y	Y	Y	Y	Y
(6) Did the review authors perform data extraction in duplicate?	Y	Y	Y	Y	Y	Y
(7) Did the review authors provide a list of excluded studies and justify the exclusions?	Y	Y	Y	Y	Y	Y
(8) Did the review authors describe the included studies in adequate detail?	Y	Y	Y	Y	Y	Y
(9) Did the review authors use a satisfactory technique for assessing the risk of bias (RoB) in individual studies that were included in the review?	Y	Y	Y	Y	Y	Y
(10) Did the review authors report on the sources of funding for the studies included in the review?	N	N	N	N	N	N
(11) If meta-analysis was performed did the review authors use appropriate methods for statistical combination of results?	Y	Y	Y	Y	Y	Y
(12) If meta-analysis was performed, did the review authors assess the potential impact of RoB in individual studies on the results of the meta-analysis or other evidence synthesis?	Y	Y	Y	Y	Y	Y
(13) Did the review authors account for RoB in individual studies when interpreting/discussing the results of the review?	Y	Y	Y	Y	Y	Y
(14) Did the review authors provide a satisfactory explanation for, and discussion of, any heterogeneity observed in the results of the review?	Y	Y	Y	Y	Y	Y
(15) If they performed quantitative synthesis did the review authors carry out an adequate investigation of publication bias (small study bias) and discuss its likely impact on the results of the review?	Y	Y	Y	Y	Y	Y
(16) Did the review authors report any potential sources of conflict of interest, including any funding they received for conducting the review?	Y	Y	Y	Y	Y	Y
Total	15	15	15	15	15	15

Abbreviations: Y = Yes, N = No.

The evidence map findings were divided into two categories: (1) non-pharmacological interventions and (2) pharmacological interventions. Table 3 provides an overview of evidence map finding for non-pharmacological interventions for TBI. Table 4 provides an overview of evidence map finding for pharmacological interventions for TBI.

Table 3. Evidence map of non-pharmacological interventions.

Intervention	Comparison	Outcome	GRADE			
			H	M	L	VL
Cognitive rehabilitation	No treatment	Return to work				⊗
		Community integration			⊗	
	Conventional Therapy	Return to work			⊗	
		Community integration			⊗	
		Activities of daily living				⊗
Hospital-based cognitive rehabilitation	Home-based cognitive rehabilitation	Return to work		⊗		
Cognitive didactic therapy	Functional experiential therapy	Return to work		⊗		
		Activities of daily living			⊗	
Cognitive behavioral therapy	Supportive psychotherapy	Depression				⊗
	Waitlist					⊗
Supervised exercise	Exercise as usual	Depression			⊗	
Large muscle group exercise	Usual care, non-exercise, no intervention	Cardiorespiratory fitness				✓
Repositioning splints	Traditional splints	Spasticity				?
		Adverse events				?
Electro-acupuncture + Rehabilitation training	Rehabilitation training	Modified Barthel Index (1 mo)				✓
		Modified Barthel Index (3 mo)				✗
		Fugl-MeyerAssessment (1 mo)				✓
		Fugl-MeyerAssessment (3 mo)				✓
Needle-acupuncture + Conventional medical intervention	Conventional medical intervention	Post-Treatment Glasgow Outcome Scale				✓
		Post-Treatment Glasgow Coma Score				✓
Electro-acupuncture + Conventional medical intervention	Conventional medical mntervention	Frequency of Normal Glasgow Coma Score				✓
		Mortality				⊗
Electro-acupuncture + Hyperbanic oxygen	Rehabilitation training vs. Hyperbanic oxygen and rehabilitation training	Frequency Barthel > 60				✓
		Frequency Barthel > 40				⊗

High = H; M = Moderate; Low = L; VL = Very low; No effect = ⊗, Favor Intervention = ✓, Favor Comparator = ✗, Uncertain = ?.

3.1. Quality of Evidence Mapping for Non-Pharmacological Interventions

3.1.1. Moderate Quality of Evidence

Hospital-based versus home-based cognitive rehabilitation likely has little to no effect on the return-to-work rate for moderate-to-severe TBI (1 study; n = 120) [26]. Similarly, cognitive didactic versus functional experiential therapy likely has little to no effect on the same outcome for moderate-to-severe TBI (1 study, n = 366) [26].

Table 4. Evidence map of pharmacological interventions.

Intervention	Comparison	Outcome	Grade H	Grade M	Grade L	Grade VL
Neuroprotective agents	Placebo	Early seizure			⊗	
Neuroprotective agents	Placebo	Late seizure (6 mo)	⊗			
Antiepileptic drugs	Placebo	Early seizure			✓	
Antiepileptic drugs	Placebo	Late seizure (3–24 mo)				⊗
Phenytoin	Antiepileptic drugs	Early seizure			⊗	
Phenytoin	Antiepileptic drugs	Late seizure (6–24 mo)		⊗		
Repetitive transcranial magnetic stimulation	repetitive transcranial magnetic stimulation plus tricyclic antidepressants	Depression				✗
Baclofen 50 μg	Saline placebo	Spasticity				NR
Baclofen 50 μg	Saline placebo	Adverse events				NR
Botulinum toxin A × 1 dose (500/1000 U) or botulinum toxin A × 1 dose 200 U+	Placebo	Spasticity				?
Botulinum toxin A × 1 dose (500/1000 U) or botulinum toxin A × 1 dose 200 U+	Placebo	Adverse events				?

Abbreviations: High = H; M = Moderate; Low = L; VL = Very low; No effect = ⊗; Favor Intervention = ✓; Favor Comparator = ✗; Uncertain = ?; Not reported = NR.

3.1.2. Low Quality of Evidence

Exercise using large muscle groups may have little to no effect on the cardiorespiratory fitness compared to usual care in severe and unspecified TBI severity levels (3 studies, $n = 67$) [27].

Cognitive rehabilitation may have little or no effect compared to no treatment on community integration in severe TBI (1 study; $n = 12$) [26], while it may have little to no effect relative to conventional therapy on return to work (1 study; $n = 68$) [26], and community integration (3 studies; $n = 123$) [26] in mild-to-severe TBI, respectively.

Electro-acupuncture as an adjunct treatment to rehabilitation training may have a positive effect on sensorimotor impairment (Fugl-Meyer Assessment) at 1 and 3 months, and on disability (Modified Barthel index) at 1 month, but not at 3 months, when the effects favored rehabilitation training alone (unspecified TBI severity; 1 study; $n = 150$) [23]. When added to conventional medical intervention, electro-acupuncture may make little to no difference to mortality rate, but it may increase the frequency of normal Glasgow Coma Score evaluations in coma patients with severe TBI (1 study, $n = 50$) [23]. Added to hyperbaric oxygen and rehabilitation training, electro-acupuncture may have an effect on the percentage of patients decreasing to moderate disability (Barthel Index > 60) but there is uncertainty on the effects on reducing its severity (Barthel Index > 40) (unspecified TBI severity; 1 study; $n = 122$) [23].

3.1.3. Very Low Quality of Evidence

In mild-to-moderate TBI, the true effect of cognitive rehabilitation remains uncertain on return-to-work when compared to no treatment (1 study; $n = 50$) [26]; on activities of daily living when compared to conventional therapy (unspecified TBI severity; 2 studies, $n = 41$) [26]; on depression level versus waiting list (3 studies, $n = 146$) [24] and supportive psychotherapy (1 study; $n = 48$) [24]. There is also uncertainty on the utility on spasticity (6 h post-treatment) of repositioning splints equipped with participant-specific pseudoelastic hinges versus traditional splints with fixed angle braces for pediatric TBI (unspecified TBI severity; 1 study; $n = 25$) [28].

3.2. Quality of Evidence Mapping for Pharmacological Interventions

3.2.1. High Quality of Evidence

Neuroprotective agents had little to no effect versus placebo on late seizures 6 months after the start of treatment in moderate-to-severe TBI in participants aged 14 and older (1 study; n = 498) [25].

3.2.2. Moderate Quality of Evidence

Phenytoin likely resulted in no changes in late seizures 6 to 24 months after the start of the treatment relative to other antiepileptic drugs in moderate-to-severe TBI (2 studies; n = 378) [25].

3.2.3. Low Quality of Evidence

There may be minimal effect on the frequency of early seizures (7 days) for neuroprotective agents compared to placebo, (moderate-to-severe TBI, 1 study, n = 499) [25]. Antiepileptic interventions compared with placebo may reduce the frequency of early seizures (moderate-to-severe, 5 studies, n=987) [25]. Neuroprotective agents versus other antiepileptic drugs may have minimal effect on adverse events (moderate-to-severe TBI, 2 studies, n = 431) [25].

3.2.4. Very Low Quality of Evidence

A review comparing baclofen 50 µg versus saline placebo included one study (n = 11) and examined the effects on spasticity (6 h), and adverse events [28]. The findings could not be extracted since they were not reported in the randomized control trial. The efficacy and safety of the intervention remain thereby unclear.

A review evaluated the efficacy of botulinum toxin A × 1 dose (500/1000 U) or botulinum toxin A × 1 dose of 200 U + serial casting versus placebo on spasticity (4–12 weeks post treatment), and adverse events (2 studies; n = 47) [28]. No statistically significant differences were detected between groups and the quality of evidence was rated very low. This hindered the ability to ascertain the true treatment effects of either intervention.

Evaluating 1029 participants and six studies, one CSR examined the difference in effects on late seizure occurrence (3 to 24 months after the start of the treatment) comparing between antiepileptic medications and placebo [25]. No significant differences were found for either outcome. The comparison was judged to provide very low quality of evidence, which indicates that the effects of antiepileptic interventions on these two outcomes remain uncertain.

In a total sample of 67 participants and one study, the reviewers found a significant difference in depression level between the repetitive transcranial magnetic stimulation and repetitive transcranial magnetic stimulation plus antidepressant groups (TBI severity unspecified) [24]. While the treatment effect was in favor of the comparator, repetitive transcranial magnetic stimulation plus tricyclic antidepressants, the true treatment effect remains uncertain due to the very low quality of evidence.

4. Discussion

This overview summarizes evidence on the effects of non-pharmacological and pharmacological interventions for any level of TBI severity, and reports the challenges identified in TBI research that are critical for further developing the integration and augmentation of rehabilitation services.

Amongst the options for non-pharmacological interventions, hospital-based cognitive rehabilitation and cognitive didactic therapy likely produce minimal or no changes in the return-to-work rate (moderate certainty evidence). These findings agree with published reports in the literature on neurocognitive status and the return-to-work rates, ref. [29–31] which maintain that favorable outcomes are facilitated by the inclusion of multidisciplinary/interdisciplinary rehabilitation services, and not by a monotherapy approach, such as cognitive rehabilitation or cognitive training alone [32,33]. Executive functions, especially sequencing and inhibitory control, are necessary to perform well at work and their status predicts the return-to-work rate following TBI [29]. Ensuring that available cognitive interventions and cognitive strategy training lead to improvements in cognitive functioning and are properly integrated in the rehabilitation management are crucial for increasing return-to-work rates, as well as improving life satisfaction and the wellbeing of individuals with TBI and their families.

The low-certainty of evidence found in acupuncture, splint therapy, and exercise of large muscle groups prevented us from ascertaining the role of these interventions on Glasgow Coma Scale scores, spasticity, and cardiorespiratory fitness, respectively. With respect to acupuncture, the lack of information on the etiology of the TBI from three of the four RCTs prevented us from determining whether the results are equally applicable to acquired brain injury, traumatic brain injury, and non-traumatic brain injury cases. Likewise, there is insufficient quality of evidence to support the roles of cognitive therapeutic approaches as monotherapy in improving community integration, depression, and activities of daily living (very low certainty evidence).

Amongst the pharmacological interventions used to reduce the number and frequency of late-seizure episodes (i.e., 6 months after the start of treatment; high-quality evidence), neuroprotective agents produced little to no difference on the frequency of late-seizures (high-quality evidence) and minimal differences on early seizures (low-quality evidence). The anti-convulsant drug, phenytoin, for example, appeared to have little effect on the number and frequency of late seizures (moderate quality evidence) and little to no effect on early-seizure events (low quality evidence). This finding aligns with current guidelines that support the use of phenytoin to treat early seizures or active seizures, but not late seizures [34].

Our evidence mapping shows that other antiepileptic drugs do not reduce the number and frequency of late seizure events. The literature primarily focuses on early seizures, and data on late seizures after TBI are limited. Discussions of study results typically note that no evidence supports the use of neuroprotective agents and antiepileptic drugs for late seizures, mainly due to the differences observed in studies on pathogenesis of early seizures in post-traumatic epilepsy [34,35]. This feature of post-TBI care warrants further attention since late seizure episodes may impair otherwise positive neurological and rehabilitation outcomes [36].

For the remaining two pharmacological interventions (botulinum toxin A × 1 dose (500/1000 U) or botulinum toxin A × 1 dose of 200 U + serial casting; intrathecal baclofen 50 µg), uncertainty of their effects on spasticity and adverse events remain, as the quality of evidence for these two therapies has been assessed as very low [28].

The absence and/or low quality of evidence for pharmacological interventions to reduce early- and late-seizure frequency, and improve spasticity, may be associated in part with the following situations: (1) research challenges exacerbated by the narrow window for effective intervention; (2) the inability of candidate medications to cross the blood–brain barrier; and (3) possible delays and ethical issues encountered when patients are unable to provide consent [37]. These difficulties are exacerbated among pediatric groups [38], which may explain the limited results for pediatric patients with TBI among the CSRs that analyzed pharmacological interventions.

The low to very- low quality evidence found is in accordance with past reviews that focused on clinical practice guidelines for TBI [39,40], which stressed the persistent paucity of quality evidence and the major gaps between the bench and the bedside in the context of rehabilitation interventions associated with both methodological issues and clinical complexity. The reviewers stated that few published trials examined rehabilitation outcomes, such as cognitive and physical function, with the majority of studies targeting symptom management or reduction [39,40].

For non-pharmacological trials, the primary issues concerned the number of studies and the small sample sizes (cumulative <500 participants), which affected the estimated effect sizes, heterogeneity among the respondents, and the imprecision of the results (i.e., wide 95% confidence intervals). Similar to pharmacological trials, some studies showed a lack of clarity regarding random sequence generation, blinding, and allocation concealment.

Overall, our evidence map shows that no prominent advances were reported in any of the CSRs, confirming the concerns expressed a decade ago by Maas et al. [41], who observed that randomized control trials (RCTs) fail to showcase significant recovery trajectories when assessing the effectiveness of interventions on TBI populations. Other study designs (e.g., observational) could provide additional insights when conducting systematic reviews for patients with TBI.

The landscape displayed by this evidence map places strong emphasis on the need to prioritize and augment rehabilitation research efforts for patients with TBI. Hence, we reiterate four priorities for bolstering the quality of evidence associated with rehabilitation outcomes: (1) revisit the recruitment and consent process and preserve ethical standards; (2) increase efforts and funding to support trials that examine functioning (i.e., cognitive, physical, and emotional); (3) consider multi-site recruitment options to increase participant diversity and sample sizes; (4) clearly identify the etiology of brain injury or offer disaggregate data in studies with mixed brain injury populations; and (5) promote the transparent reporting of adverse events, if applicable.

Strengths and Limitations

Evidence maps represent a novel approach that can be employed to detect broader issues, lead to research synthesis, and guide researchers in formulating both future research and studies with a narrower focus [42,43]. Evidence maps have been especially helpful in visualizing research contexts and appreciating how a specific focus fits into the broader research field [44]. In the case presented here, the evidence map aids in understanding how TBI research fits within the context of clinical research and where it stands overall in the field of rehabilitation.

A limitation that requires some discussion pertains to the search strategy. This overview exclusively analyzed systematic reviews published in the Cochrane library, which may have limited the inclusion of other high-quality systematic reviews on TBI. Nevertheless, Cochrane suggests this approach to preserve consistency in the results of the overview since the included works follow the same methodological standard [45].

We acknowledge that the evidence map developed for TBI is unable to address specific questions or nuances regarding the effectiveness of rehabilitation interventions in individuals with TBI.

Despite its limitations, the evidence map we have constructed disseminates evidence from existing literature findings on TBI, draws attention to the current challenges faced by researchers, and can provide an effective tool in guiding future research efforts and policymaking.

5. Conclusions

This work clarifies the need to expand research efforts in the context of TBI and clinical rehabilitation research to augment clinical applicability. In general, patients receiving rehabilitation services display a broad range of deficits and needs, which is particularly apparent among patients with TBI. Currently, the efficacy and safety of non-pharmacological and pharmacological interventions that are able to meet the needs of individuals with TBI remain uncertain, jeopardizing the clinical applicability of potentially effective interventions. To address the challenges experienced in clinical rehabilitation research, increasing the number of clinical and non-clinical trials performed that reflect sound methodology remains a priority.

Author Contributions: Conceptualization, V.M.Y. and C.A.; methodology, C.A.; validation, J.R.H. and S.N.; investigation, M.P.; data curation, M.P. and V.M.Y.; writing—original draft preparation, V.M.Y.; writing—review and editing, all authors.; visualization, V.M.Y. and J.R.H.; supervision, S.N.; project administration, C.A. All authors have read and agreed to the published version of the manuscript.

Funding: This research received no external funding.

Institutional Review Board Statement: Not applicable.

Informed Consent Statement: Not applicable.

Data Availability Statement: Not applicable.

Conflicts of Interest: The authors declare no conflict of interest.

References

1. Cieza, A.; Causey, K.; Kamenov, K.; Hanson, S.W.; Chatterji, S.; Vos, T. Global estimates of the need for rehabilitation based on the Global Burden of Disease study 2019: A systematic analysis for the Global Burden of Disease Study 2019. *Lancet Lond. Engl.* **2021**, *396*, 2006–2017. [CrossRef]
2. Gimigliano, F.; Negrini, S. The World Health Organization "Rehabilitation 2030: A call for action". *Eur. J. Phys. Rehabil. Med.* **2017**, *53*, 155–168. [CrossRef] [PubMed]
3. Negrini, S.; Arienti, C.; Patrini, M.; Kiekens, C.; Rauch, A.; Cieza, A. Cochrane collaborates with the World Health Organization to establish a Package of Rehabilitation Interventions based on the best available evidence. *Eur. J. Phys. Rehabil. Med.* **2021**, *57*, 478–480. [CrossRef] [PubMed]
4. Rauch, A.; Negrini, S.; Cieza, A. Toward Strengthening Rehabilitation in Health Systems: Methods Used to Develop a WHO Package of Rehabilitation Interventions. *Arch. Phys. Med. Rehabil.* **2019**, *100*, 2205–2211. [CrossRef] [PubMed]
5. Menon, D.K.; Schwab, K.; Wright, D.W.; Maas, A.I. Demographics and Clinical Assessment Working Group of the International and Interagency Initiative toward Common Data Elements for Research on Traumatic Brain Injury and Psychological Health. Position statement: Definition of traumatic brain injury. *Arch. Phys. Med. Rehabil.* **2010**, *91*, 1637–1640. [CrossRef]
6. Dewan, M.C.; Rattani, A.; Gupta, S.; Baticulon, R.E.; Hung, Y.C.; Punchak, M.; Agrawal, A.; Adeleye, A.O.; Shrime, M.G.; Rubiano, A.M.; et al. Estimating the global incidence of traumatic brain injury. *J. Neurosurg.* **2018**, *130*, 1080–1097. [CrossRef]
7. Kosty, J.A.; Stein, S.C. Measuring outcome after severe TBI. *Neurol. Res.* **2013**, *35*, 277–284. [CrossRef]
8. Wilson, J.T.; Pettigrew, L.E.; Teasdale, G.M. Structured interviews for the Glasgow Outcome Scale and the extended Glasgow Outcome Scale: Guidelines for their use. *J. Neurotrauma* **1998**, *15*, 573–585. [CrossRef]
9. James, S.L.; Theadom, A.; Ellenbogen, R.G.; Bannick, M.S.; Montjoy-Venning, W.; Lucchesi, L.R.; Abbasi, N.; Abdulkader, R.; Abraha, H.N.; Adsuar, J.C.; et al. Global, regional, and national burden of traumatic brain injury and spinal cord injury, 1990–2016: A systematic analysis for the Global Burden of Disease Study 2016. *Lancet Neurol.* **2019**, *18*, 56–87. Available online: https://www.thelancet.com/journals/laneur/article/PIIS1474-4422(18)30415-0/fulltext (accessed on 30 April 2022). [CrossRef]
10. Brain Injury Facts [Internet]. International Brain Injury Association. Available online: https://www.internationalbrain.org/resources/brain-injury-facts (accessed on 1 May 2022).
11. Iaccarino, C.; Carretta, A.; Nicolosi, F.; Morselli, C. Epidemiology of severe traumatic brain injury. *J. Neurosurg. Sci.* **2018**, *62*, 535–541. [CrossRef]
12. Traumatic Brain Injury: Hope through Research | National Institute of Neurological Disorders and Stroke. Available online: https://www.ninds.nih.gov/Disorders/Patient-Caregiver-Education/Hope-Through-Research/Traumatic-Brain-Injury-Hope-Through (accessed on 1 May 2022).
13. Chan, V.; Mollayeva, T.; Ottenbacher, K.J.; Colantonio, A. Clinical profile and comorbidity of traumatic brain injury among younger and older men and women: A brief research notes. *BMC Res. Notes* **2017**, *10*, 371. [CrossRef] [PubMed]
14. Najem, D.; Rennie, K.; Ribecco-Lutkiewicz, M.; Ly, D.; Haukenfrers, J.; Liu, Q.; Nzau, M.; Fraser, D.D.; Bani-Yaghoub, M. Traumatic brain injury: Classification, models, and markers. *Biochem. Cell Biol.* **2018**, *96*, 391–406. [CrossRef] [PubMed]
15. Hammond, F.M.; Corrigan, J.D.; Ketchum, J.M.; Malec, J.F.; Dams-O'Connor, K.; Hart, T.; Novack, T.A.; Bogner, J.; Dahdah, M.N.; Whiteneck, G.G. Prevalence of Medical and Psychiatric Comorbidities Following Traumatic Brain Injury. *J. Head Trauma Rehabil.* **2019**, *34*, E1–E10. [CrossRef] [PubMed]
16. Forslund, M.V.; Perrin, P.B.; Røe, C.; Sigurdardottir, S.; Hellstrøm, T.; Berntsen, S.A.; Lu, J.; Arango-Lasprilla, J.C.; Andelic, N. Global Outcome Trajectories up to 10 Years After Moderate to Severe Traumatic Brain Injury. *Front. Neurol.* **2019**, *10*, 219. [CrossRef]
17. Bramlett, H.M.; Dietrich, W.D. Long-Term Consequences of Traumatic Brain Injury: Current Status of Potential Mechanisms of Injury and Neurological Outcomes. *J. Neurotrauma* **2015**, *32*, 1834–1848. [CrossRef]
18. Page, M.J.; McKenzie, J.E.; Bossuyt, P.M.; Boutron, I.; Hoffmann, T.C.; Mulrow, C.D.; Shamseer, L.; Tetzlaff, J.M.; Akl, E.A.; Brennan, S.E.; et al. The PRISMA 2020 statement: An updated guideline for reporting systematic reviews. *J. Clin. Epidemiol.* **2021**, *134*, 178–189. [CrossRef]

19. Levack, W.M.M.; Rathore, F.A.; Pollet, J.; Negrini, S. One in 11 Cochrane Reviews Are on Rehabilitation Interventions, According to Pragmatic Inclusion Criteria Developed by Cochrane Rehabilitation. *Arch. Phys. Med. Rehabil.* **2019**, *100*, 1492–1498. [CrossRef]
20. Shea, B.J.; Reeves, B.C.; Wells, G.; Thuku, M.; Hamel, C.; Moran, J.; Moher, D.; Tugwell, P.; Welch, V.; Kristjansson, E.; et al. AMSTAR 2: A critical appraisal tool for systematic reviews that include randomised or non-randomised studies of healthcare interventions, or both. *BMJ* **2017**, *358*, j4008. Available online: https://www.bmj.com/lookup/doi/10.1136/bmj.j4008 (accessed on 10 February 2022). [CrossRef]
21. Guyatt, G.; Oxman, A.D.; Akl, E.A.; Kunz, R.; Vist, G.; Brozek, J.; Norris, S.; Falck-Ytter, Y.; Glasziou, P.; deBeer, H.; et al. GRADE guidelines: 1. Introduction-GRADE evidence profiles and summary of findings tables. *J. Clin. Epidemiol.* **2011**, *64*, 383–394. [CrossRef]
22. Guyatt, G.H.; Oxman, A.D.; Vist, G.E.; Kunz, R.; Falck-Ytter, Y.; Alonso-Coello, P.; Schünemann, H.J. GRADE: An emerging consensus on rating quality of evidence and strength of recommendations. *BMJ* **2008**, *336*, 924–926. Available online: https://www.bmj.com/content/336/7650/924 (accessed on 9 November 2021). [CrossRef]
23. Wong, V.; Cheuk, D.K.; Lee, S.; Chu, V. Acupuncture for acute management and rehabilitation of traumatic brain injury. *Cochrane Database Syst. Rev.* **2013**, *3*, CD007700. Available online: https://www-cochranelibrary-com.ezproxy1.lib.asu.edu/cdsr/doi/10.1002/14651858.CD007700.pub3/full (accessed on 9 November 2021). [CrossRef] [PubMed]
24. Gertler, P.; Tate, R.L.; Cameron, I.D. Non-pharmacological interventions for depression in adults and children with traumatic brain injury. *Cochrane Database Syst. Rev.* **2015**, *12*, CD009871. Available online: https://www.cochranelibrary.com/cdsr/doi/10.1002/14651858.CD009871.pub2/full/ru (accessed on 9 November 2021). [CrossRef]
25. Thompson, K.; Pohlmann-Eden, B.; Campbell, L.A.; Abel, H. Pharmacological treatments for preventing epilepsy following traumatic head injury. *Cochrane Database Syst. Rev.* **2015**, *8*, CD009900. [CrossRef] [PubMed]
26. Hassett, L.; Moseley, A.M.; Harmer, A.R. Fitness training for cardiorespiratory conditioning after traumatic brain injury. *Cochrane Database Syst. Rev.* **2017**, *12*, CD006123. Available online: https://www-cochranelibrary-com.ezproxy1.lib.asu.edu/cdsr/doi/10.1002/14651858.CD006123.pub3/full (accessed on 9 November 2021). [CrossRef] [PubMed]
27. Kumar, K.S.; Samuelkamaleshkumar, S.; Viswanathan, A.; Macaden, A.S. Cognitive rehabilitation for adults with traumatic brain injury to improve occupational outcomes. *Cochrane Database Syst. Rev.* **2017**, *6*, CD007935. Available online: https://www-cochranelibrary-com.ezproxy1.lib.asu.edu/cdsr/doi/10.1002/14651858.CD007935.pub2/full (accessed on 9 November 2021). [CrossRef]
28. Synnot, A.; Chau, M.; Pitt, V.; O'Connor, D.; Gruen, R.L.; Wasiak, J.; Clavisi, O.; Pattuwage, L.; Phillips, K. Interventions for managing skeletal muscle spasticity following traumatic brain injury. *Cochrane Database Syst. Rev.* **2017**, *11*, CD008929. Available online: https://www.cochranelibrary.com/es/cdsr/doi/10.1002/14651858.CD008929.pub2/full/pt (accessed on 9 November 2021). [CrossRef]
29. Wong, A.W.K.; Chen, C.; Baum, M.C.; Heaton, R.K.; Goodman, B.; Heinemann, A.W. Cognitive, Emotional, and Physical Functioning as Predictors of Paid Employment in People with Stroke, Traumatic Brain Injury, and Spinal Cord Injury. *Am. J. Occup. Ther.* **2019**, *73*, 7302205010p1–7302205010p15. Available online: https://www.ncbi.nlm.nih.gov/pmc/articles/PMC6436116/ (accessed on 18 November 2021). [CrossRef]
30. Drake, A.I.; Gray, N.; Yoder, S.; Pramuka, M.; Llewellyn, M. Factors predicting return to work following mild traumatic brain injury: A discriminant analysis. *J. Head Trauma Rehabil.* **2000**, *15*, 1103–1112. [CrossRef]
31. Ownsworth, T.; McKenna, K. Investigation of factors related to employment outcome following traumatic brain injury: A critical review and conceptual model. *Disabil. Rehabil.* **2004**, *26*, 765–783. [CrossRef]
32. Watanabe, S. Vocational rehabilitation for clients with cognitive and behavioral disorders associated with traumatic brain injury. *Work (Read. Mass)* **2013**, *45*, 273–277.
33. Bogdanova, Y.; Verfaellie, M. Cognitive sequelae of blast-induced traumatic brain injury: Recovery and rehabilitation. *Neuropsychol. Rev.* **2012**, *22*, 4–20. [CrossRef] [PubMed]
34. Wilson, C.D.; Burks, J.D.; Rodgers, R.B.; Evans, R.M.; Bakare, A.A.; Safavi-Abbasi, S. Early and Late Posttraumatic Epilepsy in the Setting of Traumatic Brain Injury: A Meta-analysis and Review of Antiepileptic Management. *World Neurosurg.* **2018**, *110*, e901–e906. [CrossRef] [PubMed]
35. Dang, K.; Gupta, P.K.; Diaz-Arrastia, R. Chapter 14: Epilepsy after Traumatic Brain Injury. In *Translational Research in Traumatic Brain Injury*; CRC Press: Boca Raton, FL, USA, 2016; pp. 299–313. Available online: https://www.ncbi.nlm.nih.gov/books/NBK326716/ (accessed on 16 January 2022).
36. Pingue, V.; Mele, C.; Nardone, A. Post-traumatic seizures and antiepileptic therapy as predictors of the functional outcome in patients with traumatic brain injury. *Sci. Rep.* **2021**, *11*, 4708. Available online: https://www.nature.com/articles/s41598-021-84203-y (accessed on 15 November 2021). [CrossRef] [PubMed]
37. Menon, D.K. Unique challenges in clinical trials in traumatic brain injury. *Crit. Care Med.* **2009**, *37*, S129–S135. [CrossRef]
38. Stanley, R.M.; Johnson, M.D.; Vance, C.; Bajaj, L.; Babcock, L.; Atabaki, S.; Thomas, D.; Simon, H.K.; Cohen, D.M.; Rubacalva, D.; et al. Challenges Enrolling Children Into Traumatic Brain Injury Trials: An Observational Study. *Acad. Emerg. Med.* **2017**, *24*, 31–39. [CrossRef] [PubMed]
39. Gerber, L.H.; Deshpande, R.; Moosvi, A.; Zafonte, R.; Bushnik, T.; Garfinkel, S.; Cai, C. Narrative review of clinical practice guidelines for treating people with moderate or severe traumatic brain injury. *NeuroRehabilitation* **2021**, *48*, 451–467. [CrossRef]

40. Gerber, L.H.; Bush, H.; Cai, C.; Garfinkel, S.; Chan, L.; Cotner, B.; Wagner, A. Scoping review of clinical rehabilitation research pertaining to traumatic brain injury: 1990–2016. *NeuroRehabilitation* **2019**, *44*, 207–215. [CrossRef]
41. Maas, A.I.R.; Menon, D.K.; Lingsma, H.F.; Pineda, J.A.; Sandel, M.E.; Manley, G.T. Re-orientation of clinical research in traumatic brain injury: Report of an international workshop on comparative effectiveness research. *J. Neurotrauma* **2012**, *29*, 32–46. [CrossRef]
42. Bragge, P.; Clavisi, O.; Turner, T.; Tavender, E.; Collie, A.; Gruen, R.L. The Global Evidence Mapping Initiative: Scoping research in broad topic areas. *BMC Med. Res. Methodol.* **2011**, *11*, 92. [CrossRef]
43. Katz, D.; Williams, A.-L.; Girard, C.; Goodman, J.; Comerford, B.; Behrman, A.; Bracken, M.B. The evidence base for complementary and alternative medicine: Methods of Evidence Mapping with application to CAM. *Altern. Ther. Health Med.* **2003**, *9*, 22–30.
44. Althuis, M.D.; Weed, D.L. Evidence mapping: Methodologic foundations and application to intervention and observational research on sugar-sweetened beverages and health outcomes. *Am. J. Clin. Nutr.* **2013**, *98*, 755–768. [CrossRef] [PubMed]
45. Pollock, M.; Fernandes, R.; Becker, L.; Pieper, D.; Hartling, L. Chapter V: Overviews of Reviews. In *Cochrane Handbook for Systematic Reviews of Interventions*; Version 6.2; Higgins, J.P.T., Thomas, J., Chandler, J., Cumpston, M., Li, T., Page, M.J., Welch, V.A., Eds.; Cochrane, 2021. Available online: www.training.cochrane.org/handbook (accessed on 13 December 2021).

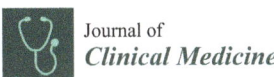

Article

In the Aftermath of Acute Hospitalization for Traumatic Brain Injury: Factors Associated with the Direct Pathway into Specialized Rehabilitation

Cathrine Tverdal [1,2,*], Nada Andelic [3,4,*], Eirik Helseth [1,2], Cathrine Brunborg [5], Pål Rønning [1], Torgeir Hellstrøm [3], Cecilie Røe [2,3,4] and Mads Aarhus [1]

1 Department of Neurosurgery, Oslo University Hospital, 0424 Oslo, Norway; ehelseth@ous-hf.no (E.H.); paroen@ous-hf.no (P.R.); madaar@ous-hf.no (M.A.)
2 Institute of Clinical Medicine, Faculty of Medicine, University of Oslo, 0318 Oslo, Norway; cecilie.roe@medisin.uio.no
3 Department of Physical Medicine and Rehabilitation, Oslo University Hospital, 0424 Oslo, Norway; uxhetz@ous-hf.no
4 Research Centre for Habilitation and Rehabilitation Models and Services (CHARM), Institute of Health and Society, Faculty of Medicine, University of Oslo, 0373 Oslo, Norway
5 Oslo Centre for Biostatistics and Epidemiology, Research Support Services, Oslo University Hospital, 0317 Oslo, Norway; uxbruc@ous-hf.no
* Correspondence: uxtvec@ous-hf.no or cathrinebt@gmail.com (C.T.); nadand@ous-hf.no (N.A.); Tel.: +47-99-224-386 (C.T.)

Abstract: Previous research has demonstrated that early initiation of rehabilitation and direct care pathways improve outcomes for patients with severe traumatic brain injury (TBI). Despite this knowledge, there is a concern that a number of patients are still not included in the direct care pathway. The study aim was to provide an updated overview of discharge to rehabilitation following acute care and identify factors associated with the direct pathway. We analyzed data from the Oslo TBI Registry—Neurosurgery over a five-year period (2015–2019) and included 1724 adults with intracranial injuries. We described the patient population and applied multivariable logistic regression to investigate factors associated with the probability of entering the direct pathway. In total, 289 patients followed the direct pathway. For patients with moderate–severe TBI, the proportion increased from 22% to 35% during the study period. Significant predictors were younger age, low preinjury comorbidities, moderate–severe TBI and disability due to TBI at the time of discharge. In patients aged 18–29 years, 53% followed the direct pathway, in contrast to 10% of patients aged 65–79 years (moderate–severe TBI). This study highlights the need for further emphasis on entering the direct pathway to rehabilitation, particularly for patients aged >64 years.

Keywords: traumatic brain injury; rehabilitation; care pathway; predictors; trauma hospital

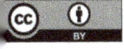

1. Introduction

The physical, cognitive and emotional consequences of traumatic brain injury (TBI) may have a substantial negative impact on daily life functioning and quality of life [1,2]. The goal of TBI rehabilitation is to maximize the final outcome and preferably restore the preinjury functional level. Specialized TBI rehabilitation is provided by multidisciplinary teams working in a coordinated effort. Ideally, such rehabilitation should start as soon as the patient is in a medically stable phase and would be part of an uninterrupted chain of treatments (direct pathway). Studies have shown improved outcomes for patients who receive more intense and early initiation of rehabilitation and follow a direct pathway into rehabilitation [3–6]. However, this goal may not be achievable in all patients. It appears that only 41–50% of patients with severe TBI are referred directly from regional acute care to brain injury rehabilitation units [7–9]. Furthermore, direct pathway interruptions may have a negative effect on functional outcomes for individuals with severe TBI [8,10].

Clinical factors positively associated with access to TBI rehabilitation include more severe injury (moderate to severe TBI), intracranial and extracranial surgery, length of stay and impaired function [11,12]. Studies determining the predictive value of demographics demonstrate that younger age is associated with discharge to rehabilitation and that the association of sex is uncertain [13]. Social factors negatively associated with access to rehabilitation are low level of education, unemployment, and substance abuse [8,11,12,14]. In stroke patients, studies suggest that reduced preinjury functional levels negatively influence the decision to refer to rehabilitation [15,16].

In 2012/2014, we published a quasi-experimental study that evaluated whether early initiation of a continuous care and rehabilitation pathway could improve functional outcomes and reduce hospitalization costs for patients with severe TBI [3,17]. We noted that patients with a continuous pathway through treatment had better functional outcomes 12 months postinjury. Across a 5-year period, TBI-related hospitalization costs were reduced, including those for inpatient rehabilitation, and improved outcomes were observed for the patients (under reasonable assumptions) [3,17]. Despite this knowledge, there is a concern that a significant number of patients are still not included in the direct care pathway. Furthermore, hospitals and patient populations are dynamic; thus, there is a constant need for evaluating clinical practice. The study aims to provide an updated overview of discharge to rehabilitation following acute traumatic intracranial injury over a 5-year period (2015–2019) and identify factors associated with a direct pathway to rehabilitation from acute care units.

2. Materials and Methods

2.1. Study Setting and Participants

Oslo University Hospital (OUH) is the only Level 1 trauma center with neurosurgical services in the southeastern region of Norway, serving 3.0 million inhabitants. OUH also serves as the primary trauma referral hospital for Oslo residents (population $\approx$ 700,000). Trauma care in Norway is organized through public hospitals with an equal access policy and is free of charge. In 2007, OUH established early specialized rehabilitation and a continuous chain of treatment for severe TBI.

Data were retrieved from the Oslo TBI Registry—Neurosurgery, a quality control database maintained by the neurosurgical department at OUH since 2015. The registration is prospective; data are derived manually from electronic medical records and stored in a Medinsight database [18]. The inclusion criteria for the Oslo TBI Registry—Neurosurgery were (i) traumatic brain injury; (ii) cerebral CT/CTA or cerebral MRI/MRA with findings of acute trauma (hemorrhage, fracture, traumatic axonal injury, vascular injury); (iii) admission to OUH within seven days postinjury; and (iv) Norwegian social security number. A more thorough description of patients in this registry has been published previously [19]. For this study, we included adult patients (age $\geq$18 years) who were residents of the southeastern region, admitted to OUH between 1 January 2015 and 31 December 2019, and discharged alive from the acute care units at OUH.

2.2. Endpoint

The endpoint in this study is discharge destination from the acute care units at OUH. Acute care units are defined as ICUs and surgical wards. Discharge destinations are categorized as home, specialized rehabilitation, local hospital, general rehabilitation, nursing home and other. The endpoint variable was binary: direct transfer to rehabilitation or not. Only patients discharged to specialized inpatient rehabilitation were categorized as "yes". All other discharge places are considered as "no". Information regarding inpatient rehabilitation at later stages of TBI was not available, thus not addressed in this study.

2.3. Independent Variables

2.3.1. Demographics and Preinjury Comorbidity

Age (stratified into 18–29 years, 30–49 years, 50–64 years, 65–79 years, 80+ years), sex, living status at the time of injury (home independent, home with assistance, or institution (e.g., nursing home)), preinjury comorbidity (as classified by the American Society of Anesthesiologists Physical Status Classification System (ASA-PS)) [20], and any preinjury substance dependence (including alcohol and/or drugs).

2.3.2. Injury Characteristics

Injury characteristics included the trauma mechanism (classified as falls, road traffic accidents (RTAs), other), whether high-energy trauma (defined as falls from a height $\geq$3 m, RTAs, or other high-energy accidents) was involved, the Glasgow Coma Scale score (GCS) (utilized lowest score documented prior to intubation or admission OUH), TBI severity according to the Head Injury Severity Score (HISS) (minimal: GCS 15 and no loss of consciousness or amnesia; mild: GCS 14 or 15 plus amnesia, or brief loss of consciousness (<5 min), or impaired alertness or memory; moderate: GCS 9–13 or loss of consciousness $\geq$5 min or focal neurological deficit; or severe: GCS $\leq$ 8) [21,22]. Computed tomography (CT) findings (primary CT head scan performed at OUH) and magnetic resonance imaging (MRI) (signs of traumatic axonal injury (TAI)) results were also collected. Minimal and mild TBI with traumatic findings on CT is referred to as complicated mild TBI [23,24].

2.3.3. Acute Treatment

Acute treatment involved the following: insertion of intracranial pressure (ICP) sensors and neurosurgical procedures including evacuation of the mass lesion (hematoma/hemorrhage), cerebrospinal fluid drainage, decompressive hemicraniectomy, repair of the dura or fractured skull (duraplasty/cranioplasty) and vascular surgery. Admission to the intensive care unit (ICU) included all patients admitted to the ICU, whereas uncomplicated short stays (<24 h) for TBI observation in the intermediate/step-down unit were registered as ward admissions. Calculation of length of stay (LOS) and days on ventilator were based on dates, with each date counted as a full day.

2.3.4. Functional Outcome

The Glasgow Outcome Score (GOS) on the day of discharge was estimated based on information from multidisciplinary medical records. The GOS is divided into 5 categories: GOS 1 dead (D), GOS 2 vegetative state (VS), GOS 3 severe disability (SD), GOS 4 moderate disability (MD) or GOS 5 good recovery (GR) [25], and only 2 through 5 were applicable in the present study population. The reasons for reduced GOSs were grouped into (i) TBI, (ii) TBI in combination with extracranial injury and/or comorbidity, and (iii) other.

2.4. Statistics

Patient characteristics are reported as frequencies (percentages) and means (standard deviations) or medians (interquartile ranges) depending on the distribution. We divided patients into two groups based on the endpoint variable. For comparisons between groups, we used t-tests or Mann–Whitney U tests for continuous variables and χ^2 tests or Fisher's exact tests for categorical variables, as appropriate. All tests were two-sided and used the 5% significance level. To examine whether the proportion of patients with moderate–severe TBI who followed the direct pathway increased over the years, logistic regression analysis was used. In the trend analysis, the year variable was treated as an ordinal score. Univariate and multivariate logistic regressions were run to examine independent predictors differentiating between patients discharged to specialized rehabilitation and patients discharged elsewhere. The first model included all patients, and the second model was a subgroup analysis that included patients with moderate–severe TBI. Independent variables were selected based on previous literature and clinical importance. Before conducting the multiple regression analysis, possible multicollinearity of the independent variables was examined. ICU LOS correlated with ICP sensor (r > 0.68), and GCS at discharge was correlated with GOS (r > 0.66); thus, ICU LOS and GCS were not included in the models. Patients with GOS 5-GR were not eligible for inpatient rehabilitation and hence were not included in the models. Evaluation of the predictive accuracy of the models was assessed by calibration and discrimination. Calibration was evaluated by the Hosmer and Lemeshow goodness-of-fit test, and a statistically nonsignificant result ($p > 0.05$) suggests that the model predicts accurately on average. Discrimination was evaluated by analysis of the area under the receiver operating characteristic curve (AUC ROC). We defined acceptable discriminatory capability as an AUC ROC greater than 0.7 [26]. The results are presented with odds ratios (ORs), 95% confidence intervals (CIs) and p-values. Data were analyzed with IBM SPSS Statistics, Version 26.0. Armonk, NY, USA: IBM Corp.

2.5. Ethics

The OUH data protection officer (DPO) approved the Medinsight database (approval number 2016/17569) and this study (approval number 18/20658).

3. Results

A total of 1887 patients ≥18 years, residents of the region and with CT-verified TBI were admitted to OUH from 2015 to 2019. Patients discharged as dead (GOS 1) were excluded (n = 163); thus, 1724 patients discharged alive from the acute care units at OUH were included in this study. The mean patient age was 57 years (SD 20), 69% were males, 87% lived independently at home, and 69% had a preinjury ASA-PS score of 1–2. The most frequent trauma mechanism was falls (56%). Head injury severity was categorized as complicated mild in 49%, moderate in 30% and severe in 21%. Further patient and injury characteristics are given in Table 1.

Table 1. Patient and injury characteristics.

	All Patients	Direct Pathway [1]	Indirect Pathway [2]	p-Value
	n = 1724 (100%)	n = 289 (100%)	n = 1435 (100%)	
Age				
In years, mean (SD)	57 (20)	45 (17)	59 (20)	
Strata				
18–29	233 (13.5)	75 (26.0)	158 (11.0)	
30–49	356 (20.6)	82 (28.4)	274 (19.1)	<0.001
50–64	438 (25.4)	94 (32.5)	344 (24.0)	
65–79	449 (26.0)	35 (12.1)	414 (28.9)	
80+	248 (14.4)	3 (1.0)	245 (17.1)	
Male	1189 (69.0)	223 (77.2)	966 (67.3)	0.001
Living status				
Home independent	1493 (86.6)	281 (97.2)	1212 (84.5)	
Home assisted	163 (9.5)	5 (1.7)	158 (11.0)	<0.001
Nursing home	46 (2.7)	0	46 (3.2)	
Other/unknown	22 (1.3)	3 (1.0)	19 (1.3)	
ASA-PS				
1 Normal healthy	696 (40.4)	170 (58.8)	526 (36.7)	
2 Mild systemic	500 (29.0)	75 (26.0)	425 (29.6)	<0.001
3 Severe systemic	506 (29.4)	44 (15.2)	421 (32.2)	
4 Life threatening	22 (1.3)	0	22 (1.5)	
Substance dependence	292 (16.9)	48 (16.6)	244 (17.0)	0.870
Trauma mechanism				
Fall	968 (56.1)	115 (39.8)	853 (59.4)	<0.001

Table 1. Cont.

	All Patients	Direct Pathway [1]	Indirect Pathway [2]	p-Value
Road traffic	390 (22.6)	93 (32.2)	297 (20.7)	
Other	366 (21.2)	81 (28.0)	285 (19.9)	
Head Injury Severity				
Minimal	106 (6.1)	1 (0.3)	105 (7.3)	
Mild	745 (43.2)	44 (15.2)	701 (48.9)	<0.001
Moderate	520 (30.2)	105 (36.3)	415 (28.9)	
Severe	353 (20.5)	139 (48.1)	214 (14.9)	
Isolated TBI	892 (51.7)	118 (40.8)	774 (53.9)	<0.001
High-energy trauma	614 (35.6)	167 (57.8)	447 (31.1)	<0.001
CT findings [3]				
Skull fracture [4]	878 (49.1)	188 (65.1)	690 (48.1)	<0.001
Acute subdural hematoma	958 (55.6)	11 (66.1)	767 (53.4)	<0.001
Epidural hematoma	244 (14.2)	62 (21.5)	182 (12.7)	<0.001
Contusion	837 (48.5)	201 (69.6)	636 (44.3)	<0.001
tSAH [5]	1021 (59.2)	207 (71.6)	814 (56.7)	<0.001
Midline shift > 5 mm	236 (13.7)	62 (21.5)	174 (12.1)	<0.001
Basal cisterns abnormal	203 (11.8)	72 (24.9)	131 (9.1)	<0.001
MRI performed	459 (26.6)	201 (69.6)	258 (18.0)	<0.001
Traumatic axonal injury	251 (14.6)	133 (46.0)	118 (8.2)	<0.001

[1] Patient discharged directly to specialized rehabilitation. [2] Patient discharged to home, local hospital, nursing home or other. [3] One patient may have more than one type of traumatic pathology. [4] Includes basilar, linear vault, depressed vault. [5] tSAH: traumatic subarachnoidal hemorrhage.

ICU admission was registered for 64% of the patients, with a median ICU stay of 3 days (IQR 2–10). A neurosurgical procedure was performed in 21% of patients, evacuation of mass lesions was the most frequently performed procedure (13%). An ICP sensor was inserted in 22%. Data on acute treatments provided are presented in Table 2.

Table 2. Acute treatment.

	All Patients	Direct Pathway [1]	Indirect Pathway [2]	p-Value
	n = 1724 (100%)	n = 289 (100%)	n = 1435 (100%)	
ICU admission	1111 (64.4)	271 (93.8)	840 (58.5)	<0.001
Days in ICU				
Median (IQR)	3 (2–10)	8 (3–22)	3 (2–6)	<0.001
Intubated	501 (29.1)	179 (61.9)	322 (22.4)	<0.001
Days on ventilator				
Median (IQR)	6 (2–15)	13 (3–22)	4 (1–11)	<0.001
Neurosurgery [3]	358 (20.8)	114 (39.4)	244 (17.0)	<0.001
Evacuation mass lesion	231 (13.4)	72 (24.9)	159 (11.1)	<0.001
Decompressive hemicraniectomy	26 (1.5)	18 (6.2)	8 (0.6)	<0.001
CSF diversion	115 (6.7)	58 (20.1)	57 (4.0)	<0.001
Duraplasty/cranioplasty	103 (6.0)	27 (9.3)	76 (5.3)	0.008
Vascular surgery	12 (0.7)	6 (2.1)	6 (0.4)	0.008
ICP-sensor	371 (21.5)	153 (52.9)	218 (15.2)	<0.001
Extracranial surgery	375 (21.8)	96 (33.2)	279 (19.4)	<0.001

[1] Patient discharged directly to specialized rehabilitation. [2] Patient discharged to home, local hospital, nursing home or other. [3] Neurosurgery includes evacuation of mass lesions, decompressive hemicraniectomy, CSF diversion, duraplasty/cranioplasty, and vascular surgery. One patient may undergo several procedures.

Functional outcomes at the time of discharge from the acute care units, measured with the GOS, indicated good recovery in 5%, moderate disability in 46%, severe disability in 46%, and a vegetative state in 3% (Table 3). In patients with good recovery as measured by the GOS, 82/83 (98.8%) were discharged directly home (one patient was discharged to "other"). The two main reasons registered for reduced functional outcome (GOS < 5) were TBI alone and a combination of TBI/extracranial injury/comorbidity. The majority of patients were discharged to their local hospital (43%), followed by home (32%) and specialized rehabilitation (17%) (Table 3). In patients with severe TBI, 39% (139/353) entered direct pathway, and 20% (105/520) of patients with moderate TBI.

Table 3. Day of discharge from acute care units at OUH: functional level and destination.

	All Patients	Direct Pathway [1]	Indirect Pathway [2]	p-Value
	n = 1724 (100%)	n = 289 (100%)	n = 1435 (100%)	
GCS 15	1136 (65.9)	128 (44.3)	1008 (70.2)	<0.001
Ventilator-dependent	125 (7.3)	1 (0.3)	124 (8.6)	—
GOS [3]				
Vegetative State	47 (2.7)	6 (2.1)	41 (2.9)	
Severe Disability	799 (46.3)	233 (80.6)	566 (39.4)	
Moderate Disability	791 (45.9)	50 (17.3)	741 (51.6)	<0.001
Good Recovery	83 (4.8)	0	83 (5.8)	
Not available	4 (0.3)	0	4 (0.3)	
Reduced GOS reason				
TBI	877 (50.9)	198 (68.5)	679 (47.3)	
TBI + extracranial injury/comorbidity	606 (35.2)	76 (26.3)	530 (36.9)	<0.001
Other	241 (14.0)	15 (5.2)	226 (15.7)	
Discharge to				
Home	554 (32.1)		554 (38.6)	
Local hospital	745 (43.3)		745 (51.9)	
Specialized rehabilitation	289 (16.8)	289 (100)	—	—
General rehabilitation	10 (0.6)		10 (0.7)	
Nursing home	105 (6.1)		105 (7.3)	
Other	21 (1.2)		21 (1.5)	

[1] Patient discharged directly to specialized rehabilitation. [2] Patient discharged to home, local hospital, nursing home or other. [3] GOS: Glasgow Outcome Score.

Tables 1–3 contain a comparison of patients discharged to specialized rehabilitation (direct pathway group) with patients discharged to other destinations (indirect pathway group). Comparing the two groups, the direct pathway group was younger, was more often male, had less comorbidity, had more severe TBI, had more intensive hospital treatment (neurosurgical procedures, ICP monitoring, ICU stay and days on ventilator), and had lower GOSs at the time of discharge.

The proportion of patients with moderate–severe TBI (N = 873) discharged directly to rehabilitation increased during the period, from 22% (36/166) in 2015 to 35% (63/180) in 2019 (Figure 1). A patient with moderate–severe TBI admitted in 2019 had higher odds for entering a direct pathway than a patient admitted in 2015 (OR 1.17, CI 1.05–2.30, ptrend = 0.004).

However, the proportions of direct pathways to rehabilitation differed substantially between age strata (moderate–severe TBI). For the youngest patient stratum (18–29 years), the proportion following the direct pathway was 53%, in contrast to patients of retirement age (65–79 years) in which it dropped to 10%, with the majority discharged to local hospitals (74%, 166/225). The distribution of discharge locations within age strata is shown in Figure 2.

To identify potential predictors for discharge directly to a rehabilitation unit, uni- and multi-variate logistic regression was performed. In univariate logistic regression, the following factors were associated with an increased likelihood of discharge directly to a rehabilitation unit: younger age, male sex, living independently, low preinjury comorbidity (ASA 1–2), increased TBI severity, placement of ICP sensors, neurosurgical procedures, extracranial surgery, lower GOS at the time of discharge, and lower GOS at discharge due to TBI and no concomitant extracranial injury. Substance dependence showed no association with direct transfer to specialized rehabilitation and hence not included in the multivariate models. In multivariate regression, the following factors remained significantly associated with an increased likelihood of discharge directly to a rehabilitation unit: younger age, living independently, low preinjury comorbidity (ASA 1–2), increased TBI severity, lower GOS at the time of discharge, and lower GOS at discharge due to TBI and no concomitant extracranial injury (Table 4). Subgroup analysis for patients with moderate–severe TBI showed similar results, except lower GOS due to TBI was not significantly associated with an increased likelihood of entering a direct pathway (Table 5).

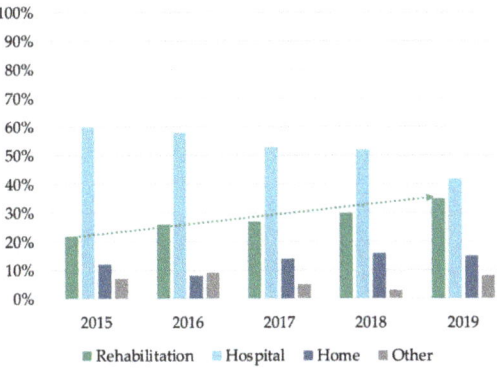

Figure 1. Direct pathway by year for patients with moderate–severe TBI (*n* = 873). The percentage of patients following the direct pathway (rehabilitation) increased during the period. "Other" includes general rehabilitation, nursing home and other.

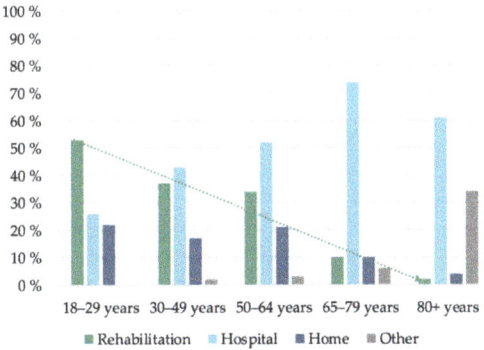

Figure 2. Direct pathway by age strata for patients with moderate–severe TBI (*n* = 873). The percentage following the direct pathway (rehabilitation) decreased with increasing age. "Other" includes general rehabilitation, nursing home and other.

Table 4. Predictors associated with discharge directly to a rehabilitation unit (n = 1724). A total of 1637 patients were included in the model; 87 were excluded (83 patients' GOS 5-GR, 4 patients' GOS not available).

Variables	Univariate			Multivariate Model [1]		
	OR	95% CI	p-Value	OR	95% CI	p-Value
Age strata						
18–29	1			1		
30–49	0.63	0.44, 0.92	0.017	0.51	0.33, 0.81	0.004
50–64	0.56	0.39, 0.81	0.002	0.44	0.28, 0.69	<0.001
65–79	0.19	0.12, 0.30	<0.001	0.15	0.09, 0.26	<0.001
80+	0.03	0.01, 0.08	<0.001	0.04	0.01, 0.13	<0.001
Sex						
Female	1			1		
Male	1.65	1.22, 2.20	0.001	1.26	0.88, 1.80	0.213
ASA						
1–2	1			1		
3–4	0.34	0.24, 0.48	<0.001	0.59	0.39, 0.90	0.014
Living status: independent						
No	1			1		
Yes	6.81	3.32, 13.96	<0.001	3.98	1.79, 8.86	0.001
HISS						
Mild	1			1		
Moderate	4.18	2.89, 6.04	<0.001	2.20	1.43, 3.39	<0.001
Severe	10.74	7.42, 15.54	<0.001	3.19	1.91, 5.32	<0.001
Neurosurgery						
No	1			1		
Yes	2.96	2.25, 3.90	<0.001	1.09	0.73, 1.61	0.682
ICP sensor						
No	1			1		
Yes	5.93	4.51, 7.79	<0.001	1.19	0.76, 1.86	0.446
Extracranial surgery						
No	1			1		
Yes	1.96	1.48, 2.59	<0.001	1.30	0.85, 1.97	0.227
GOS at discharge						
MD	1			1		
SD	6.10	4.41, 8.44	<0.001	6.78	4.39, 10.47	<0.001
VS	2.17	0.88, 5.35	0.093	1.50	0.52, 4.31	0.451
Reason for reduced GOS						
Other	1			1		
TBI	2.92	1.68, 5.09	<0.001	2.25	1.07, 4.72	0.032
TBI + extracranial injury/comorbidity	1.44	0.80, 2.57	0.224	1.30	0.65, 2.60	0.459

[1] The Hosmer and Lemeshow goodness-of-fit test was not significant, indicating a satisfactory fit of the model ($\chi^2 = 3.05$, df = 8, p = 0.93). The area under the ROC curve was 0.86 (95% CI: 0.84–0.88), indicating good discriminative ability.

Table 5. Predictors associated with discharge directly to a rehabilitation unit. Subgroup analysis of patients admitted with moderate–severe TBI (n = 873): 862 patients were included in the model; 11 were excluded (7 patients' GOS 5-GR, 4 patients' GOS not available).

Variables	Univariate			Multivariate Model [1]		
	OR	95% CI	p-Value	OR	95% CI	p-Value
Age strata						
18–29	1			1		
30–49	0.63	0.44, 0.92	0.017	0.51	0.33, 0.81	0.004
50–64	0.56	0.39, 0.81	0.002	0.44	0.28, 0.69	<0.001

Table 5. Cont.

Variables	Univariate			Multivariate Model [1]		
	OR	95% CI	p-Value	OR	95% CI	p-Value
65–79	0.19	0.12, 0.30	<0.001	0.15	0.09, 0.26	<0.001
80+	0.03	0.01, 0.08	<0.001	0.04	0.01, 0.13	<0.001
Sex						
Female	1			1		
Male	1.65	1.22, 2.20	0.001	1.26	0.88, 1.80	0.213
ASA						
1–2	1			1		
3–4	0.34	0.24, 0.48	<0.001	0.59	0.39, 0.90	0.014
Living status: independent						
No	1			1		
Yes	6.81	3.32, 13.96	<0.001	3.98	1.79, 8.86	0.001
HISS						
Mild	1			1		
Moderate	4.18	2.89, 6.04	<0.001	2.20	1.43, 3.39	<0.001
Severe	10.74	7.42, 15.54	<0.001	3.19	1.91, 5.32	<0.001
Neurosurgery						
No	1			1		
Yes	2.96	2.25, 3.90	<0.001	1.09	0.73, 1.61	0.682
ICP sensor						
No	1			1		
Yes	5.93	4.51, 7.79	<0.001	1.19	0.76, 1.86	0.446
Extracranial surgery						
No	1			1		
Yes	1.96	1.48, 2.59	<0.001	1.30	0.85, 1.97	0.227
GOS at discharge						
MD	1			1		
SD	6.10	4.41, 8.44	<0.001	6.78	4.39, 10.47	<0.001
VS	2.17	0.88, 5.35	0.093	1.50	0.52, 4.31	0.451
Reason for reduced GOS						
Other	1			1		
TBI	2.92	1.68, 5.09	<0.001	2.25	1.07, 4.72	0.032
TBI + extracranial injury/comorbidity	1.44	0.80, 2.57	0.224	1.30	0.65, 2.60	0.459

[1] The Hosmer and Lemeshow goodness-of-fit test was not significant, indicating satisfactory fit of the model ($\chi^2 = 4.14$, df = 8, $p = 0.85$). The area under the ROC curve was 0.82 (95% CI: 0.80–0.85), indicating good discriminative ability.

4. Discussion

4.1. Main Findings

In this study, we aimed to provide an overview of discharge to specialized rehabilitation following acute TBI from 2015 to 2019 and to identify factors associated with a direct pathway to rehabilitation from acute care units. We found a significant positive trend in the number of patients who followed the direct pathway during the five-year study period. Patients discharged to the direct pathway typically had the following characteristics: younger age, low preinjury comorbidity, moderate–severe TBI and disability due TBI at the time of discharge. However, the study revealed significant differences in the proportions of patients following a direct pathway among age strata.

4.2. Patient Characteristics and Direct Pathway

The study population is similar to the western TBI population in terms of the proportion of males (69%), age (mean 57 years) and the dominant trauma mechanism being falls (56%) [27,28]. Severe somatic comorbidity was found in 29% (ASA-PS 3), which is higher than in the CENTER-TBI case-mix study, which also included patients with concussions (11%) [28]. This can likely be explained by a somewhat higher mean age in our study population and no exclusion criteria based on preinjury disease. This is also reflected by the 13% of patients living with assistance at home or at a nursing home at the time of injury. We found preinjury substance dependence in 17% of patients. However, patients were not systematically assessed for substance dependence; thus, there is reason to believe the actual number is somewhat higher. By comparison, a previous study from OUH found that 26% of TBI patients had significant preinjury substance dependence (mainly alcohol) [29].

Half of the patient population was admitted with complicated mild TBI, and one-third was discharged to home. In line with previous research, patients with moderate–severe TBI dominated in the direct pathway group [11,12]. For patients with severe TBI, 39% followed the direct pathway, which was slightly lower than that in previous European studies (40–48%) [8,12,14,30]. Similar to the study by de Koning et al. [30], 20% of moderate TBI followed the direct pathway. The results from the CENTER-TBI study demonstrated different and complex care pathways in the first six months after injury, particularly for patients with severe TBI [7]. Furthermore, rehabilitation needs were reported in 90% of patients with moderate–severe TBI in the first six months after injury [31]. Our data are limited to acute treatment at a Level 1 trauma hospital, and it is likely that several patients were referred to specialized rehabilitation at a later point. However, there are different organizations and expertise in rehabilitation between local hospitals and municipalities within the health region. Thus, it is reasonable to assume that the probability of unmet rehabilitation needs increases when the direct pathway is broken.

We found a positive and significant trend for utility of the direct pathway during the five years–a result of emphasized focus on TBI rehabilitation during the past decade [3,17]. However, the situation is fragile, and it is worth mentioning that neurorehabilitation beds were periodically converted to manage the impact of COVID-19 at OUH. However, this study did not include patients injured in the 2020–2021 pandemic years. Results on the access to rehabilitation in the pandemic years will be published in a subsequent paper.

4.3. Factors Predicting the Direct Pathway

The probability of following the direct pathway increased for patients with more severe TBI, younger age, and decreased functional level at discharge as measured by the GOS. These findings are in line with previous research [13,32]. The statistical models demonstrated the striking impact of age, which is discussed in a separate paragraph. Neurosurgical procedures were significant predictors in univariate regression but not in multivariate models, which is inconsistent with the study by Jacob et al. [11]. In fact, 42% of patients following the direct pathway were treated without surgical procedures. Severe disability (GOS) was the strongest clinical positive predictor in both models, suggesting that patients are clinically assessed and prioritized for the direct pathway. In this study, TBI severity was categorized by HISS, which is mainly based on the GCS score in the acute phase. The GCS score is essential because it partly guides acute treatment [22,33,34]. The GCS score, as a measure of TBI severity, is widely used in both clinical settings and research and correlates with outcome at the group level, but it should not be used as a single injury severity predictor of TBI outcome [34]. TBI is a complex condition with substantial individual variation in outcomes. TBI can be life-threatening in the acute phase, e.g., in cases with epidural hematoma, where the patient may have rapid and good recovery if treated with immediate neurosurgery and removal of hematoma. Likewise, patients with moderate or mild TBI in the acute phase may experience long-term disability. A recent proposal in assessing the severity of TBI suggests changing from severity labels to risk assessment over time [35]. Reduced functional levels at six months are reported for patients with TBI admitted to the hospital [28]. The study identifying unmet rehabilitation needs emphasized the necessity of a more extensive and standardized assessment of functional impairments and corresponding rehabilitation needs [31]. Currently, there is no systematic assessment of rehabilitation needs at discharge from acute care units at OUH. Moreover, the decision for referral transfer to rehabilitation is not solely based on the clinical condition of patients. It can also be affected by pressure to free beds at the Level 1 trauma center, low capacity at early rehabilitation units, and professionals' knowledge about expected benefit from rehabilitation and long-term disabilities associated with TBI [12,36,37].

We found no support for the notion that patients with preinjury substance dependence are downgraded for the direct pathway, which was in contrast to findings by Jourdan et al. [12] but in line with other studies [11,13,14]. In our study, access to sociodemographic variables was limited. However, we do not believe that such variables have had an impact on the direct pathway in this study; this assumption is based on results regarding preinjury substance dependence. Nonetheless, variables such as marital status, education and employment are expected to be of importance at later stages of TBI when follow-up is more fragmented.

4.4. The Impact of Age

Age was an important explanatory variable for the direct pathway. The probability of management through the direct pathway decreased significantly with higher age, a situation not unique to our study population. In a systematic review [13], the only consistent negative predictor for discharge to specialized rehabilitation was increasing age. Preinjury comorbidity and functional impairments were highly associated with age in our study population [19]. We found these factors to have a significant negative impact on the probability of treatment in the direct pathway, similar to the literature on stroke [15,16]. Previous studies show that younger patients to a greater extent follow a direct pathway or are discharged to home, while older patients are more often discharged to general rehabilitation and rarely directly to home [13,14,38,39]. Clinical trials typically include patients aged 18–65 years and often have exclusion criteria based on comorbidities [28,40,41]. Older patients receive less aggressive therapy in the acute phase (medical and surgical) [42,43]; presumably, this may lead to directions for further treatment. Nonetheless, there is evidence that older patients with TBI may benefit from intensive inpatient rehabilitation [41]. It is clear from our results that young adults and patients of working age are prioritized for the direct pathway. Given the risk of life-long negative consequences of TBI, one can argue that it is appropriate to prioritize these patients. However, life expectancy is increasing, and in society, we observe many persons >64 years living an active life with social roles that include responsibilities with indirect socioeconomic impact (e.g., voluntary work, family obligations across generations). Moreover, it will presumably be socioeconomically beneficial if older patients regain preinjury functional levels and are able to live independently at home.

4.5. Strengths, Limitations and Future Directions

The strength of this study is the inclusion of a real-world TBI population from a defined geographical region with little migration and no exclusion criteria based on age or preinjury comorbidities. The study provides a useful overview and captures trends regarding patient flow into the direct pathway to specialized rehabilitation from a Level 1 trauma center. However, there are limitations to consider. There was no information available in the Oslo TBI Registry—Neurosurgery on later access to rehabilitation for patients not included in the direct pathway. In addition, there was a lack of information on longer-term outcomes for both groups. Thus, we cannot draw firm conclusions on the impact of direct or indirect care pathways in this study. Furthermore, the variables are crude and based on acute clinical parameters; they do not explain the multifaceted reality at the individual level. Information in the database is derived from medical records, where it is well known that information quality is variable. Moreover, database coding errors cannot be completely ruled out, although the database is continuously searched and adjusted for coding errors.

Our results highlight the importance of continued focus on optimizing and maintaining a direct TBI care pathway and systematic assessment of rehabilitation needs during the acute phase for all hospital-admitted patients with TBI. To do so, it would be beneficial to develop recommendations for clinical practice to assess rehabilitation needs before patients are discharged from acute care. Finally, future studies on TBI care pathways should focus on patients >64 years.

Author Contributions: Conceptualization, C.T., N.A., M.A. and E.H.; methodology, C.T., N.A., M.A. and E.H.; software, C.T.; validation, C.B.; formal analysis, C.T. and C.B.; investigation, C.T. and E.H.; resources, Oslo University Hospital; data curation, C.T. and E.H.; writing—original draft preparation, C.T., N.A., E.H. and M.A.; writing—review and editing, C.B., P.R., T.H. and C.R.; visualization, C.T.; supervision, N.A., E.H. and M.A.; project administration, M.A. and E.H.; funding acquisition, E.H. All authors have read and agreed to the published version of the manuscript.

Funding: This research received no external funding.

Institutional Review Board Statement: The Oslo TBI registry uses the Medinsight database and is approved by the Oslo University Hospital data protection officer (DPO) with approval number 2016/17569, and this study is approved by OUH DPO approval number 18/20658. Ethical review and approval were waived for this study because the study qualifies as a quality control study.

Informed Consent Statement: Patient consent was waived because anonymized data were retrieved from the Oslo TBI Registry—Neurosurgery.

Data Availability Statement: The data presented in this study are available on request from the corresponding author if considered appropriate. The data are not publicly available due to privacy and ethical restrictions.

Acknowledgments: Ola Fougner Skaansar, for substantial contribution in collecting data.

Conflicts of Interest: The authors declare no conflict of interest.

References

1. Forslund, M.V.; Perrin, P.B.; Sigurdardottir, S.; Howe, E.I.; van Walsem, M.R.; Arango-Lasprilla, J.C.; Lu, J.; Aza, A.; Jerstad, T.; Røe, C.; et al. Health-Related Quality of Life Trajectories across 10 Years after Moderate to Severe Traumatic Brain Injury in Norway. *J. Clin. Med.* **2021**, *10*, 157. [CrossRef]
2. Wilson, L.; Stewart, W.; Dams-O'Connor, K.; Diaz-Arrastia, R.; Horton, L.; Menon, D.K.; Polinder, S. The chronic and evolving neurological consequences of traumatic brain injury. *Lancet Neurol.* **2017**, *16*, 813–825. [CrossRef]
3. Andelic, N.; Bautz-Holter, E.; Ronning, P.; Olafsen, K.; Sigurdardottir, S.; Schanke, A.-K.; Sveen, U.; Tornas, S.; Sandhaug, M.; Roe, C. Does an early onset and continuous chain of rehabilitation improve the long-term functional outcome of patients with severe traumatic brain injury? *J. Neurotrauma* **2012**, *29*, 66–74. [CrossRef]
4. Anke, A.; Andelic, N.; Skandsen, T.; Knoph, R.; Ader, T.; Manskow, U.; Sigurdardottir, S.; Roe, C. Functional Recovery and Life Satisfaction in the First Year After Severe Traumatic Brain Injury: A Prospective Multicenter Study of a Norwegian National Cohort. *J. Head Trauma Rehabil.* **2015**, *30*, E38–E49. [CrossRef]
5. Langhorne, P.; Ramachandra, S. Organised inpatient (stroke unit) care for stroke: Network meta-analysis. *Cochrane Database of Systematic Reviews* **2020**, *4*, CD000197. [CrossRef]
6. Turner-Stokes, L.; Pick, A.; Nair, A.; Disler, P.B.; Wade, D.T. Multi-disciplinary rehabilitation for acquired brain injury in adults of working age. *Cochrane Database Syst. Rev.* **2015**, *12*, Cd004170. [CrossRef] [PubMed]
7. Borgen, I.M.H.; Røe, C.; Brunborg, C.; Tenovuo, O.; Azouvi, P.; Dawes, H.; Majdan, M.; Ranta, J.; Rusnak, M.; Eveline, J.A.W.; et al. Care transitions in the first 6 months following traumatic brain injury: Lessons from the CENTER-TBI study. *Ann. Phys. Rehabil. Med.* **2020**, *64*, 101458. [CrossRef]
8. Sveen, U.; Røe, C.; Sigurdardottir, S.; Skandsen, T.; Andelic, N.; Manskow, U.; Berntsen, S.; Soberg, H.; Anke, A. Rehabilitation pathways and functional independence one year after severe traumatic brain injury. *Eur. J. Phys. Rehabil. Med.* **2016**, *52*, 650–661 [PubMed]
9. Tverdal, C.B.; Howe, E.I.; Roe, C.; Helseth, E.; Lu, J.; Tenovuo, O.; Andelic, N. Traumatic brain injury: Patient experience and satisfaction with discharge from trauma hospital. *J. Rehabil. Med.* **2018**, *50*, 505–513. [CrossRef]
10. Tepas, J.J., 3rd; Leaphart, C.L.; Pieper, P.; Beaulieu, C.L.; Spierre, L.R.; Tuten, J.D.; Celso, B.G. The effect of delay in rehabilitation on outcome of severe traumatic brain injury. *J. Pediatr. Surg.* **2009**, *44*, 368–372. [CrossRef] [PubMed]

11. Jacob, L.; Cogné, M.; Tenovuo, O.; Røe, C.; Andelic, N.; Majdan, M.; Ranta, J.; Ylen, P.; Dawes, H.; Azouvi, P. Predictors of Access to Rehabilitation in the Year Following Traumatic Brain Injury: A European Prospective and Multicenter Study. *Neurorehabil. Neural Repair* **2020**, *34*, 814–830. [CrossRef]
12. Jourdan, C.; Bayen, E.; Bosserelle, V.; Azerad, S.; Genet, F.; Fermanian, C.; Aegerter, P.; Pradat-Diehl, P.; Weiss, J.J.; Azouvi, P. Referral to rehabilitation after severe traumatic brain injury: Results from the PariS-TBI Study. *Neurorehabil. Neural Repair* **2013**, *27*, 35–44. [CrossRef]
13. Zarshenas, S.; Colantonio, A.; Alavinia, S.M.; Jaglal, S.; Tam, L.; Cullen, N. Predictors of Discharge Destination From Acute Care in Patients With Traumatic Brain Injury: A Systematic Review. *J. Head Trauma Rehabil.* **2018**. [CrossRef]
14. Schumacher, R.; Walder, B.; Delhumeau, C.; Muri, R.M. Predictors of inpatient (neuro)rehabilitation after acute care of severe traumatic brain injury: An epidemiological study. *Brain Inj.* **2016**, *30*, 1186–1193. [CrossRef] [PubMed]
15. Hakkennes, S.; Hill, K.D.; Brock, K.; Bernhardt, J.; Churilov, L. Accessing inpatient rehabilitation after acute severe stroke: Age, mobility, prestroke function and hospital unit are associated with discharge to inpatient rehabilitation. *Int. J. Rehabil. Res.* **2012**, *35*, 323–329. [CrossRef] [PubMed]
16. Longley, V.; Peters, S.; Swarbrick, C.; Bowen, A. What factors affect clinical decision-making about access to stroke rehabilitation? A systematic review. *Clin. Rehabil.* **2019**, *33*, 304–316. [CrossRef] [PubMed]
17. Andelic, N.; Ye, J.; Tornas, S.; Roe, C.; Lu, J.; Bautz-Holter, E.; Moger, T.; Sigurdardottir, S.; Schanke, A.-K.; Aas, E. Cost-effectiveness analysis of an early-initiated, continuous chain of rehabilitation after severe traumatic brain injury. *J. Neurotrauma* **2014**, *31*, 1313–1320. [CrossRef] [PubMed]
18. Medinsight. Medinsight Database. Available online: https://medinsight.no/ (accessed on 6 June 2021).
19. Tverdal, C.; Aarhus, M.; Andelic, N.; Skaansar, O.; Skogen, K.; Helseth, E. Characteristics of traumatic brain injury patients with abnormal neuroimaging in Southeast Norway. *Injury Epidemiol.* **2020**, *7*, 45. [CrossRef]
20. American Society of Anesthesiologists. ASA Physical Status Classification System. Available online: https://www.asahq.org/standards-and-guidelines/asa-physical-status-classification-system (accessed on 11 August 2019).
21. Stein, S.C.; Spettell, C. The Head Injury Severity Scale (HISS): A practical classification of closed-head injury. *Brain Inj.* **1995**, *9*, 437–444. [CrossRef]
22. Unden, J.; Ingebrigtsen, T.; Romner, B. Scandinavian guidelines for initial management of minimal, mild and moderate head injuries in adults: An evidence and consensus-based update. *BMC Med.* **2013**, *11*, 50. [CrossRef]
23. Iverson, G.L.; Lange, R.T.; Waljas, M.; Liimatainen, S.; Dastidar, P.; Hartikainen, K.M.; Soimakallio, S.; Ohman, J. Outcome from Complicated versus Uncomplicated Mild Traumatic Brain Injury. *Rehabil. Res. Pract.* **2012**, *2012*, 415740. [CrossRef] [PubMed]
24. Williams, D.H.; Levin, H.S.; Eisenberg, H.M. Mild head injury classification. *Neurosurgery* **1990**, *27*, 422–428. [CrossRef]
25. Teasdale, G.M.; Pettigrew, L.E.; Wilson, J.L.; Murray, G.; Jennett, B. Analyzing outcome of treatment of severe head injury: A review and update on advancing the use of the Glasgow Outcome Scale. *J. Neurotrauma* **1998**, *15*, 587–597. [CrossRef] [PubMed]
26. Hosmer, D.W.; Lemeshow, S.; Sturdivant, R.X. Assessing the Fit of the Model. In *Applied Logistic Regression*, 3rd ed.; John Wiley and Sons: Hoboken, NJ, USA, 2013; pp. 153–225.
27. Peeters, W.; van den Brande, R.; Polinder, S.; Brazinova, A.; Steyerberg, E.W.; Lingsma, H.F.; Maas, A.I. Epidemiology of traumatic brain injury in Europe. *Acta Neurochir.* **2015**, *157*, 1683–1696. [CrossRef]
28. Steyerberg, E.W.; Wiegers, E.; Sewalt, C.; Buki, A.; Citerio, G.; De Keyser, V.; Ercole, A.; Kunzmann, K.; Lanyon, L.; Lecky, F.; et al. Case-mix, care pathways, and outcomes in patients with traumatic brain injury in CENTER-TBI: A European prospective, multicentre, longitudinal, cohort study. *Lancet Neurol.* **2019**, *18*, 923–934. [CrossRef]
29. Andelic, N.; Jerstad, T.; Sigurdardottir, S.; Schanke, A.K.; Sandvik, L.; Roe, C. Effects of acute substance use and pre-injury substance abuse on traumatic brain injury severity in adults admitted to a trauma centre. *J. Trauma Manag. Outcomes* **2010**, *4*, 6. [CrossRef] [PubMed]
30. de Koning, M.E.; Spikman, J.M.; Coers, A.; Schönherr, M.C.; van der Naalt, J. Pathways of care the first year after moderate and severe traumatic brain injury—Discharge destinations and outpatient follow-up. *Brain Inj.* **2015**, *29*, 423–429. [CrossRef]
31. Andelic, N.; Røe, C.; Tenovuo, O.; Azouvi, P.; Dawes, H.; Majdan, M.; Ranta, J.; Howe, E.I.; Wiegers, E.J.A.; Tverdal, C.; et al. Unmet Rehabilitation Needs after Traumatic Brain Injury across Europe: Results from the CENTER-TBI Study. *J. Clin. Med.* **2021**, *10*, 1035. [CrossRef]
32. Mellick, D.; Gerhart, K.A.; Whiteneck, G.G. Understanding outcomes based on the post-acute hospitalization pathways followed by persons with traumatic brain injury. *Brain Inj.* **2003**, *17*, 55–71. [CrossRef]
33. Carney, N.; Totten, A.M.; O'Reilly, C.; Ullman, J.S.; Hawryluk, G.W.; Bell, M.J.; Bratton, S.L.; Chesnut, R.; Harris, O.A.; Kissoon, N.; et al. Guidelines for the Management of Severe Traumatic Brain Injury, Fourth Edition. *Neurosurgery* **2017**, *80*, 6–15. [CrossRef]
34. Teasdale, G.; Maas, A.; Lecky, F.; Manley, G.; Stocchetti, N.; Murray, G. The Glasgow Coma Scale at 40 years: Standing the test of time. *Lancet Neurol.* **2014**, *13*, 844–854. [CrossRef]
35. Tenovuo, O.; Diaz-Arrastia, R.; Goldstein, L.E.; Sharp, D.J.; van der Naalt, J.; Zasler, N.D. Assessing the Severity of Traumatic Brain Injury-Time for a Change? *J. Clin. Med.* **2021**, *10*, 148. [CrossRef] [PubMed]
36. Oyesanya, T.O. Selection of discharge destination for patients with moderate-to-severe traumatic brain injury. *Brain Inj.* **2020**, *34*, 1222–1228. [CrossRef] [PubMed]
37. Norman, A.; Holloway, M.; Odumuyiwa, T.; Kennedy, M.; Forrest, H.; Suffield, F.; Dicks, H. Accepting what we do not know: A need to improve professional understanding of brain Injury in the UK. *Health Soc. Care Community* **2020**, *28*, 2037–2049. [CrossRef]

38. Chen, A.Y.; Zagorski, B.; Parsons, D.; Vander Laan, R.; Chan, V.; Colantonio, A. Factors associated with discharge destination from acute care after acquired brain injury in Ontario, Canada. *BMC Neurol.* **2012**, *12*, 16. [CrossRef]
39. Lamm, A.G.; Goldstein, R.; Giacino, J.T.; Niewczyk, P.; Schneider, J.C.; Zafonte, R. Changes in Patient Demographics and Outcomes in the Inpatient Rehabilitation Facility Traumatic Brain Injury Population from 2002 to 2016: Implications for Patient Care and Clinical Trials. *J. Neurotrauma* **2019**, *36*, 2513–2520. [CrossRef] [PubMed]
40. Gaastra, B.; Longworth, A.; Matta, B.; Snelson, C.; Whitehouse, T.; Murphy, N.; Veenith, T. The ageing population is neglected in research studies of traumatic brain injury. *Br. J. Neurosurg.* **2016**, *30*, 221–226. [CrossRef]
41. Gardner, R.C.; Dams-O'Connor, K.; Morrissey, M.R.; Manley, G.T. Geriatric Traumatic Brain Injury: Epidemiology, Outcomes, Knowledge Gaps, and Future Directions. *J. Neurotrauma* **2018**, *35*, 889–906. [CrossRef]
42. Roe, C.; Skandsen, T.; Anke, A.; Ader, T.; Vik, A.; Lund, S.B.; Mannskow, U.; Sollid, S.; Sundstrom, T.; Hestnes, M.; et al. Severe traumatic brain injury in Norway: Impact of age on outcome. *J. Rehabil. Med.* **2013**, *45*, 734–740. [CrossRef] [PubMed]
43. Skaansar, O.; Tverdal, C.; Rønning, P.A.; Skogen, K.; Brommeland, T.; Røise, O.; Aarhus, M.; Andelic, N.; Helseth, E. Traumatic brain injury-the effects of patient age on treatment intensity and mortality. *BMC Neurol.* **2020**, *20*, 376. [CrossRef]

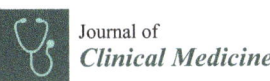

Article

Health and Well-Being of Persons of Working Age up to Seven Years after Severe Traumatic Brain Injury in Northern Sweden: A Mixed Method Study

Maud Stenberg [1,*], Britt-Marie Stålnacke [1] and Britt-Inger Saveman [2,3]

1. Department of Community Medicine and Rehabilitation, Rehabilitation Medicine, Umeå University, 901 87 Umeå, Sweden; britt-marie.stalnacke@umu.se
2. Department of Nursing, Umeå University, 901 87 Umeå, Sweden; britt-inger.saveman@umu.se
3. Centre for Research and Development in Disaster Medicine, Department of Surgical and Perioperative Sciences, Section of Surgery, Umeå University, 901 87 Umeå, Sweden
* Correspondence: maud.stenberg@rehabmed.umu.se

Abstract: Purpose: To explore the health and well-being of persons seven years after severe traumatic brain injury (STBI). Material and methods: Follow-up of 21 persons 1 and 7 years after STBI using surveys for functional outcome, anxiety/depression, health and mental fatigue. Interviews were conducted and analysed using qualitative content analysis. Convergent parallel mixed method then merged and analysed the results into an overall interpretation. Results: Good recovery, high functional outcome and overall good health were relatively unchanged between 1 and 7 years. Well-being was a result of adaptation to a recovered or changed life situation. Persons with good recovery had moved on in life. Persons with moderate disability self-estimated their health as good recovery but reported poorer well-being. For persons with severe disability, adaptation was an ongoing process and health and well-being were low. Only a few persons reported anxiety and depression. They had poorer health but nevertheless reported well-being. Persons with moderate and severe mental fatigue had low functional outcomes and overall health and none of them reported well-being. Conclusions: The life of a person who has suffered STBI is still affected to a lesser or greater degree several years after injury due to acceptance of a recovered or changed life situation. Further studies are needed on how health and well-being can be improved after STBI in the long-term perspective.

Keywords: severe traumatic brain injury; well-being; health; long-term perspective; mixed method

Citation: Stenberg, M.; Stålnacke, B.-M.; Saveman, B.-I. Health and Well-Being of Persons of Working Age up to Seven Years after Severe Traumatic Brain Injury in Northern Sweden: A Mixed Method Study. *J. Clin. Med.* 2022, *11*, 1306. https://doi.org/10.3390/jcm11051306

Academic Editors: Aaron S. Dumont, Nada Andelic, Cecilie Røe, Eirik Helseth, Emilie Isager Howe, Marit Vindal Forslund and Torgeir Hellstrom

Received: 26 January 2022
Accepted: 23 February 2022
Published: 27 February 2022

Publisher's Note: MDPI stays neutral with regard to jurisdictional claims in published maps and institutional affiliations.

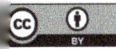

Copyright: © 2022 by the authors. Licensee MDPI, Basel, Switzerland. This article is an open access article distributed under the terms and conditions of the Creative Commons Attribution (CC BY) license (https://creativecommons.org/licenses/by/4.0/).

1. Introduction

Traumatic brain injury (TBI) is a leading cause of injury-related disabilities and mortality [1–4]. Surviving severe traumatic brain injury (STBI) often causes suffering and limitations in daily life, especially among young adults [1,2], and for some, there is a comprehensive and lifelong impact on health and well-being. Injury severity of TBI is defined according to the Glasgow Coma Score (GCS) [5]. Functional outcome following TBI and STBI is assessed using the Glasgow Outcome Scale-Extended (GOSE) [6,7]. GOSE includes functional, physical, emotional and social domains but does not measure fully how these impairments and disabilities affect health and well-being. The definition of health established by WHO in 1948 [8] has been developed with a focus on well-being and the ability to adapt and self-manage one's life [9]. Health is also described in a contemporary way as disease and disabilities co-existing together with health along a continuum from total health to total absence of health and from something temporary or limited to something more permanent [10]. Well-being covers a more individual, subjective and holistic view and is often described in narratives and interviews on the basis of, for example, personal feelings [11,12]. When the concept Health Related Quality of Life (HRQoL) is used by clinicians and researchers to define long-term satisfaction by the patient-reported outcome, it refers to how specific diseases or treatments affect life but also how they affect health after trauma [13]. Persons with STBI report lower HRQoL compared with the general population [14]. The two concepts of health and well-being are sometimes intertwined and used interchangeably. In accordance with previous research, we suggest in this paper, that health can be measured through self-reporting and described by others [15,16], while well-being is the person's own interpretation of their health, which can be described in narratives [17]. TBI is one of the most common reasons for physical, emotional and cognitive disabilities [18]. It has an impact on functioning and reintegration into society [19–21] and is linked to health and well-being [14]. In an earlier study on individuals with unemployment and disability, persons with TBI reported poor psychological well-being [22]. It is, therefore, of importance to study these areas further in order to help people into employment and to gain a better understanding of psychological well-being after TBI [23]. However, since treatment and outcome may differ between women and men, it is also important to study gender differences [24]. Initially, low GCS is in many cases not equivalent to severe outcomes, as described in other studies [25,26] and is also of interest to be studied further. Many studies have focused on responses by proxy [27], but self-reported health and well-being as described by the injured person are of importance. This can be accomplished through self-reported measures and interviews despite STBI [28]. Outcomes after STBI differ three months after STBI, and the outcomes can range from fully recovered to death [29]. However, severe cognitive impairment and impaired self-awareness are STBI consequences [30,31] that are commonly associated with disability and reduced health and well-being [32,33]. High energy trauma is prioritised in trauma triage because it is known such trauma causes more severe injury, but it is also important to be aware of low energy falls [34]. Repeated TBI is known as a risk factor for outcome [35]. Most follow-up studies on STBI have used a quantitative design with validated instruments [36], although there have also been qualitative studies [37,38]. The use of both surveys and interviews for a more complete evaluation of the outcome is recommended because validated instruments used by the injured person and proxy have a different input on what a good outcome is. Moreover, the outcome from interviews can be influenced by personal factors or the adjustment that has taken place over time [39]. A mixed-method study covering both health by self-reported surveys and well-being by narrative interviews, which enables an integration of results [40,41], can provide additional health information for trauma and STBI afflicted persons [42–44]. In order to find out what a mixed-method can add concerning similarities and differences as well as new insights in the results between surveys and interviews, the aim of this study was to explore an overall perspective of health and well-being for persons who had suffered a severe traumatic brain injury (STBI) seven years previously.

2. Material and Methods

2.1. Design

A mixed-method was chosen in order to allow the drawing of inferences from both quantitative and qualitative findings in response to the purpose of the study. A convergent parallel mixed method was conducted.

2.2. Participants

In an earlier Swedish-Icelandic multi-centre study (the Probrain study) where 5 of 6 university hospitals in Sweden and one in Iceland participated (n = 114) [29,45], 37 patients with STBI were recruited prospectively to the Regional Neurotrauma Centre in northern Sweden during 2010–2011, as part of the multi-centre study. Inclusion criteria were age 18–65 years, with acute STBI with the lowest non-sedated GCS 3–8 within 24 h post-trauma. The exclusion criterion was death within 3 weeks after injury. Initial severity in the Probrain study was GCS median 6 (3–8). The Regional Neurotrauma Centre in northern Sweden are responsible for approximately one million inhabitants in an area corresponding to almost half of Sweden with both urban and rural areas. Patients were assessed at 3 weeks, 3 months and 1 year after trauma. Of the 37 injured persons from the north of Sweden, there were 28 survivors at follow-up 7 years after injury. Two persons were not reachable. Two persons declined participation: one of them had a full recovery and the other one gave no reason. Three persons had either answered only a questionnaire or only participated in interviews and were not included. In this study, there were 21 participants, two-thirds of whom were men. For those who participated in this study, GCS was median 6 (3–8). The first author (M.S.), who had been in contact with the injured persons in earlier follow-up studies [45,46], contacted the injured person or their legal trustee and informed them verbally and in writing about the study and obtained their written consent.

2.3. Procedure

2.3.1. Mixed Method

In this study, quantitative data from questionnaires were merged with narrative interviews in a convergent parallel mixed method in order to explore aspects of health and well-being for persons who had suffered STBI 7 years earlier. Mixed method utilises the respective strengths of quantitative and qualitative research and allows the comparing or combining of results, the challenging of theoretical assumptions and the development of new theories for a better understanding and to bridge the respective weaknesses of the two methods. Parallel analysis is a widely used design in mixed method [41]. The explanatory sequential design is frequently used in trauma studies [42] but in this study we used the parallel convergent design [40]. There were 3 main methodological phases. Firstly, data collection of 2 parallel types of data on the same topic. The data were then analysed separately, and equal value was used. The results from the 2 datasets were thereafter merged and brought together into an overall interpretation. The merging step included comparing results, how they can relate to each other, i.e., the 2 results were combined to facilitate the interpretation.

2.3.2. Quantitative Data Collection and Analysis

In this study, quantitative data were collected through a questionnaire containing background questions and the following instruments: GOSE for functional outcome [6], HADS [47] for emotional health, EQ-VAS [48] as a self-report of overall perceived health, and MFS for mental fatigue [49]. All instruments had closed-ended questions and were distributed at 1-year and 7-year follow-up except MFS. The questionnaires were sent by mail in conjunction with interviews.

Instruments

Glasgow Outcome Scale-Extended, GOSE

GOSE evaluates functional outcome after STBI with regard to 8 categories, with a span from "death" (score 1) to "upper good recovery" (score 8). The categories were independence at home, shopping, work, social activities, leisure activities, family, friendship or other problems after TBI. In this study, we used good recovery (GOSE 7–8), moderate disability (GOSE 5–6) and severe disability (GOSE 3–4). The GOSE has good interrater reliability and validity [50].

Hospital Anxiety and Depression Scale, HADS

HADS is an established screening tool for anxiety and depression and has previously been used for patients with STBI [51]. It consists of 14 items organised as 7 items in 2 subscales, HADS-depression (HADS-D) and HADS-anxiety (HADS-A). Both subscales were assessed on a 4-point Likert scale (range 0–3), with the sum of each subscale as the total score (range 0–21). Cut-offs were 8 or higher for both subscales and indicate mild to severe depression and anxiety. The HADS has acceptable reliability, sensitivity and specificity in various populations [52].

Euro-QoL-Visual Analogue Scale, EQ-VAS

The EQ-VAS [41] measures self-reported overall health on a vertical visual analogue 0–100 scale, where the end points were labelled with 100 denoting the best imaginable health and zero as the worst. The EQ-VAS can be used as a quantitative measure of health outcome and is also used in studies of TBI patients (15,16). The participants were asked to mark their health status on the VAS scale. This instrument was validated and has good reliability [53].

Mental Fatigue Scale, MFS

MFS contains 15 questions about common daily activities with 4 alternatives and were associated with "affective, cognitive and sensory symptoms". It also includes questions about sleep and daily variation of symptoms. This instrument uses a rating based on "intensity, frequency and duration"; the higher the score, the more severe the symptoms [49]. In this study, we used mild (10.5–14.5), moderate (15–20) and severe (>20) mental fatigue

Statistics

Data were analysed using SPSS, version 25.0 for Windows. Data were reported as frequencies, mean or median. Non-parametric tests were used as the sample was small and/or not normally distributed. Statistical significance was set at $p < 0.05$. Wilcoxon's sign rank test was used for the study of paired observation variables. The Mann–Whitney U test was used for comparison of continuous variables. The Spearman correlation coefficient was used for the analysis of bivariate correlation.

2.3.3. Qualitative Data Collection and Analysis

A total of 21 narrative and semi-structured audio-taped interviews were performed as a family interview with the injured person together with 1–3 other family members. The interviews were transcribed verbatim. Only the texts from the injured persons were used to achieve the purpose of this study. One of the questions posed to the injured persons was how they perceived their recovery and well-being. Most interviews were carried out in the participant's home; otherwise at the participant's workplace or at the researcher's office. Three interviews were conducted by telephone or by video conference due to the great distances in northern Sweden. Qualitative content analysis was used to explore manifest interview text [54,55]. The text was read through to get a sense of the content. Then meaning units were sorted out and coded to meet the aim of the study. Thereafter, the codes were amalgamated into 2 categories, each with 3 subcategories.

2.4. Ethical Considerations

This study was approved by the Ethical Review Board, Umeå, Sweden (No. 2016/444-31). Written informed consent was obtained from the participants who were informed they were free to withdraw from the study at any time. There were no withdrawals. During the interview, some participants became emotional and even cried now and then. When this happened, they were asked if they wanted to take a break or stop the interview. No one wanted to stop the interview. A psychologist consultant was available if anyone needed it. The researchers had considered the additional burden that a mixed method study implies, i.e., that the participants were being asked to do both an interview and a survey and had taken steps to minimise that burden.

3. Results

3.1. Quantitative Results

For demographic characteristics, see Table 1. For functional outcome measured by GOSE, self-reported health by EQ-VAS, self-reported anxiety and depression by HADS measured at 1-year and 7-year follow-up, and mental fatigue MFS at 7-year follow-up, see Table 2. For injury severity in relation to functional outcome, see Figure 1.

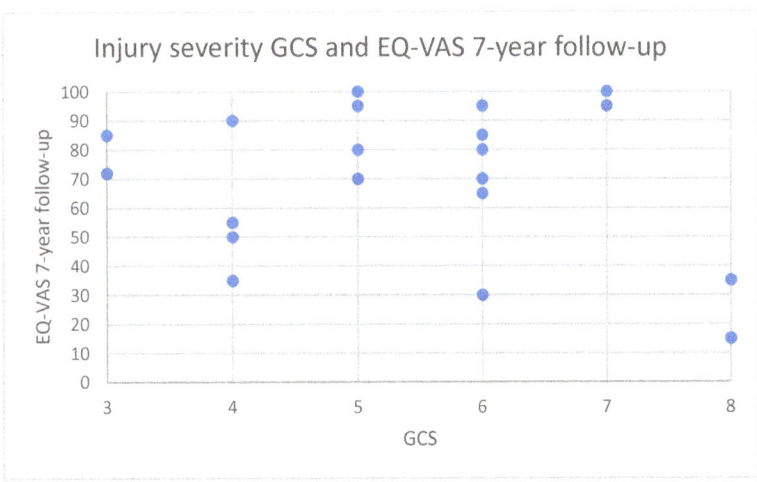

Figure 1. Injury severity on GCS at time of admission and EQ-VAS (overall health) at 7-year follow-up.

Table 1. Demographic characteristics at the time of admission and at 7-year follow-up.

	Time of Admission (n = 21)	7-Year Follow-Up (n = 21)
Gender, n (%)		
Men		14 (67)
Women		7 (33)
Age, median (min-max)		51 (27–70)
Age, mean SD		46 (13)
Men		48 (14)
Women		43 (12)
GCS, median (min-max)	6 (3–8)	
Men	6 (3–8)	
Women	5 (3–8)	
Cause of injury, High energy trauma, n (%)		
Men	2 (14)	
Women	6 (86)	
Intensive care (days), median (min-max)	14 (3–39)	
Men	13.5 (3–39)	
Women	16 (7–23)	
Inpatient rehabilitation, (days), median (min-max)	34 (0–117)	
Men	20 (0–117)	
Women	43 (34–89)	
Livelihoods, employment		
Unchanged disability pension or social insurance		2 (9.5)
Unchanged retirement pension		1 (5)
Unchanged full-time or part-time work		8 (38)
Ongoing vocational rehab or adapted work		2 (9.5)
Sick leave because of STBI		8 (38)
Other characteristics		
Known alcohol or drug abuse, n (%)	5 (24)	0 (0)
Previous brain injury, hospital stay, n (%)	7 (33)	
Post-traumatic epilepsy, n (%)	1 (5)	8 (38)
Medication for depression, n (%)		1 (5)
Co-existing spinal cord injury, n (%)		1 (5)

Table 2. HADS-A, HADS-D, EQ-VAS score, GOSE, MFS at 1-year and 7-year follow-up.

		1–Year Follow–Up (n = 21)	7–Year Follow–Up (n = 21)	p Value
HADS–A, median (min–max)		3 (0–11)	3 (0–13)	0.529
<8 n (%)		17 (81)	17 (81)	
≥8 n (%)		2 (9.5)	3 (14)	
Missing		2 (9.5)	1 (5)	
HADS–D, median (min–max)		2 (0–12)	3 (0–11)	0.391
<8 n (%)		18 (85.5)	17 (81)	
≥8 n (%)		1 (5)	3 (14)	
Missing		2 (9.5)	1 (5)	
EQ-VAS, median (min–max)		75 (10–100)	80 (15–100)	0.740
Men		90 (10–100)	87.5 (15–100)	
Women		65 (45–75)	65 (35–85)	
GOSE, median (min–max)		7 (3–8)	7 (3–8)	0.429
Men		8 (3–8)	8 (3–8)	
Women		5 (3–8)	5 (3–8)	
Severe disability	GOSE 3–4, n (%)	5 (24)	4 (19)	
Moderate disability	GOSE 5–6, n (%)	3 (14)	6 (29)	
Good recovery	GOSE 7–8, n (%)	13 (62)	11 (52)	
MFS, median (min–max)			9 (0–29)	
Men (n = 10)			3 (0–29)	
Women (n = 5)			17 (9–27)	
No mental fatigue	(<10.5), n (%)		9 (60)	
Mild mental fatigue	(10.5–14.5), n (%)		0 (0)	
Moderate mental fatigue	(15–20), n (%)		4 (27)	
Severe mental fatigue	(>20), n (%)		2 (13)	

HADS-A = Hospital Anxiety and Depression Scale—Anxiety, HADS-D = Hospital Anxiety and Depression Scale –Depression, EQ-VAS = Euro-QoL-Visual Analogue Scale, GOSE = Glasgow Outcome Scale-Extended, MFS = Mental Fatigue Scale. Wilcoxon U test sign rank test was used for the study of paired observation variables.

3.1.1. Injury Severity, High Energy Trauma and Previous Brain Injury That Required Hospitalisation Compared with Functional Outcome and Overall Health at 1-Year and 7-Year Follow-Up

There was no significant correlation between initial injury severity and overall health at 1-year and 7-year follow-up (Table 3). Six of the seven women and two of the fourteen men had suffered high-energy trauma. There was no significant difference between persons injured by high energy trauma and persons with no high energy trauma regarding health or functional outcome at 1-year and 7-year follow-up (Table 4). In addition to STBI, one person had an extra-cranial injury (incomplete thoracic spinal cord injury) with overall health rated low at both 1-year (EQ-VAS 10) and 7-year (EQ-VAS 15) follow-up. Seven persons with a previous brain injury that required inpatient care scored significantly lower health at 1-year follow-up ($p = 0.038$) and at 7-year follow-up ($p = 0.002$) compared with those without earlier brain injury that required inpatient care (Table 4).

Table 3. Correlation between EQ-VAS and GCS, GOSE, HADS-A, HADS-D and MFS at 1-year and 7-year follow-up.

1-Year Follow-Up	n	EQ-VAS 1-Year Follow-Up	7-Year Follow-Up	EQ-VAS 7-Year Follow-Up
GCS Time of admission	21	r = 0.048, p = 0.836	GCS Time of admission	R = 0.028, p = 0.903
GOSE 1-year	21	r = 0.513, p = 0.017	GOSE 7-year	r = 0.614, p = 0.003
HADS-A 1-year	19	r = −0.539, p = 0.017	HADS-A 7-year	r = −0.500, p = 0.025
HADS-D 1-year	19	r = −0.466, p = 0.044	HADS-D 7-year	r = −0.790, p < 0.001
	15		MFS 7-year	r = −0.843, p < 0.001

The Spearman correlation coefficient was used for the analysis of bivariate correlation.

Table 4. EQ-VAS and GOSE comparison between patients with and without: high energy trauma, previous brain injury with a hospital stay, changed livelihood and post-traumatic epilepsy.

	Yes/No (n) (%)	EQ–VAS 1–Year Median p Value	EQ-VAS 7–Year Median p Value	GOSE 1-Year Median p Value	GOSE 7–Year Median p Value
High energy trauma	8/13 (38/62)	yes 67.5 (10–90) no 90 (35–100) p = 0.104	yes 67.5 (15–95) no 85 (30–100) p = 0.161	yes 6 (3–8) no 8 (3–8) p = 0.374	yes 5.5 (4–8) no 8 (3–8) p = 0.414
Previous TBI, hospital stay	7/14 (33/66)	yes 45 (10–100) no 82.5 (60–99) p = 0.038	yes 35 (15–85) no 87.5 (55–100) p = 0.002	yes 7 (3–8) no 7.5 (3–8) p = 0.360	yes 5 (3–8) no 8 (4–8) p = 0.149
Changed livelihood	10/11 (48/52)	yes 67.5 (10–95) no 90 (45–100) p = 0.061	yes 60 (15–95) no 90 (50–100) p = 0.003	yes 5 (3–8) no 8 (3–8) p = 0.005	yes 5 (3–7) no 8 (3–8) p = 0.020
Post-traumatic epilepsy	8/13 (38/62)	yes 75 (35–95) no 75 (10–100) p = 0.743	yes 72 (30–95) no 82.5 (15–100) p = 0.360	yes 5 (3–8) no 8 (3–8) p = 0.046	yes 5 (3–8) no 8 (4–8) p = 0.016

Non-parametric test independent samples, Mann–Whitney U was used for comparison of continuous variables.

3.1.2. Functional Outcome and Overall Health at 1-Year and 7-Year Follow-Up

Health on EQ5D-VAS and functional outcome on GOSE for all the participants were rated high both 1 year after trauma and after 7 years (Table 2). Functional outcome 1 year after trauma was median 7 (GOSE 3–8), i.e., "lower good recovery with minor physical or mental deficit" and unchanged at 7-year follow-up (Table 2). A significant difference was found between women and men regarding functional outcome: women had lower scores both at 1-year ($p = 0.046$) and 7-year ($p = 0.046$) follow-up. There was a significant positive correlation between functional outcome and overall health at 1-year ($r = 0.513$ $p = 0.017$) and 7-year follow-up ($r = 0.614$ $p = 0.003$), which indicates that higher functional outcome is related to better overall health (Table 3). Participants that scored severe disability (GOSE 3–4) scored significantly lower for health ($p = 0.013$) compared with persons with moderate and good recovery (GOSE 5–8). There was no significant difference in health scores for persons with moderate disability (GOSE 5–6) compared with persons with good recovery (GOSE 7–8) ($p = 0.078$).

3.1.3. Changed Livelihood, Post-Traumatic Epilepsy, Mental Fatigue, Functional Outcome and Overall Health at 1-Year and 7-Year Follow-Up

Changed livelihood, such as ongoing vocational rehabilitation, adapted work or sick leave because of STBI, was relevant for five men and five women at 7-year follow-up. These persons scored a significant deterioration in health ($p = 0.003$) compared with persons with unchanged livelihood (Table 4). Eight persons had medication for post-traumatic epilepsy at 7-year follow-up (Table 1). They scored significantly lower on functional outcome, GOSE at 1-year ($p = 0.046$) and 7-year follow-up ($p = 0.016$) compared with the other participants with STBI (Table 4). Mental fatigue was reported by 40% of the participants. Persons with moderate and severe mental fatigue at 7-year follow-up had a low functional outcome

(GOSE 3–5). A significant negative correlation (r = −0.843, $p < 0.01$) at 7-year follow-up was found between mental fatigue and health, indicating that higher mental fatigue was related to poor health (Table 3).

3.1.4. Anxiety, Depression and Overall Health at 1-Year and 7-Year Follow-Up

A majority of the participants (17/21) scored <8 on HAD, indicating no anxiety or depression at both follow-ups. There was a significant negative correlation between self-reported overall health and anxiety and depression both at 1-year follow-up—anxiety (r = −0.539, $p = 0.017$), and depression (r = −0.466, $p = 0.044$), and at 7-year follow-up—anxiety (r = −0.500, $p = 0.025$), and depression (r = −0.790, $p < 0.001$). Thus, no anxiety or depression indicates high perceived health.

3.2. Qualitative Results

The qualitative results were presented as two categories, each with three subcategories. The first category was characterised by adaptation for well-being, and the second by the transformation process to well-being (Table 5).

Table 5. Perceptions 7 years after STBI.

Categories	Subcategories
Adaptation for well-being	Having the ability to adapt The difficulties of adaptation Reasonable goals as a way to adapt
The transformation process to well-being	New challenges Awareness of disability Living with a disability

3.2.1. Adaptation for Well-Being

Adaptation for well-being based on personal feelings is characterised by having the ability to adapt, being able to address the difficulties of adaptation, and setting reasonable goals.

Having the Ability to Adapt

Having a variety of strategies such as a positive outlook on life, being able to use past experiences, having the ability to use compensatory strategies, having a pragmatic lifestyle, going ahead and having a family, was described as being helpful for adaptation and well-being. There were small things that made daily life difficult, but they were accepted. Participants described being aware that life goes up and down and bearing in mind that a damaged brain finds new ways, and they also referred to themselves as being lucky. Participants described disabilities such as balance problems, hearing loss, becoming blind in one eye, mental fatigue, post-traumatic epilepsy, irritability, pain and impaired memory even though they reported good recovery. Frequently, this only came up in passing at the end of the interviews or in response to a direct question, even though they had described their recovery as being good.

> "The injuries I have are permanent and it will probably be like this for ever" … … "I'm learning to live with it," … … "I'm the sort of person who chooses to be happy about what is good instead of being sad about what is not good so I am always positive" … … "We enjoy the place where we live and do things that we usually do so we say, enjoy your life, this is quality of life. So in the future, we will continue to feel good and take care of each other. You can always find solutions to things. I don't have much to complain about—I can walk, I can eat, I can dress myself, so what's the problem? So compared with many others" … … "So it's just a matter of choosing how to act" … … "I do not attempt more difficult things than I can manage quite easily." (Female, 36 years)

The Difficulties of Adaptation

The participants described difficulties in understanding the extent of their STBI as being something life-threatening. They had no real experience of what had happened due to the initial weeks of amnesia and neuro-intensive care. Comparing how life was before STBI and how it had become afterwards impeded adaptation and well-being. Adaptation was a continuous, ongoing process for those with severe impairments. Existential changes were described, how their life had been turned upside down, how a new perspective had led to new decisions and compelling reasons to change lifestyle due to STBI with long-term disabilities and new experiences. Denying disabilities, feelings of guilt, shame, loneliness, isolation and avoidant behaviour were described as being obstacles which they had to overcome and which had affected their adaptation and well-being.

> "Yes. Umm, yes, I'm getting more and more depressed, I have become more depressed since this happened because it is always at the back of my mind, my head ruined so much for me. Otherwise I haven't noticed any other changes after my injury. I guess my memory can be a bit poor sometimes. So these days, I generally have a feeling of sadness. I have almost lost the joy of living, my life feels like that today." (Male, 27 years)

Reasonable Goals as a Way to Adapt

The participants described an ability to find new paths for themselves or for others. The ability to adapt is dependent on reasonable goals being set and that they are feasible. For most of the participants, their overall goal was to achieve independence and meaningful everyday life. Taking care of the family, achieving good home conditions, having meaningful leisure time in accordance with the new conditions, and economic independence were all important factors. Because they had been through life-threatening trauma, another successful way to move forward was to avoid drugs, alcohol and a new head injury, to invest in security and in that way reach their set goals. Participants with major disabilities described how their social situation, including their family, social network, social care interventions, housing and rehabilitation, was a prerequisite for independence and suitable goals to be achieved for well-being.

> "Yes, I was so much younger when this happened; it's completely different today. I'm not so keen on alcohol and partying and stuff like that. I'm completely different. I'm much more mature today with a family and my work . . . . So my future is to take care of the kids (laughs) and take care of my own little family." (Male, 31 years)

3.2.2. The Transformation Process to Well-Being

The participants described a transformation process with new challenges over the years: becoming aware of their disability, finding new ways in life, learning to live with a disability and then achieving well-being.

New Challenges

The participants described that returning to ordinary everyday life and achieving well-being had been a challenge over the years. Some participants said this had taken a short time, while others said it is a lifelong task, throughout the process of transformation with disabilities. Some of them described that they had left or tried to leave the incident behind them because they wanted life to move forward and STBI had been emotionally stressful. Remaining disabilities were described as a challenge and were mentioned even though some of them had described themselves initially as being completely restored. Role changes in families and in working life, difficulties in leisure time, and maintaining social relationships were described as new challenges that affected well-being. Participants with continuing severe disabilities described how daily life in itself was a challenge, how they were dependent on others, and, in many cases, did not have a meaningful everyday life.

> "But just remembering things! That's the worst! I figure it out in the end. I usually do and when I have to tell someone something, it may take several hours for me to figure things out, but I do." (Female, 55 years)

Awareness of Disability

The participants described they began the process of acceptance when they became aware of their disability instead of ignoring or not noticing it. After becoming aware, the participants described their expectations and hopes regarding improvement, a wish to go further in order to achieve well-being. No one had asked for emotional or cognitive rehabilitation, and they described that the rehabilitation they had been given had focused on physiotherapy. Now, 7 years later, it was disappointing that they had to be, as they put it, responsible for their own rehabilitation. In their opinion, more support and rehabilitation were needed in order for them to improve further and achieve well-being.

> "Yes, at the start, during the first year, I assumed I would be able to recover but 7 years later, I have realised that I will not return to the same level where I once was. I know that. I am fully aware of that." (Female, 36 years)

Living with a Disability

Living with a disability was described as being able to cope, do things differently, avoid obstacles and overcome challenges. Continuing living with a severe disability was described as frustrating, causing loneliness in everyday life, exclusion from work, social networks, leisure activities and sometimes also from the family. Striving to become more independent and to take personal responsibility was described to make it easier to accept a disability and accept changes in life and achieve well-being.

> " ... ... I can 't talk as I would like to ... nothing. Nothing. I'm so damn lonely. ... Yes, tears sometimes come when it's a little hard. Yes, but it's just a matter of accepting that this is how it is". (Male, 57 years)

3.3. Merged Results and Interpretation

The qualitative and quantitative results complement each other since the qualitative results are more explanatory than the quantitative results and cover other aspects. One way in which they differed was that the qualitative results showed an ongoing process during the years following an STBI injury, while the quantitative results showed the impact on health status at certain points in time (after 1 year and 7 years).

Participants described a process of transformation and adaptation, from being a severely injured person with STBI to striving to become an "ordinary" person with a sense of well-being, ending up either with or without a disability in a long-term perspective. Their lives were still impacted to a greater or lesser extent 7 years later by the fact they were a person with STBI. However, a good recovery, high functional outcome and overall good health were relatively unchanged between 1-year and 7-year follow-up. Well-being was described as a recovered or changed life situation that had been accepted. The family was described as being important for transformation, adaptation and well-being. Living with STBI had created opportunities for existential changes and positive outcomes, for example, that over the years, alcohol and drug abuse had ceased. Refraining from comparing their life now with how it was before the injury, having a meaningful everyday life, a positive outlook on life, and the ability to use compensatory strategies, such as making use of previous experiences of challenging events, were helpful for adaptation and well-being. These experiences and the process itself could not have been captured through any of the surveys conducted at a given point in time to measure health or functional outcome.

Changed livelihood because of STBI continued to affect health and well-being after 7 years. For persons with a severe disability, adaptation was a continuous and ongoing process and health and well-being were low. Severe disability implied impairment in all daily activities. Over the years, health and well-being decreased as isolation and loneliness increased.

For persons with moderate disability, workability and social and leisure activities were reduced. Their self-estimated health was on the same level as persons with good recovery, but they described poorer well-being. Hope for progress, being able to cope with an adapted job or find new leisure activities could compensate and improve well-being.

Good recovery was reported for just over half of the participants. High functional outcome, self-reported health and perceived well-being were found even though some of the persons still suffered from disabilities. Disabilities was not described in the interview as being a crucial factor that determined their well-being. They had moved on in life, looking for the future and put the STBI behind them. Even after 7 years, the initial disability that had changed family dynamics was still affecting their well-being and they reported that close relatives pointed out minor personality changes even though they felt completely recovered. Participants who now had a new partner in their life described how the new partner was not able to compare things with how they had been before and that was a relief.

Having an STBI caused by high energy trauma was not related to functional outcome or overall health but for the majority of those affected (6/8), low well-being was reported because it affected their ability to work, their social life and leisure time negatively. Women (6/7) were affected by high energy trauma and scored lower on functional outcome and perceived poorer well-being than men but there was no difference between women and men concerning overall health. Despite some difficulties, there were women who had become a mother but needed the support of loved ones to make daily life with children work. A lack of independence and not being able to work were obstacles that affected well-being negatively.

An earlier brain injury that had required hospitalisation was related to a low degree of overall health and perception of well-being. For persons with post-traumatic epilepsy, the functional outcome was also significantly lower compared with those who did not suffer from epilepsy. Post-traumatic epilepsy also affected well-being but not reported overall health. A few persons reported anxiety and depression and scored lower health, but nevertheless, they had a sense of well-being. Persons with moderate and severe mental fatigue had a low functional outcome and low overall health and none of them perceived well-being or were back in work.

STBI still affects the person's life to a greater or lesser extent several years after injury. Good recovery and overall good health are reported and also better well-being from interviews due to acceptance of a recovered or changed life situation.

4. Discussion

By using a mixed method, we were able to examine an overall perspective of health and well-being for persons who had suffered STBI up to seven years earlier. We found that STBI was still affecting their lives to a greater or lesser extent even though good functional outcomes and overall good health were reported. However, participants reported improved well-being due to recovery or acceptance of their changed situation.

The merged results show that a meaningful everyday life, a positive outlook on life, an ability to use compensatory strategies, such as previous experiences of challenging events, were all helpful for adaptation and well-being. These aspects were not assessed by any of the instruments used to measure health or functional outcome. The injured persons described that focusing on overall health and well-being instead of their disability, even with a remaining impairment, was one way of adapting to the new situation. The present study also found that a pragmatic lifestyle, keeping up with the family and having a meaningful everyday life were ways to overcome challenges in the transformation process for adaptation and well-being after STBI. Achieving health and well-being is connected to what each person considers to be acceptable as a normal everyday life and over the years, new perspectives have emerged.

In this study, several participants mentioned an ongoing disability even though they reported good recovery, health and well-being. This supports that it is not the absence of disease or disability that defines health [10] and that long-term follow-up of unidentified disabilities can be valuable. This was also described in an earlier study when full recovery was reported by persons with TBI after 10 years or more, even though they experienced persistent problems that affected their daily lives [56].

The only exclusion criterion at baseline was death within three weeks. One established weakness of many functional outcome instruments and health scales used in TBI studies is that if there is a pre-existing problem, such as a previous brain injury, drug or alcohol abuse, or psychiatric disorder, it is not possible to take it into account or whether there is a need for guidance when completing the questionnaire [57]. As our merged results take both self-reported health and perceived well-being into account, it is possible to see that it does not only reflect the results but also how pre-existing problems affect the situation.

The merged results show that for the participants with a severe disability, i.e., impairment in all daily activities, adaptation was a continuous, ongoing process and health and well-being were low. Over the years, health and well-being decreased as isolation and loneliness increased. Friends withdrew and sometimes their family members too, even if the family was reported to be helpful for adaptation and well-being. In other studies, STBI persons with more severe residual conditions described difficulties adapting to the new situation and highlighted the importance of having a family, close relationships and access to service and rehabilitation [58] and that feeling self-worth and maintaining self-confidence are important for well-being [59]. Severe disability is known to be related to dissatisfaction with health [28]. In a recent study of persons with STBI, it was shown how rehabilitation could help to adapt friendships and support earlier relationships for the injured person several years after the injury [60].

Participants with moderate disability had the same level of health scores as participants with good recovery but described poorer well-being because of reduced work abilities and social and leisure activities. Changed livelihood affected the health and well-being of almost half of the participants in this study. The categorisation of persons with TBI as either working or unemployed does not provide a complete picture since many people who work fewer hours than they did before the TBI are less satisfied and fail to sustain work [61]. Losing their economic independence was an obstacle and had a negative impact on well-being, especially for the women in this study. The participants in this study were in their most productive years; many of them were on sick leave because of STBI and some of them still had ongoing vocational rehabilitation. There is an obvious need for an intervention programme that is adapted to working life [14].

In this study, participants with known alcohol and drug abuse before injury had ceased all such abuse after 7 years, but none of these persons described any meaningful daily activity, thus service and support were still needed for health and well-being. In our study, the women were 10 years younger than the men. For several of them, their STBI had been caused by high energy trauma and they had lower functional outcomes than men and poorer well-being but acceptable overall health. With the exception of the age factor, our study is in line with a recent multi-centre study which found that women reported more severe outcomes, depending on TBI severity and older age [24]. A recent prediction study reported that women, persons who were unemployed before injury and persons with more severe TBI at 10-year follow-up had lower HRQL, suggesting that these persons should perhaps be targeted for regular follow-up [62]. However, there were only seven female participants in our study, and, therefore, it is not possible to draw any major conclusions regarding whether being a woman has any significance for the outcome.

The merged results showed that there was hope for progress for persons with moderate disability, to cope with work or to find new activities that could be a form of compensation and improve their well-being. Low occupational activity 10 years after TBI gives a low rating for psychosocial function [22], and in our study, we found the same for well-being. Both low life satisfaction and poorer well-being highlight the need for interventions that will promote a meaningfully productive life after TBI [23]. It was found that for up to 15 years post-injury, TBI patients experienced poorer general health, social isolation, and fewer opportunities to work compared with matched persons [63]. This is further confirmation that long-term follow-up after TBI should be considered.

Some of the participants with good recovery mentioned in passing some remaining disabilities. They had moved on in life, put the STBI behind them, reported a sense of well-being and were looking to the future. Negative and stigmatizing reactions from the environment because of earlier STBI were described in another study [64].

Persons with previous brain injury and those with post-traumatic epilepsy were affected with regard to both health and well-being and a poorer functional outcome for those with post-traumatic epilepsy. In an earlier study of persons with STBI, at 10-year follow-up, the frequency of epilepsy was nearly the same as in this study, but their scores for depression were six times higher [14]. In our study, only a few participants reported anxiety and depression at both follow-ups. However, the few who reported anxiety and depression scored lower health but nevertheless perceived well-being. In another follow-up study of survivors, 5–7 years after TBI, anxiety, depression and low self-esteem had stronger associations with persistent and new disabilities than initial severity or cognitive impairment [65]. It is, therefore, relevant to investigate these problems again a long time after the injury [65]. Persons with high scores on the mental fatigue scale had low functional outcomes and low overall health. None of them were back in work, which is in accordance with previous research that showed that higher mental fatigue was linked to low workability and employment [66]. These findings were of importance to consider and highlight the need for follow-up for persons even a long time after STBI since they could benefit from treatment and rehabilitation, including interventions for fatigue.

Strengths and Limitations

A mixed method study enables new insights to be gained concerning a heterogeneous group such as persons with STBI. The lack of depth of the information that can be gained through surveys can be compensated for through interviews. Our results show how useful it is to combine qualitative and quantitative methods whereby one gains another level of understanding where, metaphorically speaking, "one plus one become three". It is important to gain this "insider" perspective, using qualitative data and being able to understand "what it is like," realizing that both vulnerability and well-being can co-exist after STBI, thereby gaining a wider perspective [67]. In an earlier study, it was reported that the evaluation of the outcome of rehabilitation requires both subjective and objective outcome measures. In our study, well-being as a subjective outcome can be described due to adaptation to the new situation and personal factors [39].

The strengths of this study are that it was a prospective cohort study comprising a near-total regional cohort population over a period of two years of persons of working age with STBI admitted to a neuro-trauma centre. The first author (M.S.) investigated all the registered cases at 1-year and 7-year follow-up and ensured that data were precisely and completely documented, minimising the amount of missing data and ensuring it was possible for most persons to be included. Exclusion at baseline was persons who did not survive after 3 weeks. The interviews were conducted by the last author (B.-I.S.) together with the first author (M.S.), mostly in the homes of the injured persons, which represented a safe and well-known environment. The first author was well-known to the participants, which helped to make the interview situation comfortable. There was a pre-understanding among the authors, i.e., medical knowledge of STBI rehabilitation (M.S., B.-M.S.), but the last author (B.-I.S.) was unaware of the illness history of each person, thereby limiting the risk for bias.

One limitation of the study was that it was not possible to follow up on all survivors. This study included patients from a near-total regional cohort population ($n = 37$) of STBI 2010–2011 from the earlier Probrain study, and at follow-up, there were 28 survivors. A total of 21 of these answered questionnaires, which was a rather small number for statistical analyses. However, they all participated in interviews, which was then assessed as a relatively large number. With the mixed method approach using both quantitative and qualitative, the number of participants was considered sufficient. Since the age of the participants may reflect the inclusion criteria of persons of working–age, this could probably explain the results of a good recovery. However, the heterogeneity of the age (27–70 years old) of the participants made it difficult to draw any conclusions on differences due to specific age groups.

5. Conclusions

The life of a person who has suffered STBI is still affected to a lesser or greater degree several years after injury due to acceptance of a recovered or changed life situation. Further studies are needed on how the health and well-being of all persons with STBI can be improved from a long-term perspective.

Author Contributions: The three authors (M.S., B.-M.S., B.-I.S.) designed the study. The first author (M.S.) was responsible for the surveys. Two of the authors were present during the interviews (M.S., B.-I.S.) and one (B.-I.S.) performed the interviews. All three participated in the analysis. The first author (M.S.) was the main writer of the script, with contributions being made by B.-M.S. and B.-I.S. throughout the process. All authors have read and agreed to the published version of the manuscript.

Funding: This study was supported by Region Västerbotten, the Swedish Association for Survivors of Polio, Accident and Injury, and the Swedish Brain Foundation.

Institutional Review Board Statement: This study was approved by the Ethical Review Board, Umeå, Sweden (No. 2016/444-31).

Informed Consent Statement: Written informed consent was obtained from the participants who were informed they were free to withdraw from the study at any time. There were no withdrawals.

Data Availability Statement: The datasets generated and/or analysed in this study are not publicly available as the Ethical Review Board has not approved the public availability of these data.

Acknowledgments: The authors would like to thank the participating persons in this study.

Conflicts of Interest: The authors declare no conflict of interests.

References

1. Tagliaferri, F.; Compagnone, C.; Korsic, M.; Servadei, F.; Kraus, J. A systematic review of brain injury epidemiology in Europe. *Acta Neurochir.* **2005**, *148*, 255–268. [CrossRef] [PubMed]
2. Langois, J.A.; Rutland-Brown, W.; Wald, M.M. The epidemiology and impact of traumatic brain injury: A brief overview. *J. Head Trauma Rehabil.* **2006**, *21*, 375–378. [CrossRef] [PubMed]
3. Montemurro, N.; Santoro, G.; Marani, W.; Petrella, G. Posttraumatic synchronous double acute epidural hematomas: Two craniotomies, single skin incision. *Surg. Neurol. Int.* **2020**, *11*, 435. [CrossRef] [PubMed]
4. Ratilal, B.; Castanho, P.; Luiz, C.V.; Antunes, J.O. Traumatic clivus epidural hematoma: Case report and review of the literature. *Surg. Neurol.* **2006**, *66*, 200–202. [CrossRef] [PubMed]
5. Teasdale, G.; Jennet, B. Assessment of coma and impaired consciousness. A practical scale. *Lancet* **1974**, *2*, 81–84. [CrossRef]
6. Wilson, J.L.; Pettigrew, L.E.; Teasdale, G.M. Structured Interviews for the Glasgow Outcome Scale and the Extended Glasgow Outcome Scale: Guidelines for Their Use. *J. Neurotrauma* **1998**, *15*, 573–585. [CrossRef] [PubMed]
7. Weir, J.; Steyerberg, E.W.; Butcher, I.; Lu, J.; Lingsma, H.F.; McHugh, G.S.; Roozenbeek, B.; Maas, A.; Murray, G. Does the extended Glasgow Outcome Scale add value to the conventional Glasgow Outcome Scale? *J. Neurotrauma* **2012**, *29*, 53–58. [CrossRef]
8. World Health Organization. Preamble to the Constitution of the World Health Organization as Adopted by the International Health Conference, New York, NY, USA, 19–22 June 1946, and Entered into Force on 7 April 1948. In *Constitution of the World Health Organization*; World Health Organization: Geneva, Switzerland, 1948; Available online: http://www.who.int/about/definition/en/print.html (accessed on 17 June 2014).
9. Huber, M.; Knottnerus, J.A.; Green, L.W.; van der Horst, H.; Jadad, A.; Kromhout, D.; Leonard, B.; Lorig, K.; Loureiro, M.; van der Meer, J.; et al. How should we define health? *BMJ* **2011**, *343*, d4163. [CrossRef]
10. Bradley, K.L.; Goetz, T.; Viswanathan, S. Toward a Contemporary Definition of Health. *Mil. Med.* **2018**, *183*, 204–207. [CrossRef]
11. Berking, M.; Wupperman, P. Emotion regulation and mental health: Recent findings, current challenges, and future directions. *Curr. Opin. Psychiatry* **2012**, *25*, 128–134. [CrossRef]
12. American Heritage® Dictionary of the English Language, Fifth Edition. Emotional Health. (n.d.). 2011. Available online: https://www.thefreedictionary.com/Emotional+health (accessed on 9 December 2020).
13. Guyatt, G.H.; Jaeschke, R.; Feeney, D.H.; Patrick, D.L. Measurement in Clinical Trials: Choosing the Right Approach. In *Quality of Life and Pharmacoeconomics in Clinical Trials*; Spilker, B., Ed.; Lippincott-Raven: Philadelphia, PA, USA, 1996.

14. Andelic, N.; Hammergren, N.; Bautz-Holter, E.; Sveen, U.; Brunborg, C.; Røe, C. Functional outcome and health-related quality of life 10 years after moderate-to-severe traumatic brain injury. *Acta Neurol. Scand.* **2009**, *120*, 16–23. [CrossRef] [PubMed]
15. Klose, M.; Watt, T.; Brennum, J.; Feldt-Rasmussen, U. Posttraumatic Hypopituitarism Is Associated with an Unfavorable Body Composition and Lipid Profile, and Decreased Quality of Life 12 Months after Injury. *J. Clin. Endocrinol. Metab.* **2007**, *92*, 3861–3868. [CrossRef]
16. Bell, K.R.; Temkin, N.R.; Esselman, P.C.; Doctor, J.N.; Bombardier, C.H.; Fraser, R.T.; Hoffman, J.M.; Powell, J.M.; Dikmen, S. The Effect of a Scheduled Telephone Intervention on Outcome after Moderate to Severe Traumatic Brain Injury: A Randomized Trial. *Arch. Phys. Med. Rehabil.* **2005**, *86*, 851–856. [CrossRef]
17. Jumisko, E.; Lexell, J.; Söderberg, S. The meaning of feeling well in people with moderate or severe traumatic brain injury. *J. Clin. Nurs.* **2009**, *18*, 2273–2281. [CrossRef] [PubMed]
18. Rosenfeld, J.V.; Maas, A.; Bragge, P.; Morganti-Kossmann, M.C.; Manley, G.T.; Gruen, R.L. Early management of severe traumatic brain injury. *Lancet* **2012**, *22*, 1088–1098. [CrossRef]
19. Wilson, L.; Stewart, W.; Dams-O'Connor, K.; Diaz-Arrastia, R.; Mres, L.; Menon, D.; Polinder, S. The chronic and evolving neurological consequences of traumatic brain injury. *Lancet Neurol.* **2017**, *16*, 813–825. [CrossRef]
20. Polinder, S.; Haagsma, J.A.; van Klaveren, D.; Steyerberg, E.W.; Van Beeck, E.F. Health-related quality of life after TBI: A systematic review of study design, instruments, measurement properties, and outcome. *Popul. Health Metr.* **2015**, *13*, 4. [CrossRef]
21. Scholten, A.; Haagsma, J.; Andriessen, T.; Vos, P.; Steyerberg, E.; van Beeck, E.; Polinder, S. Health-related quality of life after mild, moderate and severe traumatic brain injury: Patterns and predictors of suboptimal functioning during the first year after injury. *Injury* **2015**, *46*, 616–624. [CrossRef]
22. Draper, K.; Ponsford, J.; Schönberger, M. Psychosocial and Emotional Outcomes 10 Years Following Traumatic Brain Injury. *J. Head Trauma Rehabil.* **2007**, *22*, 278–287. [CrossRef]
23. Payne, L.; Hawley, L.; Ketchum, J.M.; Philippus, A.; Eagye, C.B.; Morey, C.; Gerber, D.; Harrison-Felix, C.; Diener, E. Psychological well-being in individuals living in the community with traumatic brain injury. *Brain Inj.* **2018**, *32*, 980–985. [CrossRef]
24. Mikolić, A.; van Klaveren, D.; Groeniger, J.O.; Wiegers, E.; Lingsma, H.; Zeldovich, M.; von Steinbuchel, N.; Maas, A.; van Leneep, J.; Polinder, S.; et al. CENTER-TBI Participants and Investigators. Differences between Men and Women in Treatment and Outcome after Traumatic Brain Injury. *J. Neurotrauma* **2021**, *38*, 235–251. [CrossRef]
25. Olivecrona, M.; Rodling-Wahlström, M.; Naredi, S.; Koskinen, L.-O.D. Prostacyclin treatment and clinical outcome in severe traumatic brain injury patients managed with an ICP-targeted therapy: A prospective study. *Brain Inj.* **2012**, *26*, 67–75. [CrossRef]
26. Olivecrona, M.; Koskinen, L.O.D. The IMPACT prognosis calculator used in patients with severe traumatic brain injury treated with an ICP-targeted therapy. *Acta Neurochir.* **2012**, *154*, 1567–1573. [CrossRef] [PubMed]
27. Kratz, A.L.; Sander, A.M.; Brickell, T.A.; Lange, R.; Carlozzi, N. Traumatic brain injury caregivers: A qualitative analysis of spouse and parent perspectives on quality of life. *Neuropsychol. Rehabil.* **2017**, *27*, 16–37. [CrossRef] [PubMed]
28. Machamer, J.; Temkin, N.; Dikmen, S. Health-related quality of life in traumatic brain injury: Is a proxy report necessary? *J. Neurotrauma* **2013**, *15*, 1845–1851. [CrossRef]
29. Stenberg, M.; Koskinen, L.; Levi, R.; Stålnacke, B. Severe traumatic brain injuries in Northern Sweden: A prospective 2-year study. *J. Rehabil. Med.* **2013**, *45*, 792–800. [CrossRef] [PubMed]
30. Sherer, M.; Boake, C.; Levin, E.; Silver, B.V.; Ringholz, G.; High, W.M. Characteristics of impaired awareness after traumatic brain injury. *J. Int. Neuropsychol. Soc.* **1998**, *4*, 380–387. [CrossRef]
31. Sasse, N.; Gibbons, H.; Wilson, L.; Martinez-Olivera, R.; Schmidt, H.; Hasselhorn, M.; von Steinbuchel, N. Self-Awareness and Health-Related Quality of Life After Traumatic Brain Injury. *J. Head Trauma Rehabil.* **2013**, *28*, 464–472. [CrossRef]
32. Prigatano, G.P. Disturbances of self-awareness and rehabilitation of patients with traumatic brain injury: A 20-year perspective. *J. Head Trauma Rehabil.* **2005**, *20*, 19–29. [CrossRef]
33. Hart, T.; Sherer, M.; Whyte, J.; Polansky, M.; Novack, T.A. Awareness of behavioral, cognitive, and physical deficits in acute traumatic brain injury. *Arch. Phys. Med. Rehabil.* **2004**, *85*, 1450–1456. [CrossRef]
34. Lecky, F.E.; Otesile, O.; Marincowitz, C.; Majdan, M.; Nieboer, D.; Lingsma, H.F.; Maegele, M.; Citerio, G.; Stocchetti, N.; Steyerberg, E.W.; et al. The burden of traumatic brain injury from low-energy falls among patients from 18 countries in the CENTER-TBI Registry: A comparative cohort study. *PLoS Med.* **2021**, *18*, e1003761. [CrossRef]
35. Lasry, O.; Liu, E.Y.; Powell, G.A.; Ruel-Laliberté, J.; Marcoux, J.; Buckeridge, D. Epidemiology of recurrent traumatic brain injury in the general population: A systematic review. *Neurology* **2017**, *89*, 2198–2209. [CrossRef] [PubMed]
36. Andelic, N.; Forslund, M.V.; Perrin, P.B.; Sigurdardottir, S.; Lu, J.; Howe, E.; Sveen, U.; Rasmussen, M.S.; Søberg, H.L.; Røe, C. Long-term follow-up of use of therapy services for patients with moderate-to-severe traumatic brain injury. *J. Rehabil. Med.* **2020**, *52*, jrm00034. [CrossRef]
37. Jumisko, E.; Lexell, J.; Söderberg, S. The Meaning of Living with Traumatic Brain Injury in People with Moderate or Severe Traumatic Brain Injury. *J. Neurosci. Nurs.* **2005**, *37*, 42–50. [CrossRef] [PubMed]
38. Graff, H.J.; Christensen, U.; Poulsen, I.; Egerod, I. Patient perspectives on navigating the field of traumatic brain injury rehabilitation: A qualitative thematic analysis. *Disabil. Rehabil.* **2018**, *40*, 926–934. [CrossRef] [PubMed]
39. Fuhrer, M.J. Subjectifying quality of life as a medical rehabilitation outcome. *Disabil. Rehabil.* **2000**, *22*, 481–489. [CrossRef] [PubMed]

40. Creswell, J.W.; Plano Clark, V.L. *Designing and Conducting Mixed Methods Research*; International Student, Ed.; SAGE Publications: New York, NY, USA, 2018.
41. Östlund, U.; Kidd, L.; Wengström, Y.; Rowa-Dewar, N. Combining qualitative and quantitative research within mixed method research designs: A methodological review. *Int. J. Nurs. Stud.* 2011, 48, 369–383. [CrossRef] [PubMed]
42. Creswell, J.W.; Zhang, W. The application of mixed methods designs to trauma research: The Application of Mixed Methods Designs. *J. Trauma. Stress* 2009, 22, 612–621. [CrossRef] [PubMed]
43. Lorenz, L.S.; Charrette, A.L.; O'Neil-Pirozzi, T.M.; Doucett, J.; Pharm, J. Healthy body, healthy mind: A mixed methods study of outcomes, barriers and supports for exercise by people who have chronic moderate-to-severe acquired brain injury. *Disabil. Health J.* 2018, 11, 70–78. [CrossRef]
44. Arbour, C.; Gosselin, N.; Levert, M.-J.; Gauvin-Lepage, J.; Michallet, B.; Lefebvre, H. Does age matter? A mixed methods study examining determinants of good recovery and resilience in young and middle-aged adults following moderate-to-severe traumatic brain injury. *J. Adv. Nurs.* 2017, 73, 3133–3143. [CrossRef]
45. Godbolt, A.K.; Deboussard, C.N.; Stenberg, M.; Lindgren, M. Disorders of consciousness after severe traumatic brain injury: A Swedish-Icelandic study of incidence, outcomes and implications for optimizing care pathways. *J. Rehabil. Med.* 2013, 45, 741–748. [CrossRef] [PubMed]
46. Stenberg, M.; Godbolt, A.K.; De Boussard, C.N.; Levi, R.; Stålnacke, B.-M. Cognitive Impairment after Severe Traumatic Brain Injury, Clinical Course and Impact on Outcome: A Swedish-Icelandic Study. *Behav. Neurol.* 2015, 2015, 680308. [CrossRef] [PubMed]
47. Zigmond, A.S.; Snaith, R.P. The hospital anxiety and depression scale. *Acta Psychiatr. Scand.* 1983, 67, 361–370. [CrossRef] [PubMed]
48. Kind, P.; Hardman, G.; Macran, S. *UK Population Norms for EQ-5D. Discussion Paper 172*; Centre for Health Economics, University of York: York, UK, 1999.
49. Johansson, B.; Starmark, A.; Berglund, P.; Rödholm, M.; Rönnbäck, L. A self-assessment questionnaire for mental fatigue and related symptoms after neurological disorders and injuries. *Brain Inj.* 2010, 24, 2–12. [CrossRef] [PubMed]
50. Levin, H.S.; Boake, C.; Song, J.; McCauley, S.; Contant, C.; Diaz-Marchan, P.; Brundage, S.; Goodman, H.; Kotrla, K.J. Validity and Sensitivity to Change of the Extended Glasgow Outcome Scale in Mild to Moderate Traumatic Brain Injury. *J. Neurotrauma* 2001, 18, 575–584. [CrossRef]
51. Ruet, A.; Bayen, E.; Jourdan, C.; Ghout, I.; Meaude, L.; Lalanne, A.; Pradat-Diehl, P.; Nelson, G.; Charanton, J.; Aegerter, P.; et al. A Detailed Overview of Long-Term Outcomes in Severe Traumatic Brain Injury Eight Years Post-injury. *Front. Neurol.* 2019, 10, 120. [CrossRef]
52. Bjelland, I.; Dahl, A.A.; Haug, T.T.; Neckelmann, D. The validity of the Hospital Anxiety and Depression Scale. An updated literature review. *J. Psychosom. Res.* 2002, 52, 69–77. [CrossRef]
53. Brooks, R. EuroQol: The current state of play. *Health Policy* 1996, 37, 53–72. [CrossRef]
54. Graneheim, U.H.; Lundman, B. Qualitative content analysis in nursing research: Concepts, procedures and measures to achieve trustworthiness. *Nurse Educ. Today* 2004, 24, 105–112. [CrossRef]
55. Graneheim, U.H.; Lindgren, B.M.; Lundman, B. Methodological challenges in qualitative content analysis: A discussion paper. *Nurse Educ. Today* 2017, 56, 29–34. [CrossRef]
56. Lefkovits, A.M.; Hicks, A.J.; Downing, M.; Ponsford, J. Surviving the "silent epidemic": A qualitative exploration of the long-term journey after traumatic brain injury. *Neuropsychol. Rehabil.* 2020, 31, 1582–1606. [CrossRef] [PubMed]
57. Nichol, A.D.; Higgins, A.; Gabbe, B.; Murray, L.; Cooper, D.; Cameron, P. Measuring functional and quality of life outcomes following major head injury: Common scales and checklists. *Injury* 2011, 42, 281–287. [CrossRef] [PubMed]
58. Stenberg, M.; Stålnacke, B.-M.; Saveman, B.-I. Family experiences up to seven years after a severe traumatic brain injury–family interviews. *Disabil. Rehabil.* 2020, 44, 1774668. [CrossRef] [PubMed]
59. Douglas, J.M. Conceptualizing self and maintaining social connection following severe traumatic brain injury. *Brain Inj.* 2013, 27, 60–74. [CrossRef] [PubMed]
60. Douglas, J. Loss of friendship following traumatic brain injury: A model grounded in the experience of adults with severe injury. *Neuropsychol. Rehabil.* 2020, 30, 1277–1302. [CrossRef]
61. Watkin, C.; Phillips, J.; Radford, K. What is a 'return to work' following traumatic brain injury? Analysis of work outcomes 12 months post TBI. *Brain Inj.* 2020, 34, 68–77. [CrossRef]
62. Forslund, M.; Perrin, P.; Sigurdardottir, S.; Howe, E.; van Walsem, M.; Arango-Lasprilla, J.; Lu, J.; Aza, A.; Jerstad, T.; Røe, C.; et al. Health-Related Quality of Life Trajectories across 10 Years after Moderate to Severe Traumatic Brain Injury in Norway. *J. Clin. Med.* 2021, 10, 157. [CrossRef]
63. Hawthorne, G.; Kaye, A.H.; Gruen, R. Traumatic brain injury and long-term quality of life: Findings from an Australian study. *J. Neurotrauma* 2009, 26, 1623–1633. [CrossRef]
64. Gerard, A.; Riley, G.A.; Hagger, B.F. Disclosure of a stigmatized identity: A qualitative study of the reasons why people choose to tell or not tell others about their traumatic brain injury. *Brain Inj.* 2015, 29, 1480–1489.
65. Whitnall, L.; McMillan, T.M.; Murray, G.D.; Teasdale, G.M. Disability in young people and adults after head injury: 5–7 year follow up of a prospective cohort study. *J. Neurol. Neurosurg. Psychiatry* 2006, 77, 640–645. [CrossRef]

66. Palm, S.; Rönnbäck, L.; Johansson, B. Long-term mental fatigue after traumatic brain injury and impact on employment status. *J. Rehabil. Med.* **2017**, *49*, 228–233. [CrossRef] [PubMed]
67. Toombs, S.K. *Handbook of Phenomenology and Medicine*; Springer: London, UK, 2002; Volume 68.

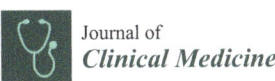

Article

Impact of Somatic Vulnerability, Psychosocial Robustness and Injury-Related Factors on Fatigue following Traumatic Brain Injury—A Cross-Sectional Study

Daniel Løke [1,2,*], Nada Andelic [3,4], Eirik Helseth [5,6], Olav Vassend [2], Stein Andersson [2,7], Jennie L. Ponsford [8,9], Cathrine Tverdal [5,6], Cathrine Brunborg [10] and Marianne Løvstad [1,2]

1. Department of Research, Sunnaas Rehabilitation Hospital, Bjørnemyrveien 11, 1453 Nesoddtangen, Norway; marianne.lovstad@sunnaas.no
2. Department of Psychology, Faculty of Social Sciences, University of Oslo, 0316 Oslo, Norway; olav.vassend@psykologi.uio.no (O.V.); stein.andersson@psykologi.uio.no (S.A.)
3. Department of Physical Medicine and Rehabilitation, Oslo University Hospital, Ullevål, 0424 Oslo, Norway; nadand@ous-hf.no
4. Institute of Health and Society, Center for Habilitation and Rehabilitation Models and Services (CHARM), University of Oslo, 0316 Oslo, Norway
5. Department of Neurosurgery, Oslo University Hospital, Ullevål, 0424 Oslo, Norway; ehelseth@ous-hf.no (E.H.); uxtvec@ous-hf.no (C.T.)
6. Institute of Clinical Medicine, Faculty of Medicine, University of Oslo, 0316 Oslo, Norway
7. Psychosomatic and CL Psychiatry, Division of Mental Health and Addiction, Oslo University Hospital, 0424 Oslo, Norway
8. Turner Institute for Brain and Mental Health, School of Psychological Sciences, Monash University, Clayton, VIC 3800, Australia; jennie.ponsford@monash.edu
9. Monash-Epworth Rehabilitation Research Centre, Epworth Healthcare, Richmond, VIC 3121, Australia
10. Oslo Centre for Biostatistics and Epidemiology, Research Support Services, Oslo University Hospital, 0424 Oslo, Norway; uxbruc@ous-hf.no
* Correspondence: danloe@sunnaas.no

Abstract: Fatigue is a common symptom after traumatic brain injuries (TBI) and a crucial target of rehabilitation. The subjective and multifactorial nature of fatigue necessitates a biopsychosocial approach in understanding the mechanisms involved in its development. The aim of this study is to provide a comprehensive exploration of factors relevant to identification and rehabilitation of fatigue following TBI. Ninety-six patients with TBI and confirmed intracranial injuries were assessed on average 200 days post-injury with regard to injury-related factors, several patient-reported outcome measures (PROMS) of fatigue, neuropsychological measures, and PROMS of implicated biopsychosocial mechanisms. Factor analytic approaches yielded three underlying factors, termed Psychosocial Robustness, Somatic Vulnerability and Injury Severity. All three dimensions were significantly associated with fatigue in multiple regression analyses and explained 44.2% of variance in fatigue. Post hoc analyses examined univariate contributions of the associations between the factors and fatigue to illuminate the relative contributions of each biopsychosocial variable. Implications for clinical practice and future research are discussed.

Keywords: fatigue; rehabilitation; traumatic brain injury; neuropsychological function; PROMS

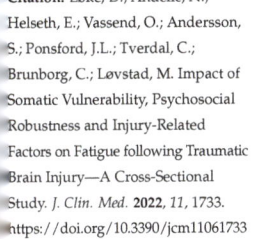

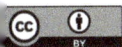

1. Introduction

Fatigue is a common symptom following traumatic brain injury (TBI) [1], with potentially severe impact on participation and quality of life [2], even when controlling for injury severity [3]. TBI is defined as "an alteration in brain function, or other evidence of brain pathology, caused by an external force" [4]. TBI is associated with increased mortality [5], and survivors may suffer from severe functional impairment, of which fatigue is often reported as a persistent problem in sub-acute and chronic phases following injury [6].

Fatigue is often defined as "an awareness of a decreased capacity for physical or mental activity, due to a perceived imbalance in the availability, utilization or restoration of energy that is needed to perform activities" [7]. A large number of heterogenous patient-reported outcome measures (PROMS) have been developed to evaluate subjectively experienced severity, characteristics and consequences of fatigue [8]. PROMS are, however, vulnerable to an assortment of potential biases [9], and there is currently no consensus for a single gold standard measure. A recent study evaluated the content overlap between items included in various fatigue PROMS often used in patients with stroke [10], showing that items from different PROMS may measure severity, characteristics, management or consequences of fatigue to varying degrees. Items from the Fatigue Severity Scale (FSS) [11], which is commonly used in patients with TBI, pertain primarily to the perceived consequences of fatigue. For a comprehensive measurement of fatigue, it is therefore necessary to expand the measurement using other PROMS and to establish whether fatigue can be construed as a unidimensional phenomenon across measures.

Conceptual models for the development and maintenance of fatigue after TBI and in other neurological disorders emphasize the heterogeneity in associated factors, spanning from premorbid characteristics, through primary injury-related factors, to secondary exacerbating factors [1,8]. The complex nature of fatigue and the abundance of implicated biopsychosocial factors necessitates an investigation of potential unifying mechanisms underlying the relationships between fatigue and associated constructs.

1.1. Mechanisms Associated with Fatigue

Demographic factors play an uncertain role in fatigue following TBI. Earlier studies have shown minimal or nonsignificant associations between fatigue, age and female gender [1,12–14], and a recent larger cohort study showed small but positive associations between fatigue, younger age, and female gender through the first six months post-injury [15]. This study further demonstrated an interaction between age and fatigue trajectory, with patients above 48 years of age reporting increasing, and younger patients decreasing, rates over the first 6 months. Of interest, injury severity does not seem to be consistently related to fatigue [1], with the caveat that most studies include a majority of patients with mild TBI. Cognitive deficits such as slowed information processing and attentional deficits have however been shown to be associated with increased levels of fatigue [16,17]. The coping hypothesis put forward by van Zomeren et al. [18] is one plausible explanation, in that cognitive deficits might result in increased energy expenditure during mental and physical exertion, which in turn may contribute to fatigue.

Beyond the direct effect of cognitive and other injury-related factors, an abundance of biopsychosocial mechanisms are implicated in onset and maintenance of fatigue. A conceptual model by Mollayeva et al. [1] emphasized the role of both TBI-specific as well as generic, non-injury-related mechanisms. A recent review [19] likewise established that there are several common risk factors for fatigue across neurological disorders, such as pre- and comorbid psychiatric symptoms, pain, sleep problems, and genetics.

Pain commonly co-occurs with fatigue after TBI [20,21] and is implicated as a central mechanism in fatigue across etiologies [22]. Beaulieu-Bonneau and Ouellet [23] found that pain was associated with fatigue 4 and 8 but not 12 months post TBI, indicating that this relationship may vary as an effect of time since injury.

Psychological distress (i.e., symptoms of depression and anxiety) is also related to fatigue following TBI [24–28]. While fatigue may by itself be a depressive symptom, fatigue may occur in isolation from depression in TBI and acquired brain injury [26], suggesting that the two are related, but distinguishable. Beaulieu-Bonneau and Ouellet [23] found depression to be associated with fatigue at 4, 8 and 12 months post-injury, indicating that these symptoms are intertwined over time. Symptoms of anxiety have also been linked with fatigue in isolation, although anxiety and depression frequently co-occur [27,29].

In addition to symptoms that may vary over time, people differ in their stable proneness for negative affect. Trait neuroticism as a five-factor personality trait has been extensively implicated as a possible precipitating mechanism in relation to fatigue in other populations, in epidemiological studies [30–33] and in mild TBI [34]. Merz et al. [34] also found negative associations between fatigue and trait agreeableness, conscientiousness and extraversion in patients with mild TBI. The role of neuroticism and other personality traits have, however, not been examined in relation to fatigue following more severe TBI. Trait optimism, furthermore, has been linked to better cognitive functioning after TBI [35], but has, to the best of our knowledge, not been examined in relation to post-TBI fatigue.

Daytime sleepiness and insomnia have been extensively studied in relation to fatigue following TBI [27,36,37]. For instance, Cantor et al. [14] demonstrated that fatigue and insomnia frequently co-occur, but that post-TBI fatigue may also occur without insomnia. Insomnia without post-TBI fatigue, however, was rare. As expected, daytime sleepiness was reported more frequently in patients with fatigue.

Motivational propensities for reward and punishment might additionally contribute to the development of fatigue. Behavioral inhibition (i.e., a tendency to be motivated by avoidance of unpleasant stimuli) and behavioral activation (i.e., a tendency to be motivated by the attainment of pleasure and reward) systems (BIS/BAS) were initially described by Carver and White [38]. A greater propensity for being motivated by avoidance of aversive stimuli and lower degree of reward responsiveness has been linked to fatigue in, e.g., multiple sclerosis [39]. The impact of BIS/BAS-propensities on fatigue has not, to the best of our knowledge, been examined in TBI.

Feelings of loneliness and isolation predict later development of both fatigue, pain and depression in non-TBI populations [40]. While loneliness has not been examined specifically as a risk factor for fatigue after TBI, loneliness is a common issue for people living with the chronic effects of TBI [41], leaving this factor of interest to explore.

Psychosocial resilience has been shown to predict increased participation following mild-severe TBI [42], and to predict longitudinal decreases in fatigue following mild TBI [43] but has not been studied extensively with regard to post-TBI fatigue.

1.2. Clinical Complexity

In summary, fatigue following TBI has a demonstrable impact on quality of life and functional recovery, and an abundance of mechanisms could potentially be implicated in the precipitation, initiation and maintenance of fatigue following TBI. The factors involved may act in isolation, their effects may be summed, and they may interact with each other in dynamic ways. An obstacle in studies involving vulnerability and protective factors is that inferences drawn from models incorporating only a few factors may not provide a comprehensive understanding of possible underlying constructs. A clearer picture of the underlying clustering of vulnerability and protective factors, however, may inform further research in selection of the most essential constructs in fatigue models, and inform clinical decision making.

1.3. Study Aims

The primary aim of this study was to enhance our theoretical understanding of the relationship between fatigue and injury-related, cognitive and self-reported biopsychosocial factors. A factor analytic approach was used to (1) examine if fatigue could be construed as one single outcome across several measures, and (2) examine potential underlying dimensionality of several injury-related, cognitive and psychosocial measures commonly associated with fatigue. Finally, we aimed to (3) explore the relevance of these dimensions to fatigue 6 months after TBI.

2. Materials and Methods

2.1. Recruitment

The study includes the first wave from a prospective observational study of patients with TBI conducted from 2018–2021. Included patients were injured between January 2018 and April 2020 and admitted to the Neurosurgery department at Oslo University Hospital

(OUH). OUH is the only Level I trauma center with neurosurgical services in the southeastern region of Norway with a population base of more than half of the Norwegian population (i.e., 2.9 million).

Injury characteristics and clinical data from the acute hospital stay were retrieved from the Oslo TBI Registry—Neurosurgery, a quality database at OUH [44]. The remaining variables were measured approximately 6 months post-injury. Inclusion criteria were patients between 18–65 years of age, admitted with TBI (ICD-10 diagnoses S06.1–S06.9), herein defined as patients presenting with intracranial injury (as confirmed by computed tomography (CT) or magnetic resonance imaging (MRI)) during the acute phase, and who have survived until six months post-injury. Exclusion criteria were pre- and comorbid diagnoses of severe mental illness or neurological disorders, ongoing substance or alcohol abuse, non-fluency in Norwegian or English, and severe functional impairment hindering completion of the study protocol (i.e., disorders of consciousness, persistent severe anosognosia and severe motor deficits). Patients were identified prospectively after admission to the Neurosurgical department at OUH. Patients were recruited through clinical follow-up consultations at Sunnaas Rehabilitation Hospital and the Department of Physical Medicine and Rehabilitation at OUH. Patients not followed up at these institutions received an invitation to participate by mail.

2.2. Injury Characteristics

Pre-injury physical health status was scored using the American Society of Anesthesiologists' physical status classification (ASA-PS), with scores ranging from 1 to 6 depending on the absence or presence of various severities of systemic disease premorbid to injury [45], with increasing scores indicating more severe disease.

Several indicators of injury severity were included. Lowest Glasgow Coma Scale (GSC) score ranged from 3–15 registered at injury site, or admission to hospital pre-intubation was registered, as well as GCS upon discharge from the acute hospital. Rotterdam CT score is a prognostic classification of traumatic brain injuries scored on the basis of grade of compression of the basal cisterns, the presence of a midline shift, epidural mass lesion, and intraventricular blood or tSAH [46], with higher scores indicating more severe injuries. The Head Abbreviated Injury Scale (AIS_head) version 1998 [47] was used to describe the anatomical severity of injury. AIS classifies injuries to various body regions ranging from minor (1) to fatal (6). We dichotomized AIS_head scores into AIS < 4 (less severe) and AIS $\geq$ 4 (very severe injury) for descriptive analyses but used the ordinal scale scores in subsequent analyses. Finally, discharge destination from the acute hospital was registered. For this study, a dichotomous dummy variable was generated for those who were referred through a direct pathway into rehabilitation units.

2.3. Measures

2.3.1. Fatigue

The Fatigue Severity Scale (FSS) [11] contains 9 items and asks the participants to rate the degree of interference from fatigue in various functional domains on a Likert scale from 1 to 7, with higher scores indicating higher degree of fatigue interference. Norwegian norms adjusted for age, gender and education are available [48]. The FSS has good psychometric qualities [48].

Chalder Fatigue Scale (CFQ) [49], has been applied primarily in research into chronic fatigue syndrome (CFS) and myalgic encephalomyelitis (ME), but also in neurological populations such as stroke [50]. Patients are asked to rate 11 items pertaining to physical and cognitive/mental symptoms of fatigue within the last month. The CFQ uses a four-point response scale where 0 = "less than usual", 1 = "no more than usual", 2 = "more than usual" and 3 = "much more than usual". Normative data from the general population exist, grouped by age and gender [51].

The fatigue subscale of Giessen Subjective Complaints List (GSCL) [52] has been used within psychosomatic and epidemiological studies. The fatigue subscale includes 6 items, rating the presence of fatigue symptoms in general on a five-point scale from 0 = "not at all" to 4 = "strongly".

Finally, one item from the Rivermead Post-Concussion Symptoms Questionnaire (RPQ) [53] asks the participants to rate the presence of fatigue on a scale from 0 to 4, where 0 = "not a problem", 1 = "no longer a problem", 2 = "a mild problem", 3 = "a moderate problem", and 4 = "a severe problem". This single item is often used to assess fatigue in patients with concussion and TBI in clinical settings, and a recent multicenter TBI study employed it as a primary outcome measure of fatigue [15].

2.3.2. Neuropsychological Tests

Cognitive functioning was assessed with the following neuropsychological measures:

The Matrix Reasoning and Similarities subtests from Wechsler's Abbreviated Scale of Intelligence (WASI) [54] were included as measures of abstract reasoning abilities. Auditory attention and working memory were assessed with Digit Span from Wechsler's Adult Intelligence Scale IV (WAIS-IV) [55]. Psychomotor speed was assessed with Trail Making Test (TMT) subtests 2–3 and Color-Word Interference Test (CWIT) subtests 1–2 from Delis–Kaplan Executive Function System (D-KEFS) [56]. Subtest 4 from the TMT and subtests 3–4 from the CWIT furthermore provide measures of executive function/mental flexibility. The Conners Continuous Performance Test III (CPT-III) [57] was included as a measure of sustained and focused attention. The change in coefficient of variation (CoV), a measure of increase in intraindividual variability in reaction times from the first to the second half of the test, was computed. CoV is calculated by dividing the standard deviation of reaction times (RT) by the average RT within the individual [58], and the measure of change in CoV was calculated by subtracting the CoV for the first three blocks from the last three blocks (CoV block change).

2.3.3. Secondary PROMS

Psychological distress over the last two weeks was measured using a 10-item short version of Hopkins Symptom Checklist [59,60], with subscales for (1) depressive and (2) anxiety symptoms.

Five-factor personality traits were measured using the NEO Five Factor Inventory 3 (NEO-FFI-3) [61], which provides gender-corrected normative scores on trait neuroticism, conscientiousness, extroversion, agreeableness and openness to experience. The inventory contains 60 items, with 12 items pertaining to each personality trait.

Behavioral inhibition and activation tendencies were measured using The Behavioral Inhibition System/Behavioral Activation System (BIS/BAS) Scale [38], which contains one subscale for BIS, and three subscales for the BAS, namely (1) reward responsiveness, (2) drive, and (3) fun seeking.

Loneliness was measured using three items from the UCLA Loneliness Scale, Version 3 [62].

Trait optimism was measured with six items from the optimism subscale of the Life Orientation Test Revised (LOT-R) [63].

Resilience was measured with the Resilience Scale for Adults (RSA) [64], with subscales for facets of resilience, namely (1) planned future, (2) social competence, (3) family cohesion, (4) perception of self, (5) social resources, and (6) structured style.

Somatic symptom burden was assessed with subscales from Giessen Subjective Complaints List (GSCL) [52], regarding the presence of (1) gastrointestinal symptoms, (2) musculoskeletal symptoms, and (3) cardiovascular symptoms. Pain localization was assessed using a pain drawing [65], with higher scores indicating generalized pain dispersed across several bodily regions. Pain severity across the last two weeks was assessed with Numerical Rating Scales (0–10, where 10 indicates most severe pain) [66], asking the participants to rate (1) the lowest pain severity, (2) the highest pain severity, (3) the average pain severity, and (4) the current pain severity.

Daytime sleepiness was measured with the Epworth Sleepiness Scale [67], which asks respondents to rate the probability of falling asleep throughout a range of daily activities. Subjective sleep deficits were measured with the Insomnia Severity Index [68], which rates the presence of difficulties with falling asleep, staying asleep, early awakening, and the functional impact of sleep problems.

2.3.4. Functional Outcome

Global functional impairment upon discharge from the acute hospital stay was estimated with the five-level Glasgow Outcome Scale (GOS) [69], while functional outcome 6 months post-injury was assessed with the eight-level Glasgow Outcome Scale Extended (GOSE) [70], which categorizes patients based on their degree of return to work, vocational and leisure activities, social and emotional symptoms and a variety of other persistent complaints following injury. Lower scores indicate greater functional impairment.

2.4. Analyses

All analyses were conducted in SPSS, version 27 [71]. Preliminary Pearson correlation analyses were conducted to evaluate bivariate relations between the various measures of fatigue, sociodemographic variables, injury-related factors, neuropsychological measures and self-reported psychosocial constructs.

2.4.1. Dimension Reduction

In order to ascertain a fatigue factor possibly reflecting a unidimensional phenomenon in our TBI sample, a factor analysis was conducted on FSS, CFQ, the fatigue subscale from GSCL, and the fatigue item from RPQ. Items pertaining specifically to cognitive complaints (CFQ items 8–11 and GSCL item 15) and daytime sleepiness (CFQ item 3 and GSCL item 4 and 14) were excluded from these analyses to avoid item overlap between fatigue and independent variables.

Furthermore, an exploratory factor analysis was conducted on all variables (PROMS, neuropsychological and injury-related) with significant ($p < 0.05$) bivariate associations with either one or several of the fatigue measures. Due to the exploratory aim of the study, variables approaching significance (i.e., $p < 0.08$) were also included. Factors with eigenvalues above 1 were first generated in line with the Kaiser Guttman criterion. A scree plot was generated and inspected according to Cattell's criterion [72]. Parallel analyses were performed to generate significant eigenvalues for factor retention [73], which has been shown to be a more consistently accurate method for factor retention decisions [74]. Oblimin oblique rotation was conducted to allow factors to correlate. Saliency of factor loadings was evaluated for significance ($p < 0.05$) according to the formula proposed by Norman and Streiner (2014), providing a cut-off for salient loadings at 0.40. Variables not loading significantly on any of the factors were removed, and the analyses were repeated without them. In the case of cross-loading variables, variables were selected on the basis of the strength of their loadings, as well as their conceptual alignment with the factor on the whole. New factor analyses were then conducted for each factor, including only those variables saliently loading on the factor. Factor scores were generated through regression.

Factor reliability was assessed for all resulting factors, through the calculation of Cronbach's alpha with standardized variables, with negatively loading variables reversed. Alpha values of 0.70 or higher were deemed acceptable, and values of 0.90 or higher were considered excellent.

2.4.2. Multiple Regression

In order to evaluate the relations between fatigue and the factors derived from the previous step, the fatigue factor was regressed on the factor scores from associated constructs. Variables were entered into the linear regression model blockwise. Sociodemographic variables were entered first, with age (centered around the sample mean of 45), educational attainment (centered around the sample mean of 13 years), and gender (female) as baseline covariates. The factors from the previous step were then added to examine if they contributed significantly to the model. Changes in F-scores were evaluated for significance in model improvement across each block. Bootstrapping was conducted to evaluate the robustness of the regression coefficients, and a 95% confidence interval (CI) was produced based on 2000 random draws from the sample. The results from linear regression analyses are reported with unstandardized regression coefficients (B) with bootstrapped standard errors (SE), 95% confidence intervals (CI), standardized regression coefficients (β) and explained variance (adjusted R^2).

Partial regression plots were generated to evaluate the impact of potential outliers. Residual plots were also inspected to evaluate deviance from assumptions of normality, homoscedasticity and linearity. Residual scores were finally checked for associations with variables not included in previous factor analyses, to evaluate potential residual effects not captured by this model. Post hoc analyses were then conducted to evaluate the potential additional explanatory value of these variables. Finally, univariate regression analyses were conducted post hoc to evaluate the associations between individual variables contained within each factor, and the fatigue factor.

3. Results

3.1. Sample Characteristics

A total of 96 patients were included. See Figure 1 for an overview of the exclusion and inclusion process.

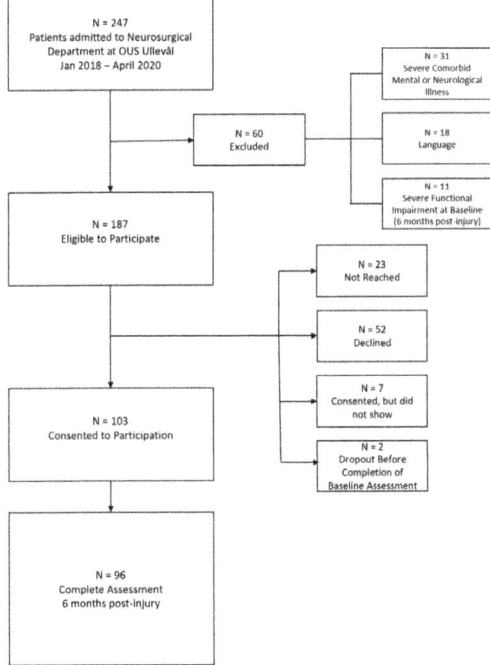

Figure 1. Flow chart of the inclusion and exclusion process. From a sample of 187 eligible patients, 103 participants (55%) consented to participate, and 96 ended up with a complete dataset.

The average age was 45.3 (SD = 13.9), with a mean educational attainment of 13.5 years (SD = 2.3). The sample consisted of 77 (80.2%) males and 19 (19.8%) females.

On the ASA-PS, 69 patients (71.9%) were classified as healthy prior to injury, 19 (19.8%) as having moderate organic disease not impairing function, and eight patients (8.3%) as having severe organic disease.

The sample mean of GCS registered at injury site or at admission to the hospital pre-intubation was 10.7 (SD = 3.6), while GCS registered upon discharge from the acute hospital was 14.4 (SD = 0.9). The sample mean Rotterdam CT score was 2.8 (SD = 0.9). Using the dichotomized AIS_head classification, 18 patients (18.8%) were classified within the less severe category, and 78 (81.3%) within the very severe category. Upon discharge from the acute hospital, GOS ratings based on medical records classified 39 patients (40.6%) with moderate disability, 56 (58.3%) with severe disability, and one patient (1.1%) as being in a vegetative state.

Fifteen patients (15.6%) were discharged directly to their homes, 32 (33.3%) to a local hospital, and 49 (51%) were referred to a rehabilitation unit.

The study assessment was conducted on average 205 days (SD = 28) since injury.

3.2. Fatigue PROMS

The FSS demonstrated good internal consistency ($\alpha = 0.91$). The average score was 3.7, corresponding to a demographically corrected T-score of 48.8 (SD = 11.9).

CFQ demonstrated good internal consistency ($\alpha = 0.89$). The mean sum score for the total scale was 16.2, corresponding to a demographically corrected T-score of 60.8 (SD = 14.2), with comparable results on the mental/cognitive and physical subscales. Items 1 and 2 on the CFQ ask the patients to rate whether they experience increased tiredness or an increased need for rest within the last month compared to their habitual function, and 58 (60.4%) and 59 (61.5%) patients, respectively, endorsed the presence of these problems as compared to their habitual function.

The GSCL subscale demonstrated good internal consistency ($\alpha = 0.89$). On the GSCL fatigue subscale, the mean score was approximately 1 (SD = 0.9), corresponding to the response category "somewhat a problem".

On the RPQ fatigue item, 47 patients (49%) reported at least mild problems with fatigue, and 27 (28.1%) reported moderate-severe problems. For an overview over bivariate correlations between fatigue PROMS, see the Supplementary Materials (Table S1).

3.3. Fatigue and Associated Factors

Overall, fatigue as measured with several PROMS was consistently associated with several biopsychosocial PROMS and functional outcome, while the associative patterns were less consistent for injury-related and neuropsychological variables. There were no bivariate associations between demographic variables (age, gender, education) and any of the fatigue measures. The Head Abbreviated Injury Scale (AIS_head), length of acute hospital stay, GOS at discharge from acute hospital, and having a direct pathway to rehabilitation were associated with higher Physical Fatigue on CFQ. GCS at discharge trended toward significance ($p < 0.08$) in its relationship with the Physical Fatigue subscale from CFQ. No other measure of fatigue was significantly associated with variables from the acute phase.

Fatigue scores (FSS, CFQ, GSCL and RPQ) were positively associated with depression, anxiety, trait neuroticism, daytime sleepiness, insomnia, behavioral inhibition (BIS), all measures of pain, loneliness, and somatic (musculoskeletal/gastrointestinal/cardiovascular) symptom burden, albeit with some variation across measures. Trait openness was positively associated with the RPQ fatigue item only.

Fatigue was negatively associated with two resilience subscales (perception of self and planned future) on most fatigue PROMS, and trending toward significance ($p < 0.08$) for trait optimism in association with the FSS. Trait extraversion was negatively associated with the GSCL fatigue subscale only, and trait conscientiousness was trending toward significance ($p < 0.08$) for a negative association with the FSS.

Fatigue was negatively associated with performance on the CWIT 4—Switching Condition (a measure of mental flexibility) for the FSS and CFQ, and FSS was negatively associated with performance on measure of intraindividual stability of sustained reaction times on the CPT-III. The mental fatigue subscale on the CFQ was negatively associated with performance on several neuropsychological measures. However, this subscale probes about subjective cognitive complaints such as memory and word-finding difficulties, and these associations are not taken into account in the following analyses.

All measures of fatigue were negatively associated with functional outcome 6 months post-injury as measured by GOSE.

For a complete overview of bivariate associations between fatigue and included variables, see the Supplementary Materials (Tables S2–S4).

3.4. Dimension Reduction

In the factor analysis of the items from the included fatigue outcome measures, three factors were initially generated with an eigenvalue above 1. Both an inspection of the scree plot and parallel analysis of critical threshold for significant eigenvalues provided support for a one-component solution. Items 1 and 2 from the FSS were excluded following the primary factor analysis due to non-salient loadings on the generated factor. All remaining items loaded saliently on the single component (see Table 1). The factor demonstrated excellent reliability (Cronbach's alpha = 0.95) and thus provided an opportunity to examine relationships between the other variables and one single and robust fatigue measure.

Table 1. Factor loadings of items from fatigue measures. All items load saliently on the component at significance level of $p < 0.05$, i.e., loadings above 0.40.

	Fatigue
	Component
FSS Item 3	0.80
FSS Item 4	0.44
FSS Item 5	0.76
FSS Item 6	0.73
FSS Item 7	0.80
FSS Item 8	0.78
FSS Item 9	0.82
CFQ Item 1	0.81
CFQ Item 2	0.70
CFQ Item 4	0.63
CFQ Item 5	0.80
CFQ Item 6	0.56
CFQ Item 7	0.54
GSCL Item 1	0.61
GSCL Item 12	0.85
GSCL Item 17	0.69
RPQ Item 6	0.81
Extraction Sum of Squared Loadings (% of variance)	8.9 (52.4%)
Cronbach's alpha	0.95

For the factor analysis of all associated constructs, seven components were initially generated with an eigenvalue above 1. While the inspection of the scree plot of eigenvalues might suggest retention of either three or four components according to Cattell's criterium, the thresholds from the parallel analysis supported the retention of only the first three components. The component matrix was obliquely rotated using Oblimin rotation, which allows for correlated components. The neuropsychological measures (CWIT-4 and CPT-III CoV Block Change) and trait openness did not load saliently on any of the three factors, and the analysis was repeated without these variables included.

Based on the salient positive loadings from resilience subscales, trait optimism, trait extraversion and trait conscientiousness on Factor 1, this component was designated as a Psychosocial Robustness factor. Factor 1 also has salient negative loadings from trait neuroticism, behavioral inhibition, symptoms of depression and anxiety, loneliness, and gastrointestinal and cardiovascular symptoms, confirming that robustness is a combination of presence of positive protective factors, but is also an absence of risk factors. Factor 2 had salient loadings from all measures of pain, somatic symptom burden (musculoskeletal, cardiovascular and gastrointestinal), daytime sleepiness, subjective sleep complaints, as well as symptoms of depression and anxiety. This factor was thus designated as a somatic vulnerability factor. Factor 3 had salient loadings from all five variables from the acute phase, with negative loadings from GCS and GOS at discharge from the acute hospital, and positive loadings from length of ICU stay, AIS_head and a direct pathway to rehabilitation. This factor was designated as an injury severity factor.

New factor analyses were conducted, one for each factor. Anxiety and depression were cross-loaded on factors 1 and 2 and were selected for inclusion in the psychosocial robustness factor due to stronger loadings. Likewise, the GSCL subscales for gastrointestinal and cardiovascular symptoms were cross-loaded on factors 1 and 2 and were selected for inclusion in the somatic vulnerability factor due to higher loadings and more conceptual overlap. The final factor analyses supported the unidimensionality of the three factors, and the factors demonstrated good to adequate factor reliability. See Table 2 for final factor loadings and reliability indicators.

Table 2. Factor loadings for the final unidimensional factor analyses of self-reported independent variables (N = 96). Squared loadings and explained variance therefore refer to only those variables included in each of the three factor analyses. For an overview of the primary factor analyses, see the Supplementary Materials (Table S5).

	Factors		
	Psychosocial Robustness	Somatic Vulnerability	Injury Severity
Behavioral Inhibition	−0.55		
Trait Neuroticism	−0.90		
Trait Extraversion	0.63		
Trait Conscientiousness	0.56		
Trait Optimism	0.69		
Loneliness	−0.70		
Anxiety Symptoms	−0.64		
Depressive Symptoms	−0.76		
Resilience–Perception of Self	0.84		
Resilience–Planned Future	0.64		
Daytime Sleepiness		0.48	
Insomnia Severity Index		0.48	
Pain–Affected Regions		0.74	
Strongest Pain		0.84	
Weakest Pain		0.64	
Average Pain		0.88	
Current Pain		0.73	
Gastrointestinal Symptoms		0.61	
Musculoskeletal Symptoms		0.84	
Cardiovascular Symptoms		0.53	
AIS_head			0.58
Length of ICU Stay (days)			0.58
GCS at Discharge			−0.67
GOS at Discharge			−0.77
Direct Pathway to Rehabilitation			0.71
Extraction Sums of Squared Loadings (% of variance in included variables)	4.9 (49.0%)	4.8 (48.0%)	2.2 (44.4%)
Cronbach's alpha	0.91	0.89	0.80

3.5. Multiple Regression

Results from the blockwise multiple linear regression of fatigue in the sample with complete data are shown in Table 3. Age, education and gender had no significant associations with the fatigue factor (Model 1), and the model explains a non-significant amount of variance in fatigue. The injury severity factor did not in isolation contribute significantly to the model in the second regression block.

Table 3. Blockwise multiple linear regression (N = 96). Unstandardized (B) and standardized coefficients (β) are reported. Adjusted R^2 shows the model-explained variance, and the F change-statistic is a test of the improvement from the previous model. Standard errors (SE) shown are calculated from bootstrapping. The final column shows the 95% confidence interval for the unstandardized coefficients (B) in Model 3. ns not significant, * $p < 0.05$, *** $p < 0.001$.

	Model 1		Model 2		Model 3		95% CI	
	β	B (SE)	β	B (SE)	β	B (SE)	Lower	Upper
Constant		−0.08 (0.14)		−0.08 (0.11)		−0.08 (0.09)	(−0.25	0.09)
Age (Centered)	0.01	0.00 (0.01)	0.00	0.00 (0.01)	−0.01	−0.00 (0.01)	(−0.01	0.01)
Education (Centered)	0.00	0.00 (0.04)	0.01	0.00 (0.01)	0.10	0.05 (0.04)	(−0.02	0.13)
Female	0.17	0.41 (0.26)	0.17	0.40 (0.27)	0.12	0.29 (0.18)	(−0.08	0.65)
Injury Severity			0.13	0.14 (0.11)	0.16 *	0.18 (0.08)	(0.01	0.34)
Psychosocial Robustness					−0.17 *	−0.17 (0.09)	(−0.34	−0.01)
Somatic Vulnerability					0.59 ***	0.60 (0.08)	(0.46	75)
Adjusted R^2		0.001		0.001		0.442		
F Change		0.89 ns		1.65 ns		36.8 ***		

In Model 3, psychosocial robustness was significantly negatively associated with fatigue, and somatic vulnerability showed a strong positive association with fatigue. The injury severity factor entered in the previous block now showed a barely statistically significant effect. While the effects for the psychosocial robustness factor and the injury severity factor were significant, the confidence intervals bootstrapped for their coefficients border on zero, and as such, demonstrate less robust effects than the somatic vulnerability factor. This final model explains 44.2% of the variance in the fatigue factor.

3.6. Post Hoc Analyses

Due to the non-inclusion of the neuropsychological measures in the factors derived from earlier steps, correlations between the residuals of the regression analysis and the neuropsychological measures were inspected. The residual from the final regression model was negatively associated with mental flexibility (CWIT-4, n = 90, r = −0.27) and sustained attention (CPT-III CoV block change, n = 95, r = −0.20). For exploratory purposes, a composite score of these two measures was added in a final block in the blockwise regression (n = 89). The results overlapped considerably with those from the primary regression model. The addition of the neuropsychological composite variable in the final block led to a significant increase in explained variance up to 51.6%. However, the neuropsychological composite score was negatively associated with the injury severity factor (n = 89, r = −0.23), and its inclusion suppressed the association of the injury severity factor below significance (see Table S6 in the Supplementary Materials).

Finally, the relative importance of each variable loading upon the three factors was explored in univariate regression models, with the fatigue factor as the dependent variable. For univariate regression coefficients and explained variance, see Tables S7–S9 in the Supplementary Materials. The anxiety, depression and the resilience subscale, planned future, had the strongest univariate impact on fatigue in the psychosocial robustness factor. In the somatic vulnerability factor, all variables explained a significant amount of variance in fatigue, but the GSCL musculoskeletal symptoms subscale demonstrated the strongest positive association. Finally, for the injury severity factor, effects were in general weak, and only the Direct Pathway to Rehabilitation and AIS_head demonstrated significant univariate associations with fatigue.

4. Discussion

The present study aimed to explore dimensions underlying various biopsychosocial constructs commonly associated with fatigue six months following TBI. In line with the notion of fatigue as being influenced by both injury-specific and general risk factors, this study examined the relationship between a multitude of variables that have previously been associated with fatigue after TBI, and several fatigue outcome measures. The results highlight that three underlying factors related to psychosocial robustness, somatic vulnerability and injury severity can be identified, providing a clearer picture of the somewhat fragmented literature on protective and risk factors for post-TBI fatigue.

4.1. Unidimensionality of Post-TBI Fatigue

Regarding fatigue levels, our findings confirm variations between measures. On the FSS, the patients reported similar levels of fatigue interference as those seen in the general population [48]. On the CFQ, however, the sample reported fatigue symptoms approximately one standard deviation above the normative average [51], and on specific items, 60% reported increases in tiredness and their need for rest. Our findings support the notion that the majority of patients with TBI experience increased levels of fatigue, while many, despite their symptoms, report little to no interference from fatigue during the first 6 months. This aligns with the findings by Kjeverud et al. [38] in stroke patients, which were interpreted as a dissociation between fatigue severity and fatigue interference. Some patients may experience more fatigue following injury but are able to compensate successfully such that it does not interfere with the roles and activities pertinent to their daily life. Additionally, many patients were still on sick leave at the time of measurement, which could contribute to a low degree of functional interference due to decreased environmental demands.

Despite these variations, the items from the included fatigue PROMS demonstrated good reliability and considerable unidimensionality in our factor analytic approach, indicating that the measures seem to measure a uniform concept. The single fatigue item from the RPQ also demonstrated good correspondence with the other measures, which support the utility of this single item in clinical practice, and items from the GSCL fatigue subscale also aligned well along the unidimensional fatigue factor. Items 1 and 2 from the FSS did not load saliently on the fatigue factor, in line with previous studies of the FSS in patients with, e.g., stroke [75], and were thus not included.

4.2. Biopsychosocial Dimensions-Relevance for Fatigue

Through factor analyses, we evaluated overlap and underlying dimensionality among self-reported PROMS of biopsychosocial constructs often associated with fatigue. Two salient factors were extracted, which we termed psychosocial robustness and somatic vulnerability. These factors showed some overlap with regard to anxiety and depression, as well as gastrointestinal and cardiovascular symptoms, showing that there are some commonalities between them despite the parsimonious structure selected. A third factor was found, termed as an injury severity factor based on strong loadings from injury-related severity indices from an acute hospital stay. In the subsequent multivariate regression analyses, somatic vulnerability, psychosocial robustness and injury severity factors all demonstrated significant associations with fatigue, explaining 44.2% of variance in fatigue 6 months after TBI.

Somatic vulnerability demonstrated a particularly strong and robust association with fatigue, in line with the literature linking pain and fatigue as central comorbidities [22,76], and earlier studies in the TBI population [23,25]. This factor explained 39% of the variance in fatigue in isolation, in essence contributing most of the explained variance in the multivariate regression models. Subsequent univariate post hoc regression analyses showed that all the variables underlying this dimension contributed significantly to the association between somatic vulnerability and fatigue. Notably, the GSCL subscale for musculoskeletal symptoms explained more variance in fatigue than the somatic vulnerability factor in large, indicating that nonspecific musculoskeletal pains are particularly crucial markers for somatic vulnerability and the factor's association with fatigue in this sample.

The association between psychosocial robustness and fatigue supports earlier findings linking resilience with less fatigue after TBI [77]. Trait extraversion, conscientiousness and optimism seemed to align with resilience factors in this protective dimension, while trait neuroticism, loneliness, behavioral inhibition and psychological distress were placed on the opposite side of this dimension, confirming that absence of negative emotionality is a prominent feature of psychosocial robustness. Associations between high neuroticism, low extraversion and low conscientiousness and fatigue have been demonstrated in mild TBI [34] and other populations [78]; thus, these findings are in line with previous findings. While trait extraversion, trait conscientiousness and trait optimism did load heavily on this protective dimension, they were not significantly associated with fatigue 6 months post-injury in isolation. Conversely, measures of state and trait negative affectivity (state depression and anxiety, and trait neuroticism to a lesser degree) and resilience (planned future, and to a lesser degree perception of self) were essential to the relevance of psychosocial robustness for fatigue in our sample. The resilience subscale for planned future pertains to the perception of the future as manageable and predictable through goal-directedness and structure, while the subscale for perception of self relates to self-efficacy and potential for growth through adversity. These constructs thus align well as opposites to anxiety and depression.

The association between fatigue and injury severity became significant when controlling for psychosocial robustness and somatic vulnerability. Among the underlying injury-related variables, only the direct pathway to rehabilitation and the AIS_head demonstrated significant univariate associations with fatigue in post hoc regression analyses, indicating that anatomical brain injury severity combined with early functional status are particularly relevant. Post hoc analyses furthermore demonstrated that a measure of mental flexibility suppressed the association between the injury severity factor and fatigue, indicating that the injury severity factor from the acute phase and the resulting cognitive deficits in mental flexibility after six months overlap in their contributions to fatigue.

A visual representation of the findings is provided in Figure 2.

4.3. Implications for Rehabilitation

The fact that fatigue was strongly associated with functional status 6 months post-injury is in line with earlier findings. The results illustrate that fatigue is associated with everyday functioning and point to the importance of addressing fatigue in rehabilitation [2]. While fatigue is a severe problem for many patients with TBI, there is nevertheless considerable heterogeneity, with some patients reporting little to no fatigue interference in everyday life. Understanding which patients are at risk of developing persistent fatigue and functional interference from fatigue, and why, is crucial in improving our care for this patient group.

While more severe injuries are accompanied by greater sensory-motor and cognitive deficits, and accordingly might necessitate greater compensatory efforts in returning to mental and cognitive activities, initial injury severity indices were inconsistently associated with fatigue in our study. Our findings showed that some brain injury severity indices and having a direct pathway to rehabilitation were weakly associated with fatigue. The latter finding may likely be interpreted as a proxy for functional status, as patients with severe symptoms were more likely to be transferred to rehabilitation, irrespective of injury severity measures. The injury severity factor was only associated with fatigue when controlling for robustness and vulnerability, confirming that other risk factors for fatigue are intertwined with injury severity initially, but can be disentangled when adjusted for. For instance, patients with relatively mild injuries, but who suffer from co- or premorbid pain or depression, may be at high risk for fatigue despite mild injuries. While having a high degree of somatic vulnerability and low degree of psychosocial robustness might contribute to an increased risk of fatigue in isolation, injury characteristics serve as an independent risk as well, although these associations are less robust.

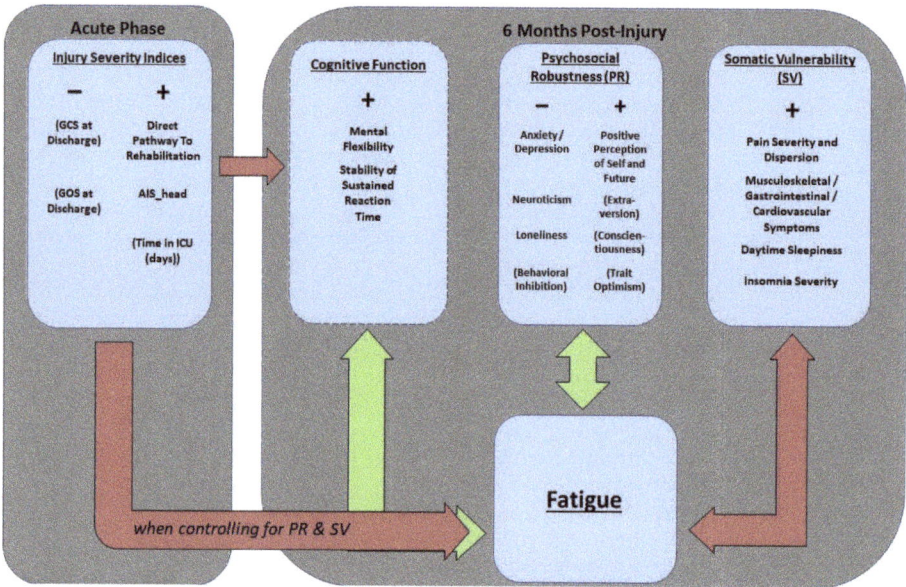

Figure 2. A visual representation of the findings from our study. Note that cognitive function is marked by a dotted box, so as to illustrate that these effects were found in post hoc analyses with a slightly smaller sample due to missing data. Double-sided arrows imply within-time associations, while one-sided arrows imply unidirectional influences. Green arrows imply positive correlations, and red arrows imply negative correlations. Parentheses signify variables with significant loadings on the factor, but with no significant contribution to fatigue when inspected in isolation.

Our findings also underline the importance of the contribution of various biopsychosocial protective and vulnerability factors. Somatic symptom burden and especially pain emerge as important associated factors with fatigue following TBI, which should be considered as central targets for rehabilitation. The exact nature of the relationship between fatigue and pain cannot be deduced based on our cross-sectional design, but until further longitudinal research sheds more light on these relationships, the possibility of temporal and bidirectional influences should be considered. Rehabilitation efforts addressing fatigue should therefore also address concurrent risk factors for fatigue. This can be achieved through holistic rehabilitation programs. New methods such as virtual reality have shown promising results in the treatment of pain, emotional symptoms, and fatigue, and should be explored [79,80].

This study furthermore demonstrates the importance of taking into account protective factors which might buffer against fatigue. Aspects of resilience such as perceiving the future as manageable and predictable, and self-efficacy in the face of adversity, were negatively associated with fatigue. On the opposite side of the same dimension, lower levels of loneliness and negative effects are positively associated with fatigue. The findings indicate that rehabilitation efforts aimed at helping patients re-establish a coherent sense of self and their future, and to reconnect with social resources, might lessen their risk of fatigue in the early stages of rehabilitation. This latter point was supported in a recent qualitative study [81], in which the use of social support was identified as a promising treatment angle for breaking vicious cycles for perpetuation and exacerbation of fatigue after brain injury.

4.4. Limitations

This study examined cross-sectional associations between fatigue and related constructs but did not allow for inferences regarding directional influences. Furthermore, while dimensions derived from factor analyses provide a parsimonious structure to the relations between various predictors of fatigue, one cannot eliminate possible within- and between-factor dynamics, such as premorbid trait neuroticism influencing the post-injury development of anxiety and depression, which could again influence fatigue. Our post hoc analyses furthermore demonstrated that the variable loading on each factor contributed to different degrees of fatigue when viewed in isolation. Finally, our study has a relatively modest sample size, and generalizations of the results to other cohorts should be made with caution. Of 450 patients with intracranial injury admitted to the Neurosurgery department in the study period, we assessed 55% for eligibility and included 21.3% of the total population. The mean age and the gender ratio included are in line with the TBI population included in the quality database [44]. However, our sample is weighted toward moderate and severe injuries (77%) compared with those included in the quality database (57%). Thus, the results may not be generalizable to those with milder intracranial injuries.

Ideally, a somewhat larger sample would have to be investigated to provide better estimates of essential parameters (particularly factor loadings and regression coefficients) in the population in question. However, while the parameter estimates could be more accurate, and small sample sizes tend to increase the liability to Type II errors, and we see no reason to doubt the general pattern of findings from the study.

5. Conclusions

Through the exploration of factors associated with fatigue following TBI, this study has demonstrated that factors related to fatigue after TBI might be described along three dimensions, i.e., psychosocial robustness, somatic vulnerability and injury-related factors. Within these factors, somatic symptom burden (especially pain), depression, anxiety, positive perceived prospects for the future, loneliness daytime sleepiness, subjective insomnia, anatomical severity of injury and being referred directly to rehabilitation services all demonstrated relevance for fatigue 6 months post-injury. These factors, while having varying importance, illustrate the breadth of biopsychosocial underpinnings for fatigue following TBI.

The findings illuminate potential tangible treatment targets in rehabilitation of fatigue after TBI and may guide future research aimed at establishing evidence-based treatment options. More research is needed to understand potential dynamic interactions between fatigue and the associated vulnerability and protective factors, and to understand how these may develop over time.

Supplementary Materials: The following supporting information can be downloaded at: https://www.mdpi.com/article/10.3390/jcm11061733/s1, Table S1: Bivariate correlations between PROMS of fatigue. Table S2: Bivariate associations between fatigue PROMS, sociodemographic variables and injury-related factors. Table S3: Bivariate correlations between fatigue PROMS and neuropsychological measures. Table S4: Bivariate correlations between fatigue PROMS and PROMS of related constructs. Table S5: Structure matrix with variable loadings for the primay factor analysis after oblique rotation (Oblimin), with factor correlations. Table S6: Post-Hoc Blockwise multiple regression. Table S7: Coefficients and explained variance in the fatigue factor (outcome variable) from univariate regression models with the Psychosocial Robustness factor and the individual variables loading onto this factor. Table S8: Coefficients and explained variance in the fatigue factor (outcome variable) from univariate regression models with the Somatic Vulnerability factor and the individual variables loading onto this factor. Table S9: Coefficients and explained variance in the fatigue factor (outcome variable) from univariate regression models with the Injury Severity factor and the individual variables loading onto this factor, as well as the neuropsychological measures and their composite.

Author Contributions: Conceptualization and methodology: D.L., M.L., O.V., N.A., S.A. and J.L.P.; recruitment and data collection: D.L., N.A., E.H., C.T. and M.L.; project management: D.L., M.L. and N.A.; data analysis: D.L., C.B., O.V., N.A. and M.L.; writing—first draft: D.L., M.L., N.A. and C.B.; writing—review and editing: D.L., N.A., E.H., O.V., S.A., J.L.P., C.B., C.T. and M.L. All authors have read and agreed to the published version of the manuscript.

Funding: The doctoral research fellowship of the corresponding author was funded by Stiftelsen Dam (grant FO202360) in collaboration with the user organization Personskadeforbundet LTN.

Institutional Review Board Statement: The project was approved by the Regional Ethical Committee for Medical and Health Research, Norway (application 2018/144).

Informed Consent Statement: Informed consent was obtained from all subjects included in the study.

Data Availability Statement: Due to the sensitive nature of the data involved in this project, the data have not been made publicly available. Interested parties may contact the corresponding author (D.L.) for requests for data access.

Acknowledgments: We would like to thank all participants for their contributions to this study, and the user organization Personskadeforbundet LTN for their collaboration and support in our research.

Conflicts of Interest: The authors declare no conflict of interest.

References

1. Mollayeva, T.; Kendzerska, T.; Mollayeva, S.; Shapiro, C.M.; Colantonio, A.; Cassidy, J.D. A systematic review of fatigue in patients with traumatic brain injury: The course, predictors and consequences. *Neurosci. Biobehav. Rev.* **2014**, *47*, 684–716. [CrossRef] [PubMed]
2. Cantor, J.B.; Ashman, T.; Gordon, W.; Ginsberg, A.; Engmann, C.; Egan, M.; Spielman, L.; Dijkers, M.; Flanagan, S. Fatigue after traumatic brain injury and its impact on participation and quality of life. *J. Head Trauma Rehabil.* **2008**, *23*, 41–51. [CrossRef] [PubMed]
3. Juengst, S.; Skidmore, E.; Arenth, P.M.; Niyonkuru, C.; Raina, K.D. Unique contribution of fatigue to disability in community-dwelling adults with traumatic brain injury. *Arch. Phys. Med. Rehabil.* **2013**, *94*, 74–79. [CrossRef] [PubMed]
4. Menon, D.K.; Schwab, K.; Wright, D.W.; Maas, A.I. Position statement: Definition of traumatic brain injury. *Arch. Phys. Med. Rehabil.* **2010**, *91*, 1637–1640. [CrossRef] [PubMed]
5. Fazel, S.; Wolf, A.; Pillas, D.; Lichtenstein, P.; Långström, N. Suicide, fatal injuries, and other causes of premature mortality in patients with traumatic brain injury: A 41-year Swedish population study. *JAMA Psychiatry* **2014**, *71*, 326–333. [CrossRef]
6. Ponsford, J.L.; Downing, M.G.; Olver, J.; Ponsford, M.; Acher, R.; Carty, M.; Spitz, G. Longitudinal follow-up of patients with traumatic brain injury: Outcome at two, five, and ten years post-injury. *J. Neurotrauma* **2014**, *31*, 64–77. [CrossRef] [PubMed]
7. Aaronson, L.S.; Teel, C.S.; Cassmeyer, V.; Neuberger, G.B.; Pallikkathayil, L.; Pierce, J.; Press, A.N.; Williams, P.D.; Wingate, A. Defining and measuring fatigue. *Image J. Nurs. Scholarsh.* **1999**, *31*, 45–50. [CrossRef]
8. Hjollund, N.H.; Andersen, J.H.; Bech, P. Assessment of fatigue in chronic disease: A bibliographic study of fatigue measurement scales. *Health Qual. Life Outcomes* **2007**, *5*, 12. [CrossRef] [PubMed]
9. Choi, B.C.; Pak, A.W. Peer reviewed: A catalog of biases in questionnaires. *Prev. Chronic Dis.* **2005**, *2*, A13.
10. Skogestad, I.J.; Kirkevold, M.; Indredavik, B.; Gay, C.L.; Lerdal, A. Lack of content overlap and essential dimensions–A review of measures used for post-stroke fatigue. *J. Psychosom. Res.* **2019**, *124*, 109759. [CrossRef]
11. Krupp, L.B.; LaRocca, N.G.; Muir-Nash, J.; Steinberg, A.D. The fatigue severity scale: Application to patients with multiple sclerosis and systemic lupus erythematosus. *Arch. Neurol.* **1989**, *46*, 1121–1123. [CrossRef] [PubMed]
12. Norup, A.; Svendsen, S.W.; Doser, K.B.; Ryttersgaard, T.O.; Frandsen, N.; Gade, L.; Forchhammer, H.B. Prevalence and severity of fatigue in adolescents and young adults with acquired brain injury: A nationwide study. *Neuropsychol. Rehabil.* **2017**, *29*, 1113–1128. [CrossRef] [PubMed]
13. Ziino, C.; Ponsford, J. Measurement and prediction of subjective fatigue following traumatic brain injury. *J. Int. Neuropsychol. Soc.* **2005**, *11*, 416–425. [CrossRef] [PubMed]
14. Cantor, J.B.; Bushnik, T.; Cicerone, K.; Dijkers, M.P.; Gordon, W.; Hammond, F.M.; Kolakowsky-Hayner, S.A.; Lequerica, A.; Nguyen, M.; Spielman, L.A. Insomnia, fatigue, and sleepiness in the first 2 years after traumatic brain injury: An NIDRR TBI model system module study. *J. Head Trauma Rehabil.* **2012**, *27*, E1–E14. [CrossRef]
15. Andelic, N.; Røe, C.; Brunborg, C.; Zeldovich, M.; Løvstad, M.; Løke, D.; Borgen, I.M.; Voormolen, D.C.; Howe, E.I.; Forslund, M.V.; et al. Frequency of fatigue and its changes in the first 6 months after traumatic brain injury: Results from the CENTER-TBI study. *J. Neurol.* **2021**, *268*, 61–73. [CrossRef]
16. Johansson, B.; Berglund, P.; Rönnbäck, L. Mental fatigue and impaired information processing after mild and moderate traumatic brain injury. *Brain Inj.* **2009**, *23*, 1027–1040. [CrossRef]

17. Ziino, C.; Ponsford, J. Selective attention deficits and subjective fatigue following traumatic brain injury. *Neuropsychology* **2006**, *20*, 383. [CrossRef]
18. van Zomeren, A.H.; Brouwer, W.H.; Deelman, B.G. Attentional deficits: The riddles of selectivity, speed and alertness. In *Closed Head Injury: Psychological, Social, and Family Consequences*; Brooks, N., Ed.; Oxford University Press: Oxford, UK, 1984; pp. 74–107.
19. Penner, I.-K.; Paul, F. Fatigue as a symptom or comorbidity of neurological diseases. *Nat. Rev. Neurol.* **2017**, *13*, 662–675. [CrossRef]
20. Bushnik, T.; Englander, J.; Katznelson, L. Fatigue after TBI: Association with neuroendocrine abnormalities. *Brain Inj.* **2007**, *21*, 559–566. [CrossRef]
21. Cantor, J.B.; Gordon, W.; Gumber, S. What is post TBI fatigue? *NeuroRehabilitation* **2013**, *32*, 875–883. [CrossRef]
22. Wyller, V.B.B. Pain is common in chronic fatigue syndrome–current knowledge and future perspectives. *Scand. J. Pain* **2019**, *19*, 5–8. [CrossRef] [PubMed]
23. Beaulieu-Bonneau, S.; Ouellet, M.-C. Fatigue in the first year after traumatic brain injury: Course, relationship with injury severity, and correlates. *Neuropsychol. Rehabil.* **2017**, *27*, 983–1001. [CrossRef] [PubMed]
24. Sigurdardottir, S.; Andelic, N.; Roe, C.; Schanke, A. Depressive symptoms and psychological distress during the first five years after traumatic brain injury: Relationship with psychosocial stressors, fatigue and pain. *J. Rehabil. Med.* **2013**, *45*, 808–814. [CrossRef]
25. Ponsford, J.L.; Ziino, C.; Parcell, D.L.; Shekleton, J.A.; Roper, M.; Redman, J.R.; Phipps-Nelson, J.; Rajaratnam, S.M.W. Fatigue and sleep disturbance following traumatic brain injury—their nature, causes, and potential treatments. *J. Head Trauma Rehabil.* **2012**, *27*, 224–233. [CrossRef]
26. Holmqvist, A.; Lindstedt, M.; Möller, M. Relationship between fatigue after acquired brain injury and depression, injury localization and aetiology: An explorative study in a rehabilitation setting. *J. Rehabil. Med.* **2018**, *50*, 725–731. [CrossRef] [PubMed]
27. Ponsford, J.; Schönberger, M.; Rajaratnam, S.M.W. A Model of Fatigue Following Traumatic Brain Injury. *J. Head Trauma Rehabil.* **2015**, *30*, 277–282. [CrossRef]
28. Englander, J.; Bushnik, T.; Oggins, J.; Katznelson, L. Fatigue after traumatic brain injury: Association with neuroendocrine, sleep, depression and other factors. *Brain Inj.* **2010**, *24*, 1379–1388. [CrossRef]
29. Ouellet, M.C.; Morin, C.M. Fatigue following traumatic brain injury: Frequency, characteristics, and associated factors. *Rehabil. Psychol.* **2006**, *51*, 140. [CrossRef]
30. Sindermann, C.; Saliger, J.; Nielsen, J.; Karbe, H.; Markett, S.; Stavrou, M.; Montag, C. Personality and primary emotional traits: Disentangling multiple sclerosis related fatigue and depression. *Arch. Clin. Neuropsychol.* **2018**, *33*, 552–561. [CrossRef]
31. Vassend, O.; Roysamb, E.; Nielsen, C.S.; Czajkowski, N.O. Fatigue symptoms in relation to neuroticism, anxiety-depression, and musculoskeletal pain. A longitudinal twin study. *PLoS ONE* **2018**, *13*, e0198594. [CrossRef]
32. Charles, S.T.; Gatz, M.; Kato, K.; Pedersen, N.L. Physical Health 25 Years Later: The Predictive Ability of Neuroticism. *Health Psychol.* **2008**, *27*, 369–378. [CrossRef] [PubMed]
33. Lau, C.G.; Tang, W.K.; Liu, X.X.; Liang, H.J.; Liang, Y.; Mok, V.; MSocSc, A.W.; Ungvari, G.S.; Kutlubaev, M.A.; Wong, K.S. Neuroticism and fatigue 3 months after ischemic stroke: A cross-sectional study. *Arch. Phys. Med. Rehabil.* **2017**, *98*, 716–721. [CrossRef]
34. Merz, Z.C.; Zane, K.; Emmert, N.A.; Lace, J.; Grant, A. Examining the relationship between neuroticism and post-concussion syndrome in mild traumatic brain injury. *Brain Inj.* **2019**, *33*, 1003–1011. [CrossRef]
35. Lee, E.; Jayasinghe, N.; Swenson, C.; Dams-O'Connor, K. Dispositional optimism and cognitive functioning following traumatic brain injury. *Brain Inj.* **2019**, *33*, 985–990. [CrossRef] [PubMed]
36. Schönberger, M.; Herrberg, M.; Ponsford, J. Fatigue as a cause, not a consequence of depression and daytime sleepiness: A cross-lagged analysis. *J. Head Trauma Rehabil.* **2014**, *29*, 427–431. [CrossRef] [PubMed]
37. Ouellet, M.-C.; Beaulieu-Bonneau, S.; Morin, C.M. Sleep-wake disturbances after traumatic brain injury. *Lancet Neurol.* **2015**, *14*, 746–757. [CrossRef]
38. Carver, C.S.; White, T.L. Behavioral Inhibition, Behavioral Activation, and Affective Responses to Impending Reward and Punishment: The BIS/BAS Scales. *J. Personal. Soc. Psychol.* **1994**, *67*, 319–333. [CrossRef]
39. Pardini, M.; Capello, E.; Krueger, F.; Mancardi, G.L.; Uccelli, A. Reward responsiveness and fatigue in multiple sclerosis. *Mult. Scler. J.* **2013**, *19*, 233–240. [CrossRef]
40. Jaremka, L.M.; Andridge, R.R.; Fagundes, C.P.; Alfano, C.M.; Povoski, S.P.; Lipari, A.M.; Agnese, D.; Arnold, M.; Farrar, W.B.; Yee, L.D.; et al. Pain, depression, and fatigue: Loneliness as a longitudinal risk factor. *Health Psychol.* **2014**, *33*, 948–957. [CrossRef]
41. Jumisko, E.; Lexell, J.; Söderberg, S. The meaning of living with traumatic brain injury in people with moderate or severe traumatic brain injury. *J. Neurosci. Nurs.* **2005**, *37*, 42–50. [CrossRef]
42. Wardlaw, C.; Hicks, A.J.; Sherer, M.; Ponsford, J.L. Psychological resilience is associated with participation outcomes following mild to severe traumatic brain injury. *Front. Neurol.* **2018**, *9*, 563. [CrossRef]
43. Losoi, H.; Wäljas, M.; Turunen, S.; Brander, A.; Helminen, M.; Luoto, T.M.; Rosti-Otajärvi, E.; Julkunen, J.; Öhman, J. Resilience is associated with fatigue after mild traumatic brain injury. *J. Head Trauma Rehabil.* **2015**, *30*, E24–E32. [CrossRef] [PubMed]
44. Tverdal, C.; Aarhus, M.; Andelic, N.; Skaansar, O.; Skogen, K.; Helseth, E. Characteristics of traumatic brain injury patients with abnormal neuroimaging in Southeast Norway. *Inj. Epidemiol.* **2020**, *7*, 45. [CrossRef]

45. Doyle, D.J.; Garmon, E.H. American Society of Anesthesiologists classification (ASA class). In *StatPearls [Internet]*; StatPearls Publishing: Treasure Island, FL, USA, 2021. Available online: https://www.ncbi.nlm.nih.gov/books/NBK441940 (accessed on 17 March 2022).
46. Maas, A.I.; Hukkelhoven, C.W.; Marshall, L.F.; Steyerberg, E.W. Prediction of outcome in traumatic brain injury with computed tomographic characteristics: A comparison between the computed tomographic classification and combinations of computed tomographic predictors. *Neurosurgery* **2005**, *57*, 1173–1182. [CrossRef] [PubMed]
47. Association for the Advancement of Automotive Medicine. *Abbreviated Injury Scale*; 1990 Revision: Update 98 [Manual]; Association for the Advancement of Automotive Medicine: Barrington, IL, USA, 1998.
48. Lerdal, A.; Wahl, A.K.; Rustoen, T.; Hanestad, B.R.; Moum, T. Fatigue in the general population: A translation and test of the psychometric properties of the Norwegian version of the fatigue severity scale. *Scand. J. Public Health* **2005**, *33*, 123–130. [CrossRef]
49. Chalder, T.; Berelowitz, G.; Pawlikowska, T.; Watts, L.; Wessely, S.; Wright, D.; Wallace, E.P. Development of a Fatigue Scale. *J. Psychosom. Res.* **1993**, *37*, 147–153. [CrossRef]
50. Kjeverud, A.; Andersson, S.; Lerdal, A.; Schanke, A.K.; Østlie, K. A cross-sectional study exploring overlap in post-stroke fatigue caseness using three fatigue instruments: Fatigue Severity Scale, Fatigue Questionnaire and the Lynch's Clinical Interview. *J. Psychosom. Res.* **2021**, *150*, 110605. [CrossRef]
51. Loge, J.H.; Ekeberg, Ø.; Kaasa, S. Fatigue in the general Norwegian population: Normative data and associations. *J. Psychosom. Res.* **1998**, *45*, 53–65. [CrossRef]
52. Brähler, E.; Scheer, J.W. *Der Gießener Beschwerdebogen: (GBB)*; Huber: Bern, Switzerland, 1983.
53. King, N.S.; Crawford, S.; Wenden, F.J.; Moss, N.E.G.; Wade, D.T. The Rivermead Post Concussion Symptoms Questionnaire: A measure of symptoms commonly experienced after head injury and its reliability. *J. Neurol.* **1995**, *242*, 587–592. [CrossRef]
54. Wechsler, D. *Wechsler Abbreviated Scale of Intelligence*; The Psychological Corporation: Harcourt Brace & Company: New York, NY, USA, 1999.
55. Wechsler, D. *Wechsler Adult Intelligence Scale–Fourth Edition (WAIS–IV)*; NCS Pearson: San Antonio, TX, USA, 2008.
56. Delis, D.C.; Kaplan, E.; Kramer, J.H. Delis-Kaplan executive function system. *APA PsycTests* **2001**. [CrossRef]
57. Conners, C.K. *Conners Continuous Performance Test 3rd Edition, Technical Manual*; Multi-Health Systems Inc.: Toronto, ON, Canada, 2014.
58. Flehmig, H.C.; Steinborn, M.; Langner, R.; Scholz, A.; Westhoff, K. Assessing intraindividual variability in sustained attention: Reliability, relation to speed and accuracy, and practice effects. *Psychol. Sci.* **2007**, *49*, 132.
59. Derogatis, L.R.; Lipman, R.S.; Rickels, K.; Uhlenhuth, E.H.; Covi, L. The Hopkins Symptom Checklist (HSCL): A self-report symptom inventory. *Behav. Sci.* **1974**, *19*, 1–15. [CrossRef]
60. Strand, B.H.; Dalgard, O.S.; Tambs, K.; Rognerud, M. Measuring the mental health status of the Norwegian population: A comparison of the instruments SCL-25, SCL-10, SCL-5 and MHI-5 (SF-36). *Nord. J. Psychiatry* **2003**, *57*, 113–118. [CrossRef] [PubMed]
61. McCrae, R.R.; Costa, P.T. *NEO Inventories for the NEO Personality Inventory-3 (NEO-PI-3), NEO Five-Factor Inventory-3 (NEO-FFI-3), NEO Personality Inventory-Revised (NEO PI-R): Professional Manual*; Psychological Assessment Resources: Lutz, FL, USA, 2010.
62. Russell, D.W. UCLA Loneliness Scale (Version 3): Reliability, validity, and factor structure. *J. Personal. Assess.* **1996**, *66*, 20–40. [CrossRef]
63. Scheier, M.F.; Carver, C.S.; Bridges, M.W. Distinguishing Optimism from Neuroticism (and Trait Anxiety, Self-Mastery, and Self-Esteem): A Reevaluation of the Life Orientation Test. *J. Personal. Soc. Psychol.* **1994**, *67*, 1063–1078. [CrossRef]
64. Hjemdal, O.; Friborg, O.; Braun, S.; Kempenaers, C.; Linkowski, P.; Fossion, P. The Resilience Scale for Adults: Construct validity and measurement in a Belgian sample. *Int. J. Test.* **2011**, *11*, 53–70. [CrossRef]
65. Kuorinka, I.; Jonsson, B.; Kilbom, A.; Vinterberg, H.; Biering-Sørensen, F.; Andersson, G.; Jørgensen, K. Standardised Nordic questionnaires for the analysis of musculoskeletal symptoms. *Appl. Ergon.* **1987**, *18*, 233–237. [CrossRef]
66. Williamson, A.; Hoggart, B. Pain: A review of three commonly used pain rating scales. *J. Clin. Nurs.* **2005**, *14*, 798–804. [CrossRef]
67. Johns, M.W. A new method for measuring daytime sleepiness: The Epworth sleepiness scale. *Sleep* **1991**, *14*, 540–545. [CrossRef] [PubMed]
68. Bastien, C.H.; Vallières, A.; Morin, C.M. Validation of the Insomnia Severity Index as an outcome measure for insomnia research. *Sleep Med.* **2001**, *2*, 297–307. [CrossRef]
69. Teasdale, G.M.; Pettigrew, L.E.; Wilson, J.L.; Murray, G.; Jennett, B. Analyzing outcome of treatment of severe head injury: A review and update on advancing the use of the Glasgow Outcome Scale. *J. Neurotrauma* **1998**, *15*, 587–597. [CrossRef] [PubMed]
70. Wilson, J.L.; Pettigrew, L.E.; Teasdale, G.M. Structured interviews for the Glasgow Outcome Scale and the extended Glasgow Outcome Scale: Guidelines for their use. *J. Neurotrauma* **1998**, *15*, 573–585. [CrossRef]
71. IBM Corp. *IBM SPSS Statistics for Windows*; IBM Corp: Armonk, NY, USA, 2020.
72. Cattell, R.B. The scree test for the number of factors. *Multivar. Behav. Res.* **1966**, *1*, 245–276. [CrossRef] [PubMed]
73. Patil, V.H.; Singh, S.N.; Mishra, S.; Donavan, D.T. *Parallel Analysis Engine to Aid in Determining Number of Factors to Retain Using R [Computer Software]*; School of Business Administration Spokane, Gonzaga University: Spokane, WA, USA, 2017; Available online: https://analytics.gonzaga.edu/parallelengine/ (accessed on 25 October 2021).
74. Norman, G.R.; Streiner, D.L. *Streiner, Biostatistics: The Bare Essentials*, 4th ed.; People's Medical Publishing House: Shelton, CO, USA, 2014.
75. Lerdal, A.; Kottorp, A. Psychometric properties of the Fatigue Severity Scale—Rasch analyses of individual responses in a Norwegian stroke cohort. *Int. J. Nurs. Stud.* **2011**, *48*, 1258–1265. [CrossRef] [PubMed]

76. van Damme, S.; Becker, S.; Van Der Linden, D. Tired of pain? Toward a better understanding of fatigue in chronic pain. *Pain* **2018**, *159*, 7–10. [CrossRef]
77. Neils-Strunjas, J.; Paul, D.; Clark, A.N.; Mudar, R.; Duff, M.C.; Waldron-Perrine, B.; Bechtold, K.T. Role of resilience in the rehabilitation of adults with acquired brain injury. *Brain Inj.* **2017**, *31*, 131–139. [CrossRef] [PubMed]
78. De Vries, J.; Van Heck, G.L. Fatigue: Relationships with basic personality and temperament dimensions. *Personal. Individ. Differ.* **2002**, *33*, 1311–1324. [CrossRef]
79. Ioannou, A.; Papastavrou, E.; Avraamides, M.N.; Charalambous, A. Virtual reality and symptoms management of anxiety, depression, fatigue, and pain: A systematic review. *SAGE Open Nurs.* **2020**, *6*, 2377960820936163. [CrossRef]
80. Aida, J.; Chau, B.; Dunn, J. Immersive virtual reality in traumatic brain injury rehabilitation: A literature review. *NeuroRehabilitation* **2018**, *42*, 441–448. [CrossRef]
81. Ezekiel, L.; Field, L.; Collett, J.; Dawes, H.; Boulton, M. Experiences of fatigue in daily life of people with acquired brain injury: A qualitative study. *Disabil. Rehabil.* **2021**, *43*, 2866–2874. [CrossRef]

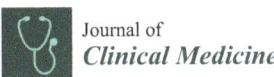

Article

Cognitive Reserve, Early Cognitive Screening, and Relationship to Long-Term Outcome after Severe Traumatic Brain Injury

Natascha Ekdahl [1,2,*], Alison K. Godbolt [2,3], Catharina Nygren Deboussard [2,3], Marianne Lannsjö [1,4], Britt-Marie Stålnacke [5], Maud Stenberg [5], Trandur Ulfarsson [6] and Marika C. Möller [2,3]

1. Centre for Research and Development, Uppsala University/County Council of Gävleborg, 801 88 Gävle, Sweden; marianne.lannsjo@regiongavleborg.se
2. Department of Clinical Sciences, Karolinska Institutet, 182 88 Stockholm, Sweden; alison.godbolt@regionstockholm.se (A.K.G.); catharina.nygren-deboussard@regionstockholm.se (C.N.D.); marika.moller@ki.se (M.C.M.)
3. Department of Rehabilitation Medicine, Danderyd University Hospital, 182 88 Stockholm, Sweden
4. Department of Neuroscience, Rehabilitation Medicine, Uppsala University, 751 24 Uppsala, Sweden
5. Department of Community Medicine and Rehabilitation, Umeå University, 901 85 Umeå, Sweden; brittmarie.stalnacke@rehabmed.umu.se (B.-M.S.); maud.stenberg@rehabmed.umu.se (M.S.)
6. Department of Rehabilitation Medicine, Sahlgrenska University Hospital, 405 30 Gothenburg, Sweden; trandur.ulfarsson@vgregion.se
* Correspondence: natascha.ekdahl@ki.se; Tel.: +46-2627-8023

Abstract: The objective was to investigate the relationship between early global cognitive functioning using the Barrow Neurological Institute Screen for Higher Cerebral Functions (BNIS) and cognitive flexibility (Trail Making Test (TMT), TMT B-A), with long-term outcome assessed by the Mayo-Portland Adaptability Index (MPAI-4) in severe traumatic brain injury (sTBI) controlling for the influence of cognitive reserve, age, and injury severity. Of 114 patients aged 18–65 with acute Glasgow Coma Scale 3–8, 41 patients were able to complete (BNIS) at 3 months after injury and MPAI-4 5–8 years after injury. Of these, 33 patients also completed TMT at 3 months. Global cognition and cognitive flexibility correlated significantly with long-term outcome measured with MPAI-4 total score (r_{BNIS} = 0.315; r_{TMT} = 0.355). Global cognition correlated significantly with the participation subscale (r = 0.388), while cognitive flexibility correlated with the adjustment (r = 0.364) and ability (r = 0.364) subscales. Adjusting for cognitive reserve and acute injury severity did not alter these relationships. The effect size for education on BNIS and TMT scores was large (d ≈ 0.85). Early screenings with BNIS and TMT are related to long-term outcome after sTBI and seem to measure complementary aspects of outcome. As early as 3 months after sTBI, educational level influences the scores on neuropsychological screening instruments.

Keywords: traumatic brain injury; cognition; neuropsychology; patient outcome assessment; executive function; education; prognosis

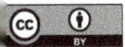

1. Introduction

Traumatic brain injury (TBI) is a major cause of lifelong disability in young adults [1,2]. The most severe form of TBI (sTBI) is characterized by great variance in outcome, from death to favorable outcome [3]. Predictors of long-term outcome for individual patients is uncertain, but long-term follow-up studies suggest that a combination of demographic, injury-related, and cognitive factors contribute [4–7]. Cognitive deficits are common following sTBI and affect work, leisure, and daily living activities [8]. Measuring cognitive deficits using a full neuropsychological assessment is time-consuming, and in the early stages after sTBI, it might not be feasible due to physical injuries and patients' lack of stamina. A shorter screening of cognitive functions might therefore be preferable, but it needs to be ensured that shorter screenings capture cognitive functions important for outcome.

One easily administered cognitive screening instrument is the Barrow Neurological Institute Screen for Higher Cerebral Functions (BNIS [9]). Previous studies have shown that BNIS is related to outcome after sTBI measured with the Glasgow Outcome Scale-Extended (GOSE) [7,10]. Since TBI may affect many areas of functioning as well as community integration and emotional adjustment, it would be of value to measure outcome with more detailed outcome scales. The Mayo-Portland Adaptability Index (MPAI-4 [11]) has been developed specifically to measure these aspects of outcome after brain injury and has been demonstrated to be a valid and reliable instrument [12,13]. To our knowledge, no studies have been published relating BNIS to more detailed measures of long-term outcome after sTBI. Additionally, BNIS does not include any specific measures of executive functions. Given that deficits in executive functions are related to functional outcome after TBI, a brief executive test, such as Trail Making Test (TMT [12]), could be used in order to complement BNIS [14,15].

Age and acute injury severity consistently play a part in outcomes after sTBI [16]. Additionally, cognitive reserve, usually approximated by educational level, has been found to influence both the score on neuropsychological tests, including BNIS, and the outcome after sTBI [10,12,16,17]. However, a relationship between cognitive reserve and a test score does not automatically imply a relationship between test score and recovery. When investigating the relationship between cognitive screening and functional outcome after sTBI, it is therefore important to take age, injury severity, and cognitive reserve into consideration. Following sTBI even though most improvement is believed to take place within the first year, changes in functional outcome, both improvements and deterioration, can continue for several years. Given that TBI often affects young individuals, who are expected to live for decades with their injury, it is important to conduct studies with a longer follow-up interval [18]. In the Swedish health care system, 3 months after injury most patients are still undergoing inpatient rehabilitation. It is at this time point that discussion about likely long-term outcomes often becomes relevant for patients and relatives as they start to plan for life after hospital care. A better understanding of factors contributing to long-term outcomes would be of use to patients, relatives, and health-care staff in planning for continued rehabilitation and support services.

In the present study, the primary aim was to investigate the relationship between findings from early cognitive screening, using BNIS and TMT, and long-term (5–8 year) outcome assessed with MPAI-4 in sTBI. A secondary aim was to investigate whether cognitive reserve, as approximated by educational level, age, and acute injury severity, influences this relationship.

2. Materials and Methods

This study is a 5–8-year prospective longitudinal observational study of patients included in the multicenter research project "Probrain". Probrain recruited patients (n = 114) during initial neurosurgical care from five neurosurgical intensive care units in Sweden and one in Iceland from January 2010 to December 2011. Follow-up was performed at the Swedish units from September 2016 to September 2018. Inclusion criteria for the Probrain study were as follows:

1. Severe nonpenetrating, TBI, with a lowest nonsedated Glasgow Coma Scale (GCS) [19] score of 3–8 in the first 24 h after injury;
2. Age at injury: 18–65 years;
3. Injury requiring neurosurgical intensive care or collaborative care with a neurosurgeon in another intensive care unit.

Exclusion criterion was death within 3 weeks of injury. For detailed methodological information, please see earlier published studies [10].

Inclusion for patients in this study was a completed BNIS assessment at 3 months after injury and a completed MPAI-4 assessment at follow-up 5–8 years after injury.

2.1. Participants

In the long-term follow-up, 63 patients from the five neurotrauma centers from Sweden participated. Due to logistical reasons, two centers followed up a randomized sample of patients, resulting in seven patients not being invited to participate in the 5–8-year follow-up. MPAI-4 was completed by 54 patients, of whom 41 had completed BNIS 3 months after injury. For more details, see Figure 1.

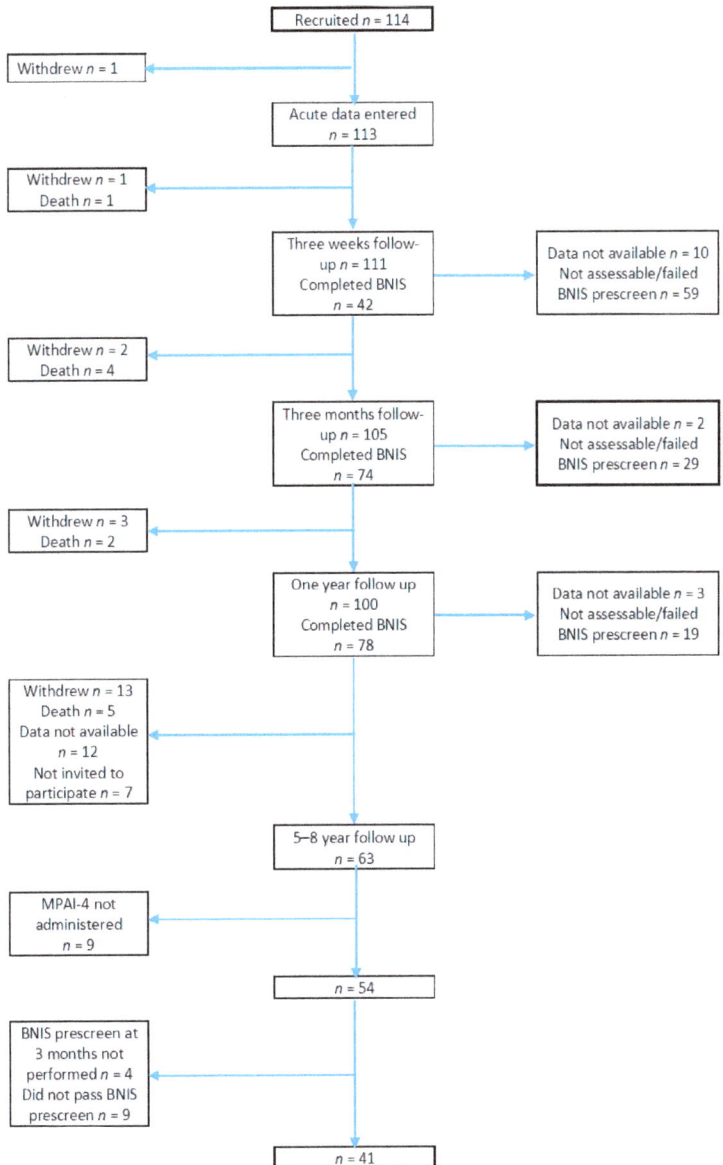

Figure 1. Flowchart of the Probrain long-term follow-up study.

There were no significant differences in age, gender, or educational level between the 41 patients included in the current study and the 73 excluded patients. However, the included patients had significantly higher acute GCS scores compared with those excluded.

2.2. Procedure

Patients were evaluated at 3 weeks, 3 months, 1 year, and 5–8 years after injury (mean of 6.6 years). In the current study, data from the 3-month screening and the 5- to 8-year follow-up were used. The 3-month time point was chosen as an earlier time point would result in too few patients being able to complete screening, and a later time point would be less relevant from a clinical standpoint, as patients are more likely to be discharged from the hospital at 1 year after injury. Furthermore, a previous article from the Probrain project found that cognition was rather stable between the 3-month follow-up and the 1-year follow-up, thus making it redundant to use data from both time points [10]. Assessments took place in the patient's current care setting or in a local rehabilitation outpatient department. The 5- to 8-year follow-ups were conducted either in combination with a visit to the local outpatient department or by post. Data regarding education were obtained by interviews with patients and/or significant others. Educational level was dichotomized as high ($\geq$12 years) and low (<12 years). At the 3-month screening, patients were interviewed, and the BNIS was administered, by either a clinical neuropsychologist or a physician specializing in rehabilitation medicine. GOSE was assessed, and MPAI-4 was administered at the 5- to 8-year follow-up. In case MPAI-4 was administered both in connection with a visit to the care facilities and by post, the highest score was chosen.

2.3. Instruments

2.3.1. BNIS

The BNIS is a cognitive screening test of global cognitive functioning, encompassing speech and language function, orientation, attention/concentration, visuospatial and visual problem solving, memory, affect, and awareness [9]. The test includes a prescreen test with a maximum score of 9, and patients must achieve at least two points on each of the items for the assessment to continue. A full BNIS has a maximum score of 50, where higher scores reflect a higher level of functioning. If the total BNIS score is below 47, further cognitive investigation is recommended. BNIS takes approximately 15–20 min to complete.

2.3.2. TMT

TMT assesses attention, processing speed, sequencing, mental flexibility, and visual-motor skills [12]. TMT contains two parts: In part A, numbers are required to be connected as fast as possible in numerical order. Part B is similar, but now the subject is required to alternate between numbers and letters, adding a component of executive functioning. The primary outcome variable is completion time. By calculating the difference between the completion time of TMT B and TMT A, a measure of cognitive flexibility is produced [20]. TMT has been proven to be sensitive to neurological impairment [12].

2.3.3. MPAI-4

MPAI-4 consists of 30 questions aimed at assessing commonly occurring difficulties after brain injury. The score ranges from 0 to 111, where a lower score indicates better recovery. The instrument consists of three subscales: ability index, adjustment index, and participation index. The ability index measures sensory, motor, and cognitive abilities; the adjustment index measures mood and interpersonal interaction; and the participation index measures social contacts, initiation, work/school, and money management. Previous studies have demonstrated good person reliability (0.92) and item reliability (0.94) [11]. MPAI-4 is linked to the International Classification of Functioning, Disability, and Health and is an established tool for investigating long-term functional outcome after TBI [21]. The instrument covers areas of physical, cognitive, emotional, behavioral, and social problems that persons with brain injury can encounter and furthermore contains assessments of areas where problems commonly arise when patients are reintegrated in society [11].

2.3.4. CRASH Model

In order to control for acute injury severity, the acute injury composite (corticosteroid randomization after significant head injury, CRASH) was used, representing a % risk of unfavorable outcome at 6 months, as calculated and used in previously published studies on the Probrain material [22]. The crash composite score includes data collected within the first 24 h regarding GCS, pupillary reaction, presence of major extracranial injury, age, country, and five CT-brain features [23]. A higher score indicates a greater risk of unfavorable outcome.

2.3.5. GOSE

GOSE score spans from 1 (dead) to 8 (upper good recovery). Traditionally, a score in the range of 1–4 is considered an unfavorable outcome, and a score in the range of 5–8 is considered a favorable outcome. The GOSE has good interrater reliability and validity and is an established measure of global outcome after traumatic brain injury [24]. GOSE was included as a descriptive variable in order to more fully depict the patient group.

2.4. Analysis

Statistical analyses were computed using the Jamovi statistical software [25]. A significance level of 0.05 was used for all statistical tests. Differences in demographic characteristics between groups were analyzed with Student's t-test for parametric data and a Mann–Whitney and χ^2 test for nonparametric data. For measures of effect size, Cohen's d was used, where 0.2 is considered a small effect size, 0.5 medium, and 0.8 large. In order to analyze the relationship between results on neuropsychological screening and outcome according to MPAI-4, correlation analysis with Spearman's rho was used. To investigate the effect of the controlling variables on the relationship between results on neuropsychological tests and outcome, linear regression was used. Since the MPAI-4 subscales are not independent of each other, linear regression on the total score was not used. Three linear regressions were computed for BNIS and cognitive flexibility separately, one for each MPAI-4 subscale score, which was used as the dependent variable, in total six models. CRASH and educational level were added as independent variables to adjust for age, injury severity, and cognitive reserve. Age is included in the CRASH model and, therefore, not entered separately in the linear regression model.

2.5. Ethics

The study was approved by the Regional Ethics Committee of Stockholm (numbers 2009/1644/31/3 and 2016/1465-31/4). The patient gave written informed consent in cases where he or she had the capacity to do so. In the majority of cases, the patient lacked capacity, and the patient's nearest relative gave consent.

3. Results

3.1. Demographics

At 3 months, 74 patients were able to complete BNIS, and out of these, 41 patients also completed MPAI-4 at the long-term follow-up (Figure 1). Of these 41 patients, 38 had data on educational level, and 33 of them also had TMT data. MPAI-4 was completed by the patients themselves in 22 cases and in 13 cases by rehabilitation personnel. For 6 patients, MPAI-4 was completed both by rehabilitation personnel and the patients themselves. In these cases, the differences between scores were usually small (median = 2 points).

Descriptive statistics of demographic variables, neuropsychological screening scores, MPAI-4, and GOSE for the included patients are presented in Table 1. The high education group was significantly younger than the low education group. No other significant differences were found between educational groups, although according to Cohen's *d*, there was a large effect size of educational level on BNIS and TMT scores.

Table 1. Descriptive statistics for all participants, separated by educational level.

	Total *n* = 41	Low Education *n* = 13	High Education *n* = 25	Effect Size Cohen's *d*
Age *	35.6 (13.7)	46.5 (11.2)	35.6 (13.7)	0.85
Gender (M/F)	30/11	11/2	17/8	
CRASH	73 (55.5–83)	76 (49–80)	66 (56–85)	0.006
BNIS total score *	42 (35–46)	39 (34–42)	44 (39–47)	0.66
Cognitive Flexibility (TMTB-TMTA) **	53 (32–82)	68 (32–97)	43 (32–59)	0.85
MPAI-4 total score **	21 (5–36)	19 (5–40)	22 (3–31)	0.20
MPAI-4 ability **	7 (2–16)	4 (2–13)	6 (2–14)	0.06
MPAI-4 adjustment **	8 (1–17)	7 (1–18)	8 (1–15)	0.08
MPAI-4 participation *	5 (0–8)	6 (0–12)	4 (0–7)	0.30
GOSE **	7 (5–8)	6 (5–8)	7 (5–8)	0.04

Note: Values are displayed as median and interquartile range (IQR) for nonparametric data and mean and standard deviation for parametric data (age). TMT missing data are 2 in the low education group and 6 in the high education group. Mann–Whitney was used for examining differences between the groups, except for age, where a Student's *t*-test was used. * value at 3 months' follow-up. ** value at 5–8 years' follow-up.

3.2. Screening Instruments and MPAI-4 in Relation to Demographic Variables

Significant correlations between demographic variables and BNIS score, Cognitive Flexibility$_{(TMTB-TMTA)}$, and MPAI-4 can be seen in Table 2. There were no significant gender differences on any of the measures. In the high education group, seven patients (28%) were above the cut-off value of 47, indicating no cognitive dysfunction, compared to one patient (8%) in the low education group.

Table 2. Correlation for neuropsychological tests and MPAI-4 with age and injury-related variables.

	BNIS *n* = 41	Cognitive Flexibility$_{(TMTB-TMTA)}$ *n* = 32	MPAI-4 Total Score *n* = 41	MPAI-4 Ability *n* = 41	MPAI-4 Adjustment *n* = 41	MPAI-4 Participation *n* = 41
Age	−0.33 *	0.052	−0.14	−0.23	−0.20	0.13
GCS	0.041	0.097	0.14	−0.19	−0.053	−0.22
CRASH with CT	−0.007	0.11	−0.38 *	−0.36 *	−0.44 **	−0.26

* = *p* < 0.05, ** = *p* < 0.01.

3.3. Relationships between Neuropsychological Screening and MPAI-4

There were significant correlations between both BNIS and Cognitive Flexibility$_{(TMTB-TMTA)}$ and BNIS and total score on MPAI-4 (Table 3). Dividing MPAI-4 into subscales revealed that it was primarily the participation subscale that was related to BNIS score, while for Cognitive Flexibility$_{(TMTB-TMTA)}$, this correlation was driven by the adjustment and ability subscales.

Table 3. Correlation between MPAI and neuropsychological screening instruments.

	MPAI-4 Total Score	MPAI-4 Ability	MPAI-4 Adjustment	MPAI-4 Participation
BNIS (*n* = 42)	−0.32 *	−0.28	−0.15	−0.39 *
Cognitive flexibility$_{(TMTB-TMTA)}$ (*n* = 32)	0.36 *	0.36 *	0.36 *	0.34 §

* = *p* < 0.05, § = *p* = 0.06.

3.4. Regression Analysis

Linear regression was used to assess the independent effect of BNIS and Cognitive Flexibility$_{(TMTB-TMTA)}$ on functional outcome. When adjusting for acute injury severity and educational level (Table 4), linear regression analysis showed that BNIS was significantly and independently related to outcome according to the participation subscale on MPAI-4; Cognitive Flexibility$_{(TMTB-TMTA)}$, however, was not. For the MPAI-4 ability and adjustment subscales, Cognitive Flexibility$_{(TMTB-TMTA)}$ but not BNIS was significantly and independently related to outcome (Table 4). For the adjustment subscale, acute injury severity was also independently and significantly related to outcome in the model both with BNIS (estimate = -0.200, $p = 0.020$) and with Cognitive Flexibility$_{(TMTB-TMTA)}$ (estimate = -0.2246, $p = 0.006$). Educational level was not significantly and independently related to outcome in any of the models.

Table 4. Linear regression investigating the relationship between neuropsychological screening instruments and MPAI, adjusting for acute injury severity (including age) and educational level.

		Unadjusted		Adjusted		R-Square
		Est.	95% CI	Est.	95% CI	Adjusted Model
MPAI-4 ability	BNIS	-0.32	-0.72–0.077	-00.26	-0.73–0.20	0.12
	Cognitive Flexibility$_{(TMTB-TMTA)}$	0.060 **	0.016–0.10	0.059 *	0.0026–0.11	0.25
MPAI-4 adjustment	BNIS	-0.10	-0.50–0.30	-0.18	-0.66–0.30	0.18
	Cognitive Flexibility$_{(TMTB-TMTA)}$	0.068 **	0.020–0.12	0.076 **	0.021–0.13	0.41
MPAI-4 participation	BNIS	-0.32 *	-0.59–0.057	-0.41 *	-0.74–-0.074	0.21
	Cognitive Flexibility$_{(TMTB-TMTA)}$	0.033 *	0.00034–0.067	0.029	-0.012–0.070	0.26

* = $p < 0.05$, ** = $p < 0.01$. Separate linear regression models for BNIS and cognitive flexibility for each MPAI-4 outcome scale. In the adjusted models, CRASH and educational level are used as adjusting variables.

When Cognitive Flexibility$_{(TMTB-TMTA)}$, CRASH, and educational level were included in the model, the MPAI-4 adjustment subscale model was found to be statistically significant ($F(3,25) = 5.73$, $p = 0.004$). No other models reached statistical significance.

4. Discussion

The present study investigated the relationship between findings from early cognitive screening using BNIS and TMT and long-term outcome assessed with MPAI-4 in sTBI by considering whether this is influenced by cognitive reserve, age, and injury severity. We found that both BNIS and Cognitive Flexibility$_{(TMTB-TMTA)}$ correlated with long-term outcome after sTBI measured with a MPAI-4 total score. When considering the MPAI-4 subscales, we found that BNIS correlated with the participation subscale of MPAI-4, while Cognitive Flexibility$_{(TMTB-TMTA)}$ mainly correlated with the adjustment and ability subscale. Adjusting for cognitive reserve and acute injury severity did not significantly alter these relationships. The results also show, except for the model regarding the adjustment scale containing the variables Cognitive Flexibility$_{(TMTB-TMTA)}$, CRASH, and educational level, that very little of the variance was explained by these variables. This strongly suggests that there are other variables, besides results on cognitive screening, age, and acute injury severity, that influence outcome after sTBI.

Nonetheless, these results suggest that early screening with TMT and BNIS can be used as a tool to help predict later outcomes for patients with sTBI and that these two tests seem to measure different aspects of outcome. Scores on BNIS are related to participation, both independently and when adjusting for confounders. The participation subscale mainly reflects community integration, including a return to work, and our results are in line with previous research emphasizing the link between cognition and return to work [26]. Cognitive Flexibility$_{(TMTB-TMTA)}$ did not correlate significantly with the participation subscale.

The ability subscale in MPAI-4 measures problems with both motor and cognitive abilities and did not correlate with the BNIS score, neither on its own nor when adjusting for controlling variables. The ability scale does, however, correlate with Cognitive

Flexibility$_{(TMTB-TMTA)}$. A possible explanation is that Trail Making requires more motor skills compared with BNIS, thereby requiring more of the abilities that the ability scale is measuring. Still, one might have expected a correlation between BNIS and the ability scale since both measure cognitive abilities. The lack of relationship might be due to the fact that rating problems with cognitive abilities are not the same as measuring cognitive function. Prior research has found that subjective measures of cognitive problems have a stronger relationship with a concurrent emotional state than with objective cognitive test measures [27]. An alternative explanation is that individuals with better cognitive function participate more in daily life, according to the correlation between scores on BNIS and the MPAI participation subscale. Greater participation, for instance, more leisure activities, and higher rate of employment likely lead to greater cognitive demands and, therefore, possibly the same amount of experienced cognitive problems in spite of having higher ability.

There was no relationship between BNIS and the MPAI adjustment index, which rates problems with psychological well-being and social interaction. However, acute severity of injury (CRASH) and the score for Cognitive Flexibility$_{(TMTB-TMTA)}$ were both moderately related to outcome on the adjustment scale, acute injury severity slightly stronger than Cognitive Flexibility$_{(TMTB-TMTA)}$. The relationship between the CRASH index and the MPAI adjustment index indicates that CRASH not only can predict mortality but is also related to functional outcome, as have been seen in previous studies [28]. Impaired executive functions have also previously been demonstrated to affect functional outcome negatively, including social functions [14], and difficulties seem to increase with more severe forms of TBI [29]. Executive function is a broad concept that also encompasses aspects such as impulse control, emotion regulation, and motivational drive [12]. In this study, only one aspect of executive function was examined, namely, cognitive flexibility. In order to learn more about the relationship between executive impairments and outcome on MPAI-4 subscales, a more detailed assessment of the executive function would be needed.

We found that as early as 3 months after sTBI, a large effect, according to Cohen's *d*, could be seen between education groups on both BNIS score and Cognitive Flexibility$_{(TMTB-TMTA)}$. These results were not statistically significant, however, and probably due to a lack of power. This finding is in line with previous research, which has pointed out that the effect of education on cognitive measures is strong even in the early stages after a brain injury, increasing the possibility of misclassifying patients with longer education as having lesser consequences of their brain injury [9,10,30,31]. In our study, 28% of the patients with longer education were classified as having no obvious cognitive impairments from their brain injury 3 months after sTBI, compared with 8% (one patient) in the low education group. In the present study, there was also an age difference between the educational groups, and some of the difference in BNIS scores might be due to the high education group being younger, as there was a correlation between BNIS score and age. Taken together, our findings support the risk of misclassifying patients with longer education as having no cognitive impairments using BNIS, especially if they are also younger.

In the present study, there was no significant difference on outcome according to MPAI-4 based on the level of cognitive reserve, which differs from that of previous studies. However, several previous studies have primarily used cognitive measures as outcome variables, which are more directly influenced by cognitive reserve [32,33]. Nonetheless, other studies have found that cognitive reserve also influences long-term functional outcome after TBI, although these studies have used less detailed outcome assessments [6,34].

Study Limitations and Strengths

The main limitation of the present study is the small sample size. This limits the conclusions that can be drawn from the data, and the study cannot on its own make definite assumptions on the relationship between neuropsychological screening and long-term functional outcome. Even though all patients were followed by their local outpatient rehabilitation unit, their medical follow-up and rehabilitative efforts varied during the follow-up period. In order to as fully as possible reflect this group of patients, we were restrictive with exclusion criteria; the only one was death or expected death within 3 weeks. This, however, implies that there was less control of medical comorbidities that may have occurred during this time period. The inability to control for further life events, both medical and other, is an inherent flaw in many studies following patients over several years and also greatly restricts the conclusions that can be made from the data.

Initially, over 100 patients were recruited. When considering the incidence of sTBI and the size of the population in Sweden and Iceland, this could in comparative terms be considered a large sample, even though in absolute terms it is small. Given that not all patients could complete a neuropsychological screening and the expected drop-out rate over time, obtaining a larger sample size for a long-term follow-up of sTBI in Sweden is difficult. Drop-out analysis revealed that the only significant difference between included and excluded patients was that included patients had a less severe brain injury according to their GCS score, probably related to the fact that patients able to complete BNIS at 3 months are less severely injured. This highlights another limitation of the study; the results are only generalizable to patients able to complete BNIS at 3 months. The generalizability is also limited to Sweden or countries with a similar social welfare system. An additional weak point is the unusual age difference between the educational groups. However, age was adjusted in the linear regression analysis. A strength of the study is the prospective design; the patients were followed from time of injury until the 5- to 8-year follow-up. We also applied a more nuanced estimate of acute injury severity, using CRASH instead of GCS, thereby better controlling for this variable.

5. Conclusions

These findings indicate that for patients able to complete screening with BNIS as well as TMT 3 months after sTBI, these screening instruments are valuable tools that help estimate patients' long-term outcome after sTBI. Nevertheless, given the small sample size, the results should be interpreted with caution. The instruments measure different aspects of cognition and seem to relate to different aspects of outcome, thereby complementing each other well. Both are relatively easily administered tests that do not require extensive training to use, but consideration should be given to educational level when interpreting neuropsychological test scores. It would be of value to develop education and age-separated norms for both BNIS and TMT. As executive functions include a broad range of functions, it would also be of interest to further explore the impact of various executive impairments on long-term outcome after sTBI.

Author Contributions: Conceptualization, N.E., A.K.G., C.N.D., M.L., B.-M.S., M.S., T.U. and M.C.M.; methodology, N.E., A.K.G., C.N.D., M.L., B.-M.S., M.S., T.U. and M.C.M.; validation, A.K.G., C.N.D. and N.E.; formal analysis, N.E.; investigation, A.K.G., C.N.D., M.L., M.S. and T.U.; resources, A.K.G., C.N.D., M.L., M.S. and T.U.; data curation, A.K.G., C.N.D. and N.E.; writing—original draft preparation, N.E.; writing—review and editing, N.E., A.K.G., C.N.D., M.L., B.-M.S., M.S., T.U. and M.C.M.; visualization, N.E.; supervision, M.C.M., B.-M.S. and M.L.; project administration, A.K.G. and C.N.D.; funding acquisition, N.E., A.K.G., B.-M.S. and M.S. All authors have read and agreed to the published version of the manuscript.

Funding: This research was funded by Promobilia grant 19111; AFA insurance grants 060833 and 130095; Region Västerbotten; the Swedish Association for Survivors of Polio, Accident, and Injury; and the Swedish Brain Foundation. ALF grants from Uppsala University Hospital, Danderyd Hospital, and Umeå University Hospital.

Institutional Review Board Statement: The study was conducted in accordance with the Declaration of Helsinki and approved by the Ethics Committee of Stockholm (number 2009/1644/31/3 and 2016/1465-31/4).

Informed Consent Statement: Informed consent was obtained from all subjects involved in the study. The patient gave written informed consent in cases where he or she had the capacity to do so. In the majority of cases, the patient lacked capacity, and the patient's nearest relative gave consent.

Data Availability Statement: Data available on request due to restrictions (e.g., privacy or ethical). The data presented in this study are available on request from the corresponding author. The data are not publicly available due to the fact that the ethical board requires the data to be kept confidential in order to protect the privacy of the patients.

Acknowledgments: The authors thank the patients and their relatives. The authors also thank Marie Lindgren at the Department of Clinical Rehabilitation Medicine, County Council, Linköping, Sweden, and Richard Levi at the Department of Rehabilitation Medicine, Linköping University, Linköping, Sweden, for their part in realizing the original study. Thanks also to Catharina Apelthun at the Centre for Research and Development, Uppsala University/County Council of Gävleborg, Sweden, for her support and assistance during the statistical analyses. This study is funded by Stiftelsen Promobilia; AFA; Region Västerbotten; the Swedish Association for Survivors of Polio, Accident, and Injury; and the Swedish Brain Foundation.

Conflicts of Interest: The authors declare no conflict of interest. The funders had no role in the design of the study; in the collection, analyses, or interpretation of data; in the writing of the manuscript; or in the decision to publish the results.

References

1. Iaccarino, C.; Carretta, A.; Nicolosi, F.; Morselli, C. Epidemiology of severe traumatic brain injury. *J. Neurosurg. Sci.* **2018**, *62*, 535–541. [CrossRef] [PubMed]
2. GBD 2019 Diseases and Injuries Collaborators. Global burden of 369 diseases and injuries in 204 countries and territories, 1990–2019: A systematic analysis for the Global Burden of Disease Study 2019. *Lancet* **2020**, *396*, 1204–1222, Erratum in *Lancet* **2020**, *396*, 1562. [CrossRef]
3. Rosenfeld, J.V.; Maas, A.I.; Bragge, P.; Morganti-Kossmann, M.C.; Manley, G.T.; Gruen, R.L. Early management of severe traumatic brain injury. *Lancet* **2012**, *380*, 1088–1098. [CrossRef]
4. Vallat-Azouvi, C.; Swaenepoël, M.; Ruet, A.; Bayen, E.; Ghout, I.; Nelson, G.; Pradat-Diehl, P.; Meaude, L.; Aegerter, P.; Charanton, J.; et al. Relationships between neuropsychological impairments and functional outcome eight years after severe traumatic brain injury: Results from the PariS-TBI study. *Brain Inj.* **2021**, *35*, 1001–1010. [CrossRef] [PubMed]
5. Ponsford, J.; Draper, K.; Schönberger, M. Functional outcome 10 years after traumatic brain injury: Its relationship with demographic, injury severity, and cognitive and emotional status. *J. Int. Neuropsychol. Soc.* **2016**, *14*, 233–242. [CrossRef] [PubMed]
6. Ruet, A.; Bayen, E.; Jourdan, C.; Ghout, I.; Meaude, L.; Lalanne, A.; Pradat-Diehl, P.; Nelson, G.; Charanton, J.; Aegerter, P.; et al. A Detailed Overview of Long-Term Outcomes in Severe Traumatic Brain Injury Eight Years Post-injury. *Front. Neurol.* **2019**, *10*, 120. [CrossRef]
7. Stålnacke, B.M.; Saveman, B.I.; Stenberg, M. Long-term follow-up of disability, cognitive, and emotional impairments after severe traumatic brain injury. *Behav. Neurol.* **2019**, *2019*, 9216931. [CrossRef]
8. Rabinowitz, A.R.; Hart, T.; Whyte, J.; Kim, J. Neuropsychological Recovery Trajectories in Moderate to Severe Traumatic Brain Injury: Influence of Patient Characteristics and Diffuse Axonal Injury. *J. Int. Neuropsychol. Soc.* **2018**, *24*, 237–246. [CrossRef]
9. Denvall, V.; Elmståhl, S.; Prigatano, G.P. Replication and construct validation of the Barrow Neurological Institute Screen for Higher Cerebral Function with a Swedish population. *J. Rehabil. Med.* **2002**, *34*, 153–157. [CrossRef]
10. Stenberg, M.; Godbolt, A.K.; Nygren De Boussard, C.; Levi, R.; Stålnacke, B.M. Cognitive impairment after severe traumatic brain injury, clinical course and impact on outcome: A Swedish-icelandic study. *Behav. Neurol.* **2015**, *2015*, 680308. [CrossRef]
11. Malec, J.; Lezak, M. Manual for the Mayo-Portland Adaptability Inventory (Mpai-4) for Adults, Children And Adolescents; 2003; The center of Outcome Measurement In Brain Injury. pp. 1–84. Available online: tbims.org/combi/mpai (accessed on 30 January 2022).
12. Lezak, M.D.; Howieson, D.B.; Loring, D.W.; Hannay, J.H.; Fischer, J.S. *Neuropsychological Assessment*; Oxford University Press: New York, NY, USA, 2004.
13. Kean, J.; Malec, J.F.; Altman, I.M.; Swick, S. Rasch Measurement Analysis of the Mayo-Portland Adaptability Inventory (MPAI-4) in a Community-Based Rehabilitation Sample. *J. Neurotrauma* **2011**, *28*, 745–753. [CrossRef] [PubMed]
14. Spitz, G.; Ponsford, J.L.; Rudzki, D.; Maller, J.J. Association between cognitive performance and functional outcome following traumatic brain injury: A longitudinal multilevel examination. *Neuropsychology* **2012**, *26*, 604–612. [CrossRef] [PubMed]
15. Struchen, M.A.; Clark, A.N.; Sander, A.M.; Mills, M.R.; Evans, G.; Kurtz, D. Relation of executive functioning and social communication measures to functional outcomes following traumatic brain injury. *NeuroRehabilitation* **2008**, *23*, 185–198. [CrossRef] [PubMed]
16. Algethamy, H. Baseline Predictors of Survival, Neurological Recovery, Cognitive Function, Neuropsychiatric Outcomes, and Return to Work in Patients after a Severe Traumatic Brain Injury: An Updated Review. *Mater. Socio Med.* **2020**, *32*, 148–157. [CrossRef]
17. Hofgren, C. Screening of Cognitive Functions Evaluation of Methods and their Applicability in Neurological Rehabilitation. Ph.D. Thesis, University of Gothenburg, Gothenburg, Sweden, 2009.

18. Mostert, C.Q.B.; Singh, R.D.; Gerritsen, M.; Kompanje, E.J.O.; Ribbers, G.M.; Peul, W.C.; van Dijck, J.T.J.M. Long-term outcome after severe traumatic brain injury: A systematic literature review. *Acta Neurochir.* **2022**, *164*, 599–613. [CrossRef]
19. Teasdale, G.; Maas, A.; Lecky, F.; Manley, G.; Stocchetti, N.; Murray, G. The Glasgow Coma Scale at 40 years: Standing the test of time. *Lancet Neurol.* **2014**, *13*, 844–854. [CrossRef]
20. Drane, D.L.; Yuspeh, R.L.; Huthwaite, J.S.; Klingler, L.K. Demographic characteristics and normative observations for derived-Trail Making Test indices. *Neuropsychiatry Neuropsychol. Behav. Neurol.* **2002**, *15*, 39–43.
21. Jacobsson, L.; Lexell, J. Functioning and disability from 10 to 16 years after traumatic brain injury. *Acta Neurol. Scand.* **2020**, *141*, 115–122. [CrossRef]
22. Godbolt, A.K.; Stenberg, M.; Jakobsson, J.; Sorjonen, K.; Krakau, K.; Stålnacke, B.-M.; DeBoussard, C.N. Subacute complications during recovery from severe traumatic brain injury: Frequency and associations with outcome. *BMJ Open* **2015**, *5*, e007208. [CrossRef]
23. MRC CRASH Trial Collaborators. Predicting outcome after traumatic brain injury: Practical prognostic models based on large cohort of international patients. *BMJ* **2008**, *336*, 425–429. [CrossRef]
24. McMillan, T.; Wilson, L.; Ponsford, J.; Levin, H.; Teasdale, G.; Bond, M. The Glasgow Outcome Scale—40 years of application and refinement. *Nat. Publ. Group* **2016**, *12*, 477–485. [CrossRef] [PubMed]
25. The Jamovi Project. *Jamovi, Version 1.6*; Idaho State University: Pocatello, ID, USA, 2021.
26. Manoli, R.; Delecroix, H.; Daveluy, W.; Moroni, C. Impact of cognitive and behavioural functioning on vocational outcome following traumatic brain injury: A systematic review. *Disabil. Rehabil.* **2019**, *43*, 2531–2540. [CrossRef] [PubMed]
27. Draper, K.; Ponsford, J. Long-term outcome following traumatic brain injury: A comparison of subjective reports by those injured and their relatives. *Neuropsychol. Rehabil.* **2009**, *19*, 645–661. [CrossRef] [PubMed]
28. Bonds, B.; Dhanda, A.; Wade, C.; Diaz, C.; Massetti, J.; Stein, D.M. Prognostication of Mortality and Long-Term Functional Outcomes Following Traumatic Brain Injury: Can We Do Better? *J. Neurotrauma* **2021**, *38*, 1168–1176. [CrossRef] [PubMed]
29. Robinson, K.E.; Fountain-Zaragoza, S.; Dennis, M.; Taylor, H.G.; Bigler, E.D.; Rubin, K.; Vannatta, K.; Gerhardt, C.A.; Stancin, T.; Yeates, K. Executive Functions and Theory of Mind as Predictors of Social Adjustment in Childhood Traumatic Brain Injury. *J. Neurotrauma* **2014**, *31*, 1835–1842. [CrossRef]
30. Sherer, M.; Stouter, J.; Hart, T.; Nakase-Richardson, R.; Olivier, J.; Manning, E.; Yablon, S.A. Computed tomography findings and early cognitive outcome after traumatic brain injury. *Brain Inj.* **2006**, *20*, 997–1005. [CrossRef]
31. Fraser, E.E.; Downing, M.G.; Biernacki, K.; McKenzie, D.P.; Ponsford, J.L. Cognitive reserve and age predict cognitive recovery after mild to severe traumatic brain injury. *J. Neurotrauma* **2019**, *36*, 2753–2761. [CrossRef]
32. Stenberg, J.; Håberg, A.K.; Follestad, T.; Olsen, A.; Iverson, G.L.; Terry, D.P.; Karlsen, R.H.; Saksvik, S.B.; Karaliute, M.; Ek, J.A.; et al. Cognitive Reserve Moderates Cognitive Outcome After Mild Traumatic Brain Injury. *Arch. Phys. Med. Rehabil.* **2020**, *101*, 72–80. [CrossRef]
33. Donders, J.; Stout, J. The Influence of Cognitive Reserve on Recovery from Traumatic Brain Injury. *Arch. Clin. Neuropsychol.* **2018**, *34*, 206–213. [CrossRef]
34. Pettemeridou, E.; Constantinidou, F. The Association Between Brain Reserve, Cognitive Reserve, and Neuropsychological and Functional Outcomes in Males With Chronic Moderate-to-Severe Traumatic Brain Injury. *Am. J. Speech Lang. Pathol.* **2021**, *30*, 883–893. [CrossRef]

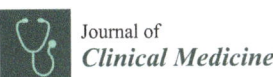

Article

Age Moderates the Effect of Injury Severity on Functional Trajectories in Traumatic Brain Injury: A Study Using the NIDILRR Traumatic Brain Injury Model Systems National Dataset

Laraine Winter [1,2,*], Janell L. Mensinger [3], Helene J. Moriarty [1,2], Keith M. Robinson [4], Michelle McKay [2] and Benjamin E. Leiby [5]

1. Nursing Service, Corporal Michael J. Crescenz Veterans Affairs Medical Center, Philadelphia, PA 19104, USA; helene.moriarty@villanova.edu
2. M. Louise Fitzpatrick College of Nursing, Villanova University, Villanova, PA 19085, USA; michelle.mckay@villanova.edu
3. Department of Clinical and School Psychology, College of Psychology, Nova Southeastern University, Fort Lauderdale, FL 33314, USA; jmensing@nova.edu or janell.mensinger@villanova.edu
4. Department of Physical Medicine and Rehabilitation, Perelman School of Medicine, University of Pennsylvania, Philadelphia, PA 19104, USA; keith.robinson@va.gov
5. Division of Biostatistics, Department of Pharmacology and Experimental Therapeutics, Sidney Kimmel Medical College, Thomas Jefferson University, Philadelphia, PA 19107, USA; benjamin.leiby@jefferson.edu
* Correspondence: laraine.winter@gmail.com

Citation: Winter, L.; Mensinger, J.L.; Moriarty, H.J.; Robinson, K.M.; McKay, M.; Leiby, B.E. Age Moderates the Effect of Injury Severity on Functional Trajectories in Traumatic Brain Injury: A Study Using the NIDILRR Traumatic Brain Injury Model Systems National Dataset. *J. Clin. Med.* **2022**, *11*, 2477. https://doi.org/10.3390/jcm11092477

Academic Editor: Giorgio Costantino

Received: 28 March 2022
Accepted: 25 April 2022
Published: 28 April 2022

Publisher's Note: MDPI stays neutral with regard to jurisdictional claims in published maps and institutional affiliations.

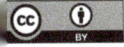

Copyright: © 2022 by the authors. Licensee MDPI, Basel, Switzerland. This article is an open access article distributed under the terms and conditions of the Creative Commons Attribution (CC BY) license (https://creativecommons.org/licenses/by/4.0/).

Abstract: Age is a risk factor for a host of poor outcomes following traumatic brain injury (TBI), with some evidence suggesting that age is also a source of excess disability. We tested the extent to which age moderates the effect of injury severity on functional trajectories over 15 years post injury. Data from 11,442 participants from the 2020 National Institute of Disability and Independent Living Rehabiitation Research (NIDILRR) Traumatic Brain Injury Model Systems (TBIMS) National Dataset were analyzed using linear mixed effects models. Injury severity was operationally defined using a composite of Glasgow Coma Scale scores, structural imaging findings, and the number of days with post-trauma amnesia. Functioning was measured using the Glasgow Outcomes Scale-Extended. Age at injury was the hypothesized moderator. Race, ethnicity, sex, education, and marital status served as covariates. The results showed a significant confounder-adjusted effect of injury severity and age of injury on the linear slope in functioning. The age effect was strongest for those with mild TBI. Thus, the effects of injury severity on functional trajectory were found to be moderated by age. To optimize outcomes, TBI rehabilitation should be developed specifically for older patients. Age should also be a major focus in TBI research.

Keywords: brain injury; traumatic; age; functional impairments; recovery trajectory; injury severity

1. Introduction

Age is a risk factor for a host of poor outcomes following traumatic brain injury (TBI), a major public health problem in the U.S. [1] and globally [2]. Older patients with TBI have a higher mortality [3,4], worse functional outcomes [5–7], weaker community reintegration [8], a greater likelihood of re-injury [4], and more emergency department visits compared to younger ones [9].

In addition to its direct effects on important outcomes, some evidence suggests a role for age in excess disability [10,11]. This refers to the phenomenon that some patients' recovery is worse than would be expected given their relatively mild degree of pathology, whereas others with more severe pathology emerge with better functional outcomes than anticipated. Thus, TBI patients' functional outcomes may seem disproportionate to their objective level of pathology. Excess disability is commonly observed and has been studied in diverse clinical populations [12,13]. Understanding the factors that account for it has important clinical implications: A factor that accounts for excess disability should be a focus of research and, if possible, intervention. Thus, if the effect of injury severity on functioning depends on the individual's age at the time of injury, such that an older age is associated with more negative trajectories, efforts to more effectively tailor rehabilitation to the needs of older TBI patients with milder injuries could help to improve rehabilitation outcomes.

The existing research provides evidence of considerable excess disability in TBI and implicates age as a major factor in it. Several studies have reported worse outcomes for older patients, despite their having milder TBIs. For example, Susman et al. [3] found a higher mortality in patients 65 or older with milder injuries compared to younger ones. Marquez de la Plata et al.'s [5] study of age and 5-year functional recovery revealed older patients to have less severe TBI upon admission but worse functional decline subsequently. Livingston and associates [14] reported a worse functional status at discharge and less improvement at one year in TBI patients 60 or older compared with younger ones. In addition, the poorer functional outcomes began to appear even in patients between 45 and 59 years.

In these studies, poorer outcomes occurred despite patients having a milder TBI upon admission. The present study extends that research by explicitly testing whether age moderates the effects of injury severity on recovery trajectories—that is, whether age interacts with injury severity to affect the trajectory of functioning.

The focus on trajectories of functioning rather than outcomes at single points in time further distinguishes the present study from previous research. Functional trajectories are important TBI-related outcomes [15], especially because TBI becomes chronic for many individuals [16]. Indeed, TBI has been called a chronic and even a dynamic condition [8,17,18]. Functional trajectories address the arc of this recovery experience. For this reason, trajectories have a particular clinical relevance in research on aging with TBI. Using the National Institute for Disability, Independent Living, and Rehabilitation Research (NIDILRR) Model Systems National Dataset [19], the present study calculated the trajectories of functional recovery [3,5,8] and examined the role of age at time of injury as a possible moderator of injury severity on these trajectories.

Investigating the role of age in TBI rehabilitation outcomes is especially important in light of the aging of the population, the growing prevalence of TBI in the older age group [20], and their relatively poor outcomes [21]. Dams-O'Connor et al. cited a 20–25 percent increase in U.S. trauma center admissions for TBI among those ≥75 years, relative to the general population, between 2007 and 2010 [22]. These trends have led to a greater recognition of TBI's importance in the older population [23]. Nevertheless, the effects of age on TBI recovery are still understudied and clinical guidelines underdeveloped [24].

The present study tested the possible moderating effect of age at injury on recovery trajectories up to 15 years post injury. This is a meaningful length of time to capture the change in functioning in chronic TBI. In addition to examining the confluence of injury severity and age of injury on the change in functioning over time, we also tested the prediction that age and severity of injury would be unique sources of change in functioning over time in persons with TBI.

2. Method

2.1. Participants

The present study utilized data from the NIDILRR Traumatic Brain Injury Model Systems (TBIMS) National Dataset. Than 17,000 were new cases collected in 2020 data base that was sufficiently severe to require hospitalization. All had received comprehensive inpatient rehabilitation services at one of the NIDILRR-funded centers in the United States. Data were collected in person at the time of injury, with follow-up interviews by telephone at one, two, and five years post injury and at five years intervals after that. To be eligible, participants must have experienced an injury-related event (e.g., external mechanical force) and met at least one criterion for moderate or severe TBI (post traumatic amnesia lasting >24 h, abnormal neuroimaging abnormalities, or Glasgow Coma Scale score < 13); been 16 years of age or older at injury; presented to a TBIMS acute care hospital within 72 h of the injury; received both acute hospital care and comprehensive rehabilitation within the TBIMS; and been able to provide consent or have a family member or legally authorized representative who could provide consent. The criteria for inclusion are described more fully elsewhere [25].

The sample size for the present analysis was 11,442. This secondary analysis was approved by the Villanova University Institutional Review Board.

2.2. Measures

Injury Severity. Classification of TBI severity (mild, moderate, severe) generally takes into account five criteria: Glasgow Coma Scale (GCS) scores [26], structural imaging findings, length of time with loss of consciousness, alternation of consciousness, and post-trauma amnesia [27]. The TBIMS dataset includes data on GCS score, structural imaging findings, and amnesia for some participants but no data for loss of consciousness or alteration of consciousness. Therefore, we used the available criteria to develop an algorithm to estimate injury severity, as follows: Patients who scored 13–15 on the GCS or had post-trauma amnesia (PTA) for less than 1 day and had no structural imaging findings were classified as mild; patients at any level of GCS who did have a positive imaging finding and had PTA for 2–6 days were classed as moderate; and those who had positive imaging findings and PTA lasting longer than 7 days or a GCS score less than 9 were classified as severe.

Functional Impairment. The Glasgow Outcomes Scale-Extended (GOS-E) is a 20-item disability scale focusing on the major areas of functioning affected by TBI (e.g., traveling independently; social and leisure activities; disruption in social relationships). It is a self-report measure administered at each follow-up interview. Wilson et al. [28] developed a structured interview to improve on the original GOS, extending the rating categories to eight levels of functional limitations, on which 8 = "no functional limitations." Deceased is coded 0. Therefore, higher scores indicate better functioning.

Sociodemographic characteristics. Sex, race, years of education, and marital status were examined as possible covariates. Race was coded White vs. non-White, and marital status as married vs. not married (single, divorced, separated, widowed).

2.3. Procedure

Initial interviews were held in the in-patient facilities where patients were treated for their TBI. Follow-up interviews were conducted by telephone.

Data Analysis. Data were analyzed using SAS 9.4 (SAS Institute, Cary, NC, USA). After performing descriptive statistics, linear mixed effects models were used to address our primary aims. First, we fit a series of unconditional growth models using the methods outlined by Singer and Willet [29] to establish the best curvature of the slope for functioning over the 15-year post-acute time period. The final model included the following fixed effects: a linear time effect (represented by years post-injury); a quadratic time effect (represented by years post-injury squared), which together represent the nonlinear form of the trajectory of change in functioning; the age of injury (representing the effect of age on functioning at the beginning of the post-acute phase); the injury severity (representing the effect of injury severity on functioning at the beginning of the post-acute phase); an age by injury severity interaction (representing the differential effects of severity on functioning by age at the beginning of the post-acute phase); an age by linear time and an age by quadratic time effect (representing the effect of age on the change in functioning over time); and an age by injury severity by linear time interaction effect and an age by injury severity by quadratic time interaction effect (representing the confluence of age and injury severity on the change in functioning over time). We also adjusted for the effects of race, marital status, education, and sex on the initial status in functioning. Random effects for the intercept and the linear slope were included in the model to allow for subject-specific differences in the initial status for functioning (represented by intercept variance) and the trajectories of change (represented by the slope variances).

Mixed effects models are an especially advantageous analytic framework for questions about the predictors of change trajectories because random effects allow one to model person-specific differences in slopes as the outcome of interest. In addition, mixed models use maximum likelihood estimation, which allows for the maintenance of all observations with complete data on the predictor variables in the analysis as long as they have at least one data point to contribute to the outcome variable. This makes them preferable to repeated measures ANOVA-methods, which use listwise deletion when a case is missing any observations on the outcome.

3. Results

Table 1 presents the sociodemographic characteristics of the participants in the study sample at the time of injury.

Table 1. Sociodemographic characteristics of sample at year 1 post injury (n =11,442).

	Mean (SD)	Range	Percent (n)
Age	40.6 (18.7)	16–88	
Sex (% male)			73.6 (8420)
Race (% White)			69.7 (7860)
Hispanic ethnicity (% Hispanic)			10.3 (1177)
Education (number of years)	12.5 (2.9)	1–20	
Marital status (% married)			33.9 (3972)

SD: Standard deviation.

In reference to the primary aim, the findings revealed a significant confounder-adjusted effect of age of injury on the linear slope in functioning over the years beyond the post-acute treatment phase. The effect of age was strongest for those with mild TBI, $\gamma = -0.0037$, SE = 0.0004 $t = -8.51$, $p < 0.001$. For those with moderate TBI (GCS scores between 9 and 12) and severe TBI (GCS < 8), the effect of age was less pronounced, $\gamma = -0.0028$, SE = 0.0005 $t = -5.28$ $p < 0.001$; and $\gamma = -0.0024$, SE = 0.0003 $t = -6.95$ $p < 0.001$, respectively, showing that the impact of injury on age is less evident for those with more severe injuries. The estimated marginal means of functioning over time for age of injury, ranging from 20 years to 80 years, in 10-year increments are shown in Figure 1, panels A, B, and C for mild, moderate, and severe injuries, respectively.

The quadratic slope also differed by age of injury in all severity groups, meaning that the curvature of the trajectory of functioning differed by age. As an inspection of Figure 1 indicates, older age led to a steeper decline in all severity groups. Inspection of the figure panels indicates that age effects are manifested across the age span, with the trajectory of recovery sloping downward by age 50 at all severity levels.

The effect was again strongest in the mild group ($\gamma = 0.0002$, SE = 0.00004 $t = 4.52$, $p < 0.001$) and smaller in the moderate and severe TBI groups ($\gamma = 0.00011$, SE = 0.00005 $t = 2.27$ $p = 0.024$; and $\gamma = 0.00010$, SE = 0.00003 $t = 2.87$ $p = 0.004$), respectively. Table 2 presents confounder-adjusted model estimates, presented in the Singer and Willet format [29].

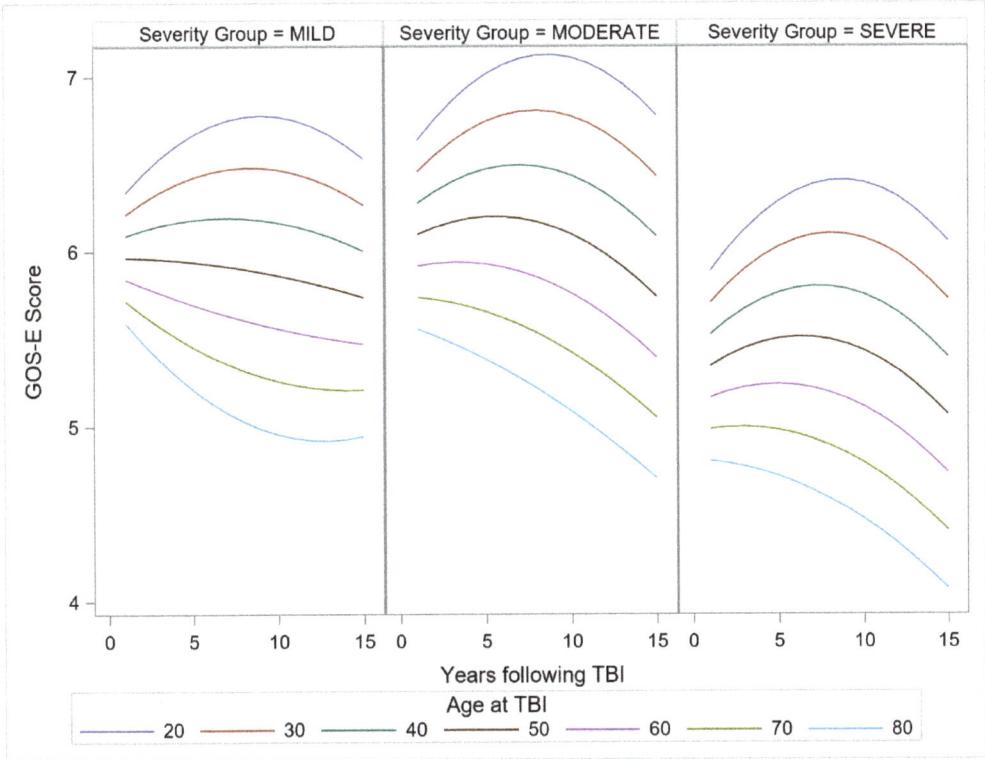

Figure 1. Functioning over time for age of injury in 10-year increments from 20 to 80 years, with the three panels representing mild, moderate, and severe injuries, respectively. TBI: traumatic brain injury; GOS-E: Glasgow Outcomes Scale-Extended.

Table 2. Confounder-adjusted mixed-effects model predicting functioning over time.

	γ (SE)	p
Fixed effects		
Model for initial status at 1 year post-acute injury		
Intercept	5.254 (0.076)	<0.001
Age at injury	−0.015 (0.001)	<0.001
Injury severity (mild)	0.691 (0.065)	<0.001
Injury severity (moderate)	0.775 (0.069)	<0.001
Injury severity (severe) [reference]	-	-
Age × injury severity (mild)	0.0056 (0.0025)	0.026
Age × injury severity (moderate)	0.00009 (0.0027)	0.972
Age × injury severity (severe) [reference]	-	-
Covariates		
Racial and/or ethnic minority	−0.407 (0.032)	<0.001
Non-Hispanic white [reference]	-	-
Female	−0.111 (0.033)	<0.001

Table 2. Cont.

	γ (SE)	p
Male [reference]	-	-
Married	0.120 (0.034)	<0.001
Nonmarried [reference]	-	-
Years of education	0.105 (0.005)	<0.001
Model for linear slope		
Intercept	0.185 (0.013)	<0.001
Age × injury severity (mild)	−0.0037 (0.0004)	<0.001
Age × injury severity (moderate)	−0.0028 (0.0005)	<0.001
Age × injury severity (severe)	−0.0024 (0.0003)	<0.001
Model for quadratic slope		
Intercept	−0.011 (0.0013)	<0.001
Age × injury severity (mild)	0.00020 (0.00004)	<0.001
Age × injury severity (moderate)	0.00011 (0.00005)	0.024
Age × injury severity (severe)	0.00010 (0.00003)	0.0041
Random effects		
Level 1	σ^2 (SE)	
Within-person	0.946 (0.032)	
Level 2	τ^2 (SE)	
Initial status	1.894 (0.037)	
Linear slope	0.0030 (0.00047)	

Notes. Total sample size after adjustments for covariate missingness, N = 11,442. SE: Standard error.

The analysis also revealed significant main effects for injury severity and age, as well as the predicted interaction effect of age injury severity, as noted. When an interaction is detected using this method, however, a main effect cannot be interpreted independently, making it difficult to make global statements about the effect of the interacting variables. Nevertheless, as is clear in the plot, there was little difference between the mild and moderate groups at baseline regardless of age. If anything, the moderate group might have had slightly higher GOS-E scores than the mild group, whereas the severe group was always lower than the other groups at baseline, regardless of age.

4. Discussion

The study findings confirm that the effect of injury severity on functional trajectory is moderated by age. Thus, the predictive validity of injury severity for functional trajectories is conditional on the individual's age at the time of injury, with older people experiencing worse functional trajectories. This indicates that excess disability (i.e., weak associations between injury severity and functional outcomes) is heavily attributable to age.

These findings are consistent with previous research documenting age effects on outcomes at specific points in time. The present study extends those findings to functional trajectories [3–5,9] as the outcome of interest and confirms the moderation-by-age hypothesis. In addition, the present data confirm the finding that age effects are already manifest in middle age [14,30]. Thus, the adverse effects of age are not limited to the oldest age groups.

How can we account for the moderating effect of age on functional trajectories? The steeper downward functional trajectories are likely to reflect normal aging processes or comorbidities of aging. In the absence of data from a non-TBI population, there is no way to assess this. In addition, data on comorbidities that may impair functioning were not available and therefore could not be examined as mediators or moderators. For example, the presence of TBI is associated with the development of neurodegenerative disease later in life [19], which may affect future functional decline. The GOS-E scale measures disability in independence, social activities, and social relationships. Research on specific areas of functioning decline measured within the GOS-E in older adults with mild TBI (mTBI) may provide further insight into where rehabilitation services should be targeted to improve functioning or prevent decline as they age.

A potential factor in age-associated excess disability may be frailty. This has various definitions [31], with common components being weakness, slowness, exhaustion, low activity, and weight loss [32]. Frailty affects fifteen percent of community-dwelling persons over 65 years of age, with another forty-five percent considered pre-frail [33]. Frailty influences not only a person's response to injury but also the response to treatment and resulting outcomes. Could older adults with mTBI (in addition to those with moderate and severe) have frailty contributing to falls that lead to more functional decline over time? In Abdulle and associates' [34] study of 161 older adults with mild TBI, fewer than a quarter fully recovered from their injuries. A majority of the frail older adults were left with a significantly worse disability compared to the non-frail.

Despite its role as a risk factor for poor rehabilitation outcomes, frailty is not always assessed clinically. Frailty is thought to be reversible, especially among those considered pre-frail [35]. In adults with TBI, the assessment of frailty at time of injury and continuously throughout the post-injury phase may be useful in predicting functional decline. Future research should investigate whether frailty screening and frailty-focused intervention can mitigate functional decline or excess disability. If so, targeted interventions may improve frailty and prevent its progression, decreasing excess disability in the TBI population. Indeed, the International Initiative for Traumatic Brain Injury Research Consortium of leading health-care professionals has argued for further understanding of the relationship between frailty and TBI [36].

A caveat when interpreting the relatively steep downward trajectories for older individuals is that the GOS-E includes several questions about employment. Retirement, more common among older individuals than younger ones, may produce spuriously low GOS-E scores for older individuals, suggesting that their functioning is lower than it actually is. A second caveat is that all individuals with mTBI in the TBIMS sample had received inpatient rehabilitation services, suggesting that they may have more problems than typical mTBI patients. Their GOS-E scores may be lower than expected in persons with mTBI.

Although older individuals overall showed worse functioning over time in all levels of TBI severity, especially steep declines were observed among those with mTBI. This was an unexpected finding. Several lines of speculation are possible. First, geriatric patients with mTBI may have received less inpatient rehabilitation than older ones with moderate and severe TBI [37]. Since inpatient rehabilitation is important for maximizing recovery, provider bias against rehabilitation for older individuals should be minimized [38]. This argues for specialized neurologic rehabilitation services for this subgroup to prevent the excessive disability that is documented in the present study.

A further consideration is that some comorbidities, especially PTSD and depression, occur more commonly in mild TBI than in moderate or severe. Clinical depression is more common after a mild TBI than after moderate or severe in patients of all ages [38,39]. PTSD is also more common in mTBI than in moderate or severe [40,41]. Such mental health sequelae of mTBI could contribute to functional decline over time, and their predominance in mTBI may help account for the worse functional trajectories in that group of older individuals. Another speculation is that many TBIs in older adults may be misdiagnosed as milder than they really are, perhaps owing to missed structural imaging findings (i.e., false negatives). Such missed findings might occur in older individuals because of age-associated biological changes such as a decrease in brain volume that may mask hemorrhaging in the brain. Thus, some patients with more severe injuries may be misclassified as mTBI [42].

Clinical Implications. Standard rehabilitation may be less beneficial for older patients than younger ones due to changes attributable to normal aging and comorbidities common in older age. Geriatric rehabilitation for TBI should differ from standard rehabilitation in specific ways [42–44]. Allowing a longer period of time may accommodate a slower trajectory of improvement. Rehabilitation may require more repetition and sustained rehearsal, especially for patients with cognitive impairment. Maintenance rehabilitation may be needed, geared toward sustaining optimal functioning over time. Activities may be directed by family caregivers, as well as self-directed.

Falls are also a major issue [9] both because they are a major cause of TBI in older adults and because of the likelihood of *recurring* falls. Medications that cause hypotension or dizziness or are dopaminergic may increase the risk of falling and should be avoided. Anticoagulant use increases the risk of serious bleeding in falls in older adults with TBI [43]. Poor balance also increases the risk of falls and should be assessed and remediated. Patients' fear of falling may have serious implications for activity engagement, risk of deconditioning, and recurring falls. A study by Bandeen-Roche and colleagues [33] revealed that half of frail older adults in the U.S. had experienced a fall in the previous year. Frailty might therefore amplify the excess disability seen in TBI.

Findings also highlight the needs of those with chronic TBI for some form of rehabilitation. By five years post injury, little rehabilitation is typically being delivered to patients [42]. Those who need continuing help are a neglected population. Rehabilitation treatments that continue into the chronic phase should be designed, tested, and implemented [45].

Research Implications. The present findings raise the question of why older patients with TBI fare worse than their injury severity would predict. The high prevalence of comorbidities in older adults with TBI may account for it. Such comorbidities are a powerful negative prognostic indicator of recovery, as several studies TBI have shown [46,47]. Kumar and colleagues' [48] study of 393 TBI patients with moderate and severe TBI evaluated the impact of physical, mental, and total health burden on functional and life satisfaction up to 10 years post injury. Their findings demonstrated the long-term impact of comorbidity on recovery from injury. Perhaps comorbidity burden or particular comorbidities mediate the effect of age on functional recovery. The TBI Model Systems Database does not include data on comorbidities that would allow additional analyses with these variables. Until mediators of age effects on TBI recovery are identified, it will be difficult to know how to intervene clinically. Therefore, a promising direction for future research should be the mediation analyses of comorbidities or other factors that could explain why age affects TBI outcomes.

5. Conclusions

The growing number of older adults in the population and their increasing representation in the TBI population highlight the importance of age as a crucial factor in TBI outcomes. These trends underscore the need for further attention to age effects on TBI recovery. This should be a major focus of research and clinical attention in the future.

Author Contributions: Conceptualization, L.W., H.J.M., J.L.M.; Formal analysis, J.L.M. and B.E.L.; Investigation, K.M.R.; Methodology, L.W.; Writing—original draft, L.W. and H.J.M.; Writing—review & editing, K.M.R., J.L.M., M.M. and B.E.L. All authors have read and agreed to the published version of the manuscript.

Funding: This research received no external funding.

Institutional Review Board Statement: Approved by the Villanova University Institutional Review Board.

Informed Consent Statement: Informed consent was obtained from all subjects involved in the study.

Data Availability Statement: Data supporting this analysis were from the NIDILRR TBI Model Systems dataset.

Conflicts of Interest: The authors declare no conflict of interest. Disclaimer: The views expressed in this article are those of the authors and do not necessarily reflect the position or policy of the Department of Veterans Affairs or the United States government.

References

1. Center for Disease Control. Traumatic Brain Injury and Concussion. Available online: https://www.cdc.gov/traumaticbraininjury/data/index.html (accessed on 17 February 2018).
2. Corrigan, J.D.; Selassie, A.W.; Langlois Orman, J.A. The epidemiology of traumatic brain injury. *J. Head Trauma Rehabil.* **2010**, *25*, 72–80. [CrossRef] [PubMed]
3. Susman, M.; DiRusso, S.M.; Sullivan, T.; Tisucci, D.; Nealson, P.; Cuff, S.; Haider, A.; Benzil, D.L. Traumatic brain injury in the elderly: Increased mortality and worse functional outcome at discharge despite lower injury severity. *J. Trauma* **2002**, *53*, 219–223. [CrossRef] [PubMed]
4. Dams-O'Connor, K.; Gibbons, L.E.; Bowen, J.D.; McCurry, S.M.; Larson, E.B.; Crane, P.K. Risk for late-life re-injury, dementia and death among individuals with traumatic brain injury: A population-based study. *J. Neurol. Neurosurg. Psychiatry* **2013**, *84*, 177–182. [CrossRef] [PubMed]
5. Marquez de la Plata, C.; Hart, T.; Hammond, F.M.; Frol, A.; Hudak, A.; Harper, C.R.; O'Neil-Pirozzi, T.; Whyte, J.; Carlile, M.; Diaz-Arrastia, R. Impact of age on long-term recovery from traumatic brain injury. *Arch Phys. Med. Rehabil.* **2008**, *89*, 896–903. [CrossRef] [PubMed]
6. Forslund, M.V.; Roe, C.; Perrin, P.; Sigurdardottir, S.; Lu, J.; Berntseng, S.; Andelic, N. The trajectories of overall disability in the first 5 years after moderate and severe traumatic brain injury. *Brain Injury* **2017**, *31*, 329–335. [CrossRef]
7. Howrey, B.T.; Graham, J.E.; Pappadis, M.R.; Ottenbacher, K.J. Trajectories of functional change following inpatient rehabilitation for traumatic brain injury. *Arch Phys. Med. Rehabil.* **2017**, *98*, 1606–1613. [CrossRef]
8. Andelic, N.; Arango-Lasprilla, C.; Perrin, P.B.; Sigurdrdottir, S.; Lu, J.; Landa, L.O.; Forslund, M.V.; Roe, C. Modeling of community integration trajectories in the first five years after traumatic brain injury. *J. Neurotrauma* **2016**, *33*, 95–100. [CrossRef]
9. Albrecht, J.S.; Hirshon, J.M.; McCunn, M.M.D.; Bechtold, K.T.; Rao, V.; Simoni-Wastila, L.; Smith, G.S. Increased rates of mild traumatic brain injury among older adults in US emergency departments, 2009–2010: Mild traumatic brain injury in older adults. *J. Head Trauma Rehabil.* **2016**, *31*, E1–E7. [CrossRef]
10. Brody, E.M.; Kleban, M.H.; Lawton, M.P.; Silverman, H.A. Excess disabilities of mentally impaired aged: Impact of individualized treatment. *Gerontologist* **1971**, *11*, 124–133. [CrossRef]
11. Dawson, P.; Kline, K.; Wainscot, D.C.; Wells, D. Preventing excess disability in patients with Alzheimer's disease. *Geriatr. Nurs.* **1998**, *7*, 298–301. [CrossRef]
12. Lawton, M.P.; Nahemow, L. Environment and other determinants of well being in older people. *Gerontologist* **1983**, *23*, 349–357. [CrossRef] [PubMed]
13. Roberts, A.H.; Sternbach, R.A.; Polich, J. Behavioral management of chronic pain and excess disability: Long-term follow-up of an outpatient program. *Clin. J. Pain* **1993**, *9*, 41–48. [CrossRef] [PubMed]
14. Livingston, D.H.; Lavery, R.F.; Mosenthal, A.C.; Knudson, M.M.; Lee, S.; Morabito, D.; Manley, G.T.; Nathens, A.; Jurkovich, G.; Hoyt, D.B.; et al. Recovery at one year following isolated traumatic brain injury: A Western Trauma Association prospective multicenter trial. *J. Trauma* **2005**, *59*, 1298–1304. [CrossRef] [PubMed]
15. Malec, J.F.; Ketchum, J.M.; Hammond, F.M.; Corrigan, J.D.; Dams-O'Connor, K.; Hart, T.; Novack, T.; Dahdah, M.; Whiteneck, G.G.; Bogner, J. Longitudinal effects of medical comorbidities on functional outcome and life satisfaction after traumatic brain injury: An individual growth curve analysis of NIDILIRR Traumatic Brain Injury Model System Data. *J. Head Trauma Rehabil.* **2019**, *34*, E24–E35. [CrossRef] [PubMed]
16. National Academies of Sciences, Engineering, and Medicine. *Traumatic Brain Injury: A Roadmap for Accelerating Progress*; The National Academies Press: Washington, DC, USA, 2022. [CrossRef]
17. Corrigan, J.D.; Hammond, F.M. Traumatic brain injury as a chronic health condition. *Arch. Phys. Med. Rehab.* **2013**, *94*, 1199–1201. [CrossRef]
18. Wilson, L.; Stewart, W.; Dams-O'Connor, K.; Diaz-Arrastia, R.; Horton, L.; Menon, D.K.; Polinder, S. The chronic and evolving neurological consequences of traumatic brain injury. *Lancet Neurol.* **2017**, *16*, 813–825. [CrossRef]
19. Traumatic Brain Injury Model Systems National Database. Traumatic Brain Injury Model Systems National Data and Statistical Center. Available online: https://osf.io/a4xzb/ (accessed on 24 April 2022). [CrossRef]
20. Peters, M.E. Traumatic brain injury in older adults: Shining light on a growing public health crisis. *Internat. Rev. Psychiat.* **2020**, *32*, 1–2. [CrossRef]
21. Schneider, A.L.C.; Wang, D.; Gottesman, R.F.; Selvin, E. Prevalence of disability associated with head injury with loss of consciousness in adults in the United States: A population-based study. *Neurology* **2021**, *97*, e124–e135. [CrossRef]
22. Dams-O'Connor, K.; Cuthbert, J.P.; Whyte, J.; Corrigan, J.D.; Faul, M.; Harrison-Felix, C. Traumatic brain injury among older adults at Level I and II trauma centers. *J. Neurotrauma* **2013**, *30*, 2001–2013. [CrossRef]
23. Flanagan, S.R.; Hibbard, M.R.; Gordon, W.A. The impact of age on traumatic brain injury. *Phys. Med. Rehabil. Clin. N. Am.* **2005**, *16*, 163–177. [CrossRef]
24. Stein, D.M.; Kozar, R.A.; Livingston, H.; Luchette, F.; Adams, S.D.; Agrawal, V.; Arbabi, S.; Ballou, J.; Barraco, R.D.; Bernard, A.C.; et al. Geriatric traumatic brain injury—What we know and what we don't. *J. Trauma Acute Care Surg.* **2018**, *85*, 788–798. [PubMed]
25. Dijkers, M.P.; Marwitz, J.H.; Harrison-Felix, C. Thirty years of National Institute on Disability, Independent Living, and Rehabilitation Research Traumatic Brain Injury Model Systems Center Research—An update. *J. Head Trauma Rehabil.* **2018**, *33*, 363. [PubMed]

26. Teasdale, G.; Jennett, B. Assessment and prognosis of coma after head injury. *Acta Neurochir.* **1976**, *34*, 45–55. [CrossRef]
27. Management of Concussion/mTBI Working Group. VA/DoD Clinical Practice Guideline for Management of Concussion/Mild Traumatic Brain Injury. *J. Rehabil. Res. Dev.* **2009**, *46*, CP1–CP68. [CrossRef]
28. Wilson, J.T.L.; Pettigrew, L.E.L.; Teasdale, G.M. Structured interviews for the Glasgow Outcome Scale and the Extended Glasgow Outcome Scale: Guidelines for Their Use. *J. Neurotrauma* **1997**, *15*, 573–585.
29. Singer, J.D.; Willett, J.B. *Applied Longitudinal Data Analysis: Modeling Change and Event Occurrence*; Oxford University Press: New York, NY, USA, 2003.
30. MRC CRASH Trial Collaborators. Predicting outcome after traumatic brain injury: Practical prognostic models based on large cohort of international patients. *Brit. Med. J.* **2008**, *336*, 425–429.
31. Walston, J.; Buta, B.; Zue, Q. Frailty syndrome and interventions: Considerations for clinical practice. *Clin. Geriatr Med.* **2018**, *34*, 25–38. [CrossRef]
32. Fried, L.P.; Tangen, C.M.; Walston, J.; Newman, A.B.; Hirsch, C.; Gottdiener, J.; Seeman, T.; Tracy, R.; Kop, W.J.; Burke, G.; et al. Frailty in older adults: Evidence for a phenotype. *J. Gerontol. A Biol. Sci. Med. Sci.* **2001**, *56*, M146–M156. [CrossRef]
33. Bandeen-Roche, K.; Seplaki, C.L.; Huang, J.; Buta, B.; Kalyani, R.R.; Varadhan, R.; Xue, Q.-L.; Walston, J.D.; Kasper, J.D. Frailty in older adults: A nationally representative profile in the United States. *Gerontol. A Biol. Sci. Med. Sci.* **2015**, *70*, 1427–1434. [CrossRef]
34. Abdulle, A.E.; de Koning, M.E.; van der Horn, H.J.; Scheenen, M.E.; Roks, G.; Hageman, G.; Spikman, J.M.; van der Naalt, J. Early predictors for long-term functional outcome after mild traumatic brain injury in frail elderly patients. *J. Head Trauma Rehabil.* **2018**, *33*, E59–E67. [CrossRef]
35. Travers, J.; Romero-Ortuno, R.; Bailey JCooney, M. Delaying and reversing frailty: A systematic review of primary care interventions. *Br. J. Gen. Pract.* **2018**, *69*, e61–e69. [CrossRef] [PubMed]
36. Maas, A.J.R.; Menon, D.K.; Adelson, P.D.; Andelic, N.; Bell, M.J.; Bragge, P.; Brazinova, A.; Büki, A.; Chesnut, R.M.; Citerio, G.; et al. Traumatic brain injury: Integrated approaches to improve prevention, clinical care, and research. *Lancet Neurol.* **2017**, *16*, 987–1048. [CrossRef]
37. Gardener, R.C.; van Dams-O'Connor, K.; Morrissey, M.R.; Manley, G.T. Geriatric traumatic brain injury: Epidemiology, outcomes, knowledge gaps and future directions. *J. Neurotrauma* **2018**, *35*, 889–906. [CrossRef] [PubMed]
38. Rapoport, M.J.; McCullach, S.; Streiner, D.; Feinstein, A. The clinical significance of major depression following mild traumatic brain injury. *Psychosomatics* **2003**, *44*, 31–37. [CrossRef] [PubMed]
39. Alexander, M.P. Neuropsychiatric correlates of persistent post-concussive syndrome. *J. Head Trauma Rehabil.* **1992**, *7*, 60–69. [CrossRef]
40. Vasterling, J.J.; Jacobs, S.N.; Rasmusson, A. Traumatic brain injury and posttraumatic stress disorder: Conceptual, diagnostic, and therapeutic considerations in the context of co-occurrence. *J. Neuropsychiat. Neurosci.* **2018**, *30*, 91–100. [CrossRef]
41. Kiraly, M.A.; Kiraly, S.J. Traumatic brain injury and delayed sequelae: A review—Traumatic brain injury and mild traumatic brain injury (concussion) are precursors to later onset brain disorders including early-onset dementia. *Sci. World J.* **2007**, *7*, 1768–1776. [CrossRef]
42. Swanson, R.; Robinson, K.E. Geriatric rehabilitation, gait in the elderly, falls prevention, and Parkinson's disease. *Med. Clin. N. Am.* **2020**, *104*, 327–343. [CrossRef]
43. Narapareddy, B.R.; Richey, L.N.; Peters, M.E. The Growing Epidemic of TBI in Older Patients. Available online: https://www.neurologylive.com/view/growing-epidemic-tbi-older-patients (accessed on 18 January 2021).
44. Peters, M.E. Traumatic brain injury (TBI) in older adults: Aging with a TBI versus incident TBI in the aged. *Internat. Psychogeriatr.* **2016**, *28*, 1931–1934. [CrossRef]
45. Mosenthal, A.C.; Livingston, D.H.; Lavery, R.F.; Knudson, M.M.; Lee, S.; Morabito, D.; Manley, G.T.; Nathens, A.; Jurkovich, G.; Hoyt, D.B.; et al. The effect of age on functional outcome in mild traumatic brain injury: 6-month report of a prospective multicenter trial. *J. Trauma* **2004**, *56*, 1042–1048. [CrossRef]
46. Thompson, H.J.; Dikmen, S.; Temkin, N. Prevalence of comorbidity and its association with traumatic brain injury and outcomes in older adults. *Res. Gerontol. Nurs.* **2012**, *5*, 17–246. [CrossRef] [PubMed]
47. Lecours, A.; Sirois, M.J.; Ouellet, M.C.; Boivin, K.; Simard, J.F. Long-term functional outcome of older adults after a traumatic brain injury. *J. Head Trauma Rehabil.* **2012**, *27*, 379–390. [CrossRef] [PubMed]
48. Kumar, R.G.; Ketchum, J.M.; Corrigan, J.D.; Hammond, F.M.; Sevigny, M.; Dams-O'Connor, K. The longitudinal effects of comorbid health burden on functional outcomes for adults with moderate to severe traumatic brain injury. *J. Head Trauma Rehabil.* **2020**; *epub ahead of print*. [CrossRef]

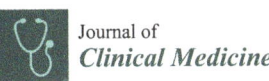

Article

Goal Attainment in an Individually Tailored and Home-Based Intervention in the Chronic Phase after Traumatic Brain Injury

Ida M. H. Borgen [1,2,*], Solveig L. Hauger [2,3], Marit V. Forslund [1], Ingerid Kleffelgård [1], Cathrine Brunborg [4], Nada Andelic [1,5], Unni Sveen [1,6], Helene L. Søberg [1,7], Solrun Sigurdardottir [8], Cecilie Røe [1,9] and Marianne Løvstad [2,3]

1. Department of Physical Medicine and Rehabilitation, Oslo University Hospital, 0424 Oslo, Norway; mavfor@ous-hf.no (M.V.F.); uxinff@ous-hf.no (I.K.); nada.andelic@medisin.uio.no (N.A.); unsvee@ous-hf.no (U.S.); h.l.soberg@medisin.uio.no (H.L.S.); cecilie.roe@medisin.uio.no (C.R.)
2. Department of Psychology, Faculty of Social Sciences, University of Oslo, 0316 Oslo, Norway; solveigl@ous-hf.no (S.L.H.); marianne.lovstad@sunnaas.no (M.L.)
3. Department of Research, Sunnaas Rehabilitation Hospital, 1453 Nesoddtangen, Norway
4. Oslo Centre for Biostatistics and Epidemiology, Oslo University Hospital, 0424 Oslo, Norway; uxbruc@ous-hf.no
5. Center for Habilitation and Rehabilitation Models and Services (CHARM), Institute of Health and Society, Faculty of Medicine, University of Oslo, 0316 Oslo, Norway
6. Department for Occupational Therapy Prosthetics and Orthotics, Faculty of Health Sciences, Oslo Metropolitan University, 0130 Oslo, Norway
7. Department of Physiotherapy, Faculty of Health Sciences, Oslo Metropolitan University, 0130 Oslo, Norway
8. Centre for Rare Disorders, Oslo University Hospital, 0424 Oslo, Norway; sosigu@ous-hf.no
9. Institute of Clinical Medicine, Faculty of Medicine, University of Oslo, 0316 Oslo, Norway
* Correspondence: idmbor@ous-hf.no

Abstract: Traumatic brain injury (TBI) is a heterogeneous condition with long-term consequences for individuals and families. Goal-oriented rehabilitation is often applied, but there is scarce knowledge regarding types of goals and goal attainment. This study describes goal attainment in persons in the chronic phase of TBI who have received an individualized, SMART goal-oriented and home-based intervention, compares goal attainment in different functional domains, and examines indicators of goal attainment. Goal attainment scaling (GAS) was recorded in the intervention group ($n = 59$) at the final session. The goal attainment was high, with 93.3% increased goal attainment across all goals at the final session. The level of goal attainment was comparable across domains (cognitive, physical/somatic, emotional, social). Gender, anxiety symptoms, self-reported executive dysfunction, and therapy expectations were indicators of goal attainment. These results indicate a potential for the high level of goal attainment in the chronic phase of TBI. Tailoring of rehabilitation to address individual needs for home-dwelling persons with TBI in the chronic phase represents an important area of future research.

Keywords: traumatic brain injury; goal-oriented rehabilitation; home-based rehabilitation; community-based rehabilitation; SMART; goal attainment scaling (GAS)

1. Introduction

Traumatic brain injury (TBI) is a costly condition with long-lasting impact for many individuals [1–3]. Persons who suffer a TBI might experience a variety of consequences, including difficulties with physical, cognitive, emotional, behavioral, vocational, and social functioning. Many experience persistently reduced quality of life and restrictions in community participation [4–9]. Families are also affected and may have to adapt to a new life with their injured family member being dependent on their assistance and support [10–14]. It has been increasingly recognized that TBI is a chronic condition with multiple and interacting effects on health and wellbeing [15–18], as a significant proportion of patients continue to experience life-long difficulties and impaired functional status [8,19–22]. A challenge in rehabilitation after TBI is the heterogeneous nature of sequelae. Moreover, the patient's specific difficulties interact with contextual and psychosocial factors [23,24]. Hence, many individuals are in need of long-term support from health care services. Evidence suggests that rehabilitation can be effective in reducing symptom burden and in improving participation and quality of life, and also for those who experience persisting symptoms [25–28]. However, evidence suggests that one-third of patients with chronic TBI have unmet needs related to cognitive, emotional, and vocational functioning [29], and that certain symptoms, such as neuropsychiatric sequelae, might often be overlooked in rehabilitation [30].

Rehabilitation efforts have become increasingly focused on enhancing patient involvement [31], and person-centered rehabilitation has been shown to have positive effects on occupational performance and rehabilitation satisfaction [32]. Goal-oriented rehabilitation with patient involvement is considered a key approach to rehabilitation [33,34], and has been shown to increase patient satisfaction and adherence [35], as well as improve self-efficacy, health-related quality of life and emotional status. There is, however, a need for more methodologically rigorous studies involving the use of individualized and specific treatment goals [36]. Although some studies have demonstrated the utility of a goal-oriented approach in tailoring rehabilitation efforts to the heterogeneous functional difficulties due to persistent TBI symptoms [37,38], more high-quality studies are needed on the effect of such approaches in the chronic phase of TBI.

Although goal-oriented rehabilitation seems promising in chronic TBI, there might also be individual differences in the suitability of the approach. Many advocate that a high level of patient involvement is necessary in goal-oriented rehabilitation [34,39–41], and that patients with cognitive impairments are susceptible to being less involved in goal setting [42]. Cognitive impairment might, thus, lead to difficulties both with setting goals and with achieving them and should be explored when evaluating goal attainment [43]. Impaired self-awareness might be a particular challenge for patients with TBI, potentially influencing goal setting and engagement in rehabilitation [44]. Some studies have identified fatigue and emotional difficulties as potential barriers to early goal-oriented rehabilitation [45]. In addition, individual factors such as self-efficacy, tenacity, and motivation have further been identified as potential moderators of goal attainment [43,46,47]. To our knowledge, a systematic investigation of the degree to which cognitive impairment, emotional distress, demographic factors (i.e., age, gender, education), and/or injury-related variables predict goal attainment in the chronic phase of TBI has not yet been explored.

Despite the focus on goal-oriented rehabilitation over the past decades, conceptual terms vary, theoretical frameworks are often lacking [48,49], and there is a need to describe goal attainment [40,50], as goal attainment is rarely reported [51]. The SMART goal approach is frequently applied, i.e., setting goals that are Specific, Measurable, Achievable, Relevant, and Timed. Furthermore, the use of goal attainment scaling (GAS) [52] to measure goal attainment seems to be the best available alternative [53]. GAS is a systematic scoring of individualized goals in specific areas, which allows comparison of goal attainment across individualized goals and patients. GAS has been shown to be reliable, valid, and to have satisfactory responsiveness, as well as being sensitive to change [54]. Recently, Trevena-Peters, McKay [55] published results from a randomized controlled trial (RCT) supporting the effectiveness of an intervention to improve activities of daily living during post-traumatic amnesia, providing detailed results from GAS. A feasibility study of a project-based intervention for acquired brain injuries also detailed goal attainment results [56]. However, the studies neither provided information on the attainability of goals in distinct domains, nor did they investigate predictors of goal attainment.

The current study is modeled after a goal-oriented, home-based rehabilitation program shown to be effective in improving TBI-specific problem areas nominated by participants and which was shown to be highly acceptable for both patients and family members [57]. The current study represents an expansion and development of this approach in a different cultural setting (i.e., Norway), in a civilian sample, and with more severe injuries. The design was expanded by including SMART goals and GAS scoring within a randomized controlled trial, resulting in the combination of an individually targeted and standardized intervention approach. In addition to reporting group-based outcomes on standardized measures in the RCT, the design allows for exploration of the functional domains where individuals with TBI report a need for rehabilitation efforts. It also allows description of the degree to which setting individualized goals within the individual problem areas results in positive goal attainment. The study thus addresses several of the weaknesses in the current literature that have been noted above.

Aims

The primary aim was to describe goal attainment in persons with persistent symptoms of TBI in the chronic phase. We hypothesized that participants would achieve goal attainment at expected levels. A second aim was to explore the functional domains of SMART goals established in the chronic phase and to determine whether goal attainment varied according to functional domains. We hypothesized that SMART goals would be related to physical/somatic, cognitive, emotional, and social problem areas typically seen in the chronic phase of TBI, and that goal attainment was achievable in all functional domains. Thirdly, we explored variables that might be associated with goal attainment, such as age, injury severity, and cognitive and emotional functioning. The existing literature does not give reason for a strong hypothesis regarding this aim; hence, this approach was considered exploratory in nature.

2. Materials and Methods

2.1. Participants

Participants were recruited from a two-group RCT conducted in Oslo, Norway. A detailed description of the study design is provided elsewhere [58]. Recruitment took place between June 2018 and December 2020. Between-group results of this trial will be published pending completion of 12 months follow-up assessments. Eligible participants were invited by letter, screened by phone, and, if eligible, invited to a baseline assessment at Oslo University Hospital (OUH). A family member was also invited if possible. Eligibility criteria were patients aged 18–72, with a TBI diagnosis with intracranial abnormalities verified by either computed tomography or magnetic resonance imaging. The participants had to be ≥ 16 years old at the time of injury, at least two years post-injury, and be living at home. Furthermore, they had to report ongoing TBI-related problems and/or reduced physical and mental health and/or difficulties with participation in their everyday life. Exclusion criteria were severe progressive neurologic or severe psychiatric disorders (including active substance abuse and violence), inability to provide informed consent, inability to participate in a goal-setting process, or insufficient fluency in Norwegian. After baseline assessment, participants were randomized 1:1 to either the control group or the intervention group by an independent researcher using a randomly generated number sequence. Participants in the control group received treatment as usual but no additional study-based treatment. Only patients randomized to the intervention group established SMART goals with subsequent GAS; hence, only results from the intervention group are reported in the current paper ($n = 60$).

2.2. Intervention

The intervention group received a home-based intervention consisting of eight contacts over a 4-month period. Initially, six home visits and two telephone calls were carried out. Due to the Covid-19 pandemic, some patients were followed up by phone only during the initial Norwegian lockdown in March–May 2020. A pragmatic solution was adapted to continue recruitment during the pandemic, and most participants included from May to December 2020 ($n = 17$) were offered one to two home visits (first, ±last), while six to seven meetings were conducted by videoconference or telephone. Figure 1 displays an overview of the intervention sessions. Four therapists delivered the intervention: a medical doctor, a psychologist, a physiotherapist, and a neuropsychologist, all four with TBI rehabilitation expertise. Each participant was followed up by the same therapist throughout the intervention.

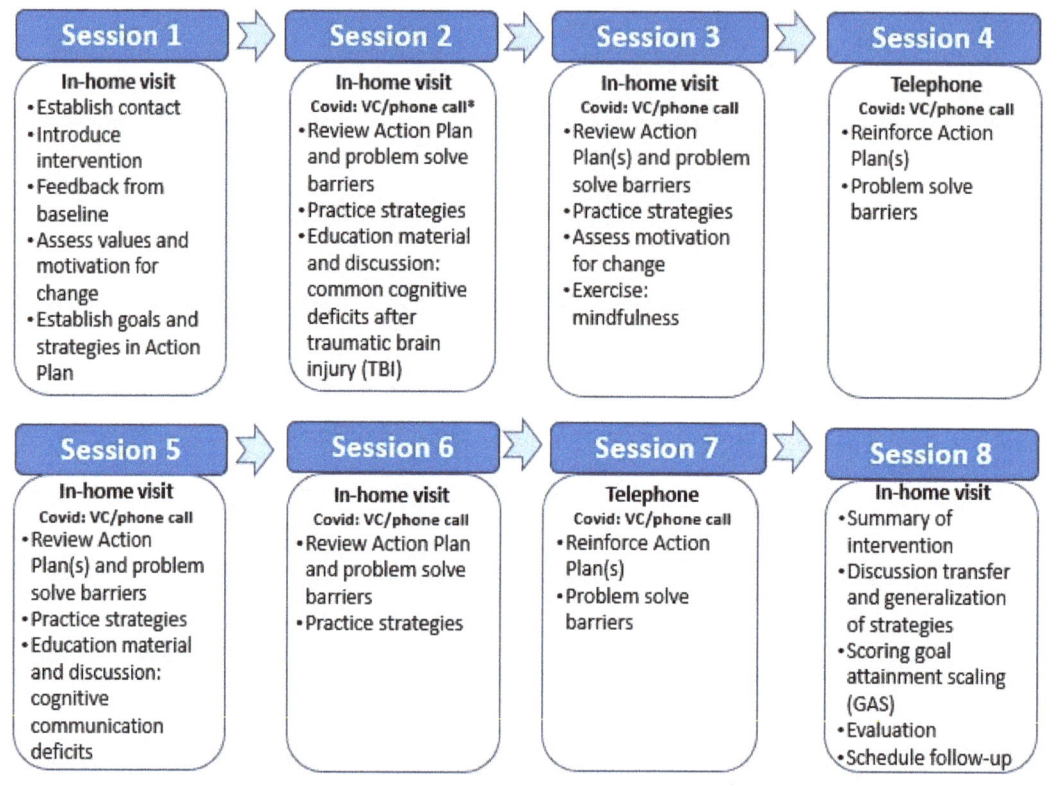

Figure 1. Overview of intervention sessions. * Delivery format was adjusted due to the Covid-19 pandemic, i.e., videoconference (VC) and phone calls replaced some home visits to reduce risk of infection.

The intervention was manualized and based on the study by Winter et al. [57]. It contained three phases: (1) identification of target problem areas, (2) establishment of SMART goals and GAS for the selected target problems, and (3) development of an Action Plan consisting of strategies to achieve the goal. Figure 2 displays an example of an action plan. Goals were established through brainstorming between the patient, therapist, and family member, and included identification of needs for support, barriers to change, and current adaptive strategies to be built upon. There was no upper limit on the number of SMART goals for each patient, but new goals were not established after session 5. The process of establishing SMART goals, GAS, and Action plans was based on recommendations for collaborative goal setting from several authors [50,59,60]. Patients were presented with visual and verbal information about the SMART approach to goal setting, and the SMART approach was applied in a flexible manner to increase patient involvement. Specific and written strategies to be employed to reach the SMART goals were established, based on collaborative interactions between participants, family members, and therapists. Therapists suggested a range of therapeutic strategies based on the current evidence base for the specific target problem area, and a list of common strategies was built up throughout the study related to recurring functional areas of SMART goals. Therapists reviewed and updated these strategies, and specific interventions were adopted to the individual needs of each patient. For details, see study protocol [58]. Team meetings were held on a regular basis, ensuring calibration of manual adherence across therapists. Ten percent of the sessions were observed by a senior professional with TBI expertise to evaluate treatment fidelity.

ACTION PLAN PARTICIPANT

TARGET OUTCOME # 1

Increased negative affect, rumination and feeling like there are no "good" days

SMART GOAL (specific, measurable, achievable, realistic/relevant, timed)

Goal 1.1: Stopping negative thoughts and focus on positive things in my everyday life

Strategies:
- Increase positive feelings:
  - Write down three positive things that have happened today before going to bed
  - List of positive activities – "positive refill" – apply at least 1 per day
- Work on my negative thoughts:
  - Learn about negative thought spirals - Read handout about rumination and mark up important topics for discussion for next session
  - Log thoughts-feelings-actions after experiencing negative emotions
  - Learn to apply distraction, distance and discussion
    - Positive supportive thoughts
    - Strategies for discussion (e.g., "ask my friend")
    - Practice recognizing cognitive distortions with reminders from spouse
    - Start positive refill activity
- Daily physical activity (walking, biking, swimming)
- Management of fatigue and sleep (see goal 2.1)

GAS score:	GAS levels
+2= A lot better than expected	Experience day as neutral or better (stopped my negative thoughts) 6–7 days per week AND 1 day or more feels like a "good day"
+1= A little better than expected	Experience day as neutral or better (stopped my negative thoughts) 6–7 days per week OR Experience day as neutral or better (stopped my negative thoughts) 4–5 days a week AND 1 day or more feels like a "good day"
0= As expected*	Experience day as neutral or better (stopped my negative thoughts) 4–5 days per week
−1= A little worse than expected	Experience day as neutral or better (stopped my negative thoughts) 2–3 days per week
−2= Much worse than expected	Experience day as neutral or better (stopped my negative thoughts) 0–1 days per week
GAS Baseline	−2	GAS Session 8	+1

Figure 2. Action plan example with SMART goal, strategies, and GAS. * "As expected" here means the level you expect to accomplish before the program ends with a reasonable amount of effort.

2.3. Outcomes

2.3.1. Goal Attainment Scaling

The main outcome measure in this study was goal attainment as measured by GAS scores, where five levels of goal attainment was agreed upon and established for each goal. GAS is, thus, subjective for each individual and goal specific. The expected level of goal attainment (scored as 0) was recorded, as well as two levels below the expected level (−1, −2; with baseline level being one of these) and two levels above the expected level (+1, +2). Baseline levels were set to −2 in cases where deterioration was impossible, and otherwise set to −1. Baseline levels were applied to evaluate change from the time at which the goal was set to GAS scoring at the last intervention session (session 8). To enhance precision, GAS levels were defined as specifically as possible, e.g., using percentages or number of days within the past week, as recommended by Malec [60]. Figure 2 displays an action plan example. At session 8, patient-reported goal attainment was registered, i.e., the patient's own evaluation of their current goal level. In cases of reduced awareness or other factors influencing the patient reporting of goal attainment, therapist and family members interacted with the patient to establish consensus.

Descriptive data are provided to depict the number of goals with goal attainment at the expected level or above, as well as goals with less than expected levels of attainment. As baseline GAS varied between −2 and −1, change scores were provided to describe goal attainment. GAS change scores were calculated as the difference between baseline and session 8 scores, and could, thus, vary between −1 (deterioration) and +4 (maximum improvement). A mean GAS score per participant was calculated by adding the raw change score for each goal and dividing the score on the number of goals for the specific individual.

2.3.2. SMART Goal Categorization

To describe the functional domains covered by SMART goals, goals were categorized by two independent researchers (authors I.M.H.B. and S.L.H.) who identified goal themes based on the wording of each SMART goal. The categories were established earlier in the study to classify the target problem areas nominated by patients and family members, based on procedures described by Winter, Moriarty [61] and the International Classification of Functioning (ICF). See Borgen, Kleffelgaard [62] for an overview of this categorization of target outcomes. Twenty-four categories were established, which covered four overarching domains: cognitive, physical/somatic, emotional, and participation/social functioning. There was full agreement on categorization for 92% of the goals, and disagreements were resolved by consensus in the research group.

2.3.3. Exploring Variables Associated with Goal Attainment

Indicators of goal attainment were chosen within the domains of demographic variables, injury characteristics, intervention-related factors, cognitive functioning, global outcome, and self-reported symptoms. The data included in this analysis were collected at our outpatient clinic by members of the research team during the baseline assessment before randomization. Demographic data, i.e., age, work status (work percentage), and years of education was collected at baseline. Injury-related factors (i.e., injury severity, time since injury, and cause of injury) were retrieved from medical records. Injury severity was classified based on the lowest unsedated Glasgow Coma Scale (GCS) score the first 24 h after injury. GCS scores 3–8 were classified as severe TBI, 9–12 as moderate, and 13–15 as mild TBI [63]. Intervention-related factors included whether a family member participated and treatment expectation, the latter measured at session 1 and 3 by asking participants to rate their expectation that the intervention would be useful for them on a Likert scale from 1–10 (not at all to a very high degree). See Table 1 for an overview of standardized measures of global functioning, cognition, and self-reported symptoms, and their scorings [64–73].

Table 1. Standardized outcomes and their applied scaling.

Assessment Domain	Measure Name	Score Used (Min.–Max.)
Global Outcome	GOSE [64]	Total score (3–8)
Cognitive functioning		
Verbal and visual abstraction/reasoning	Similarities and Matrices, WAIS-IV [65]	A dichotomized impairment variable was established, where impairment was defined as at least two test results being ≤1.5 standard deviation below the normative mean (no/yes) [66,67]
Verbal attention and working memory	Digit Span, WAIS-IV [65]	
Verbal learning and memory	CVLT-II [68]	
Processing speed, mental flexibility, and inhibition	Trail Making Tests 1–5 and Color Word Interference Tests 1–4, D-KEFS [69]	
Self-reported symptoms		
Post-concussive symptoms	RPQ [70]	Total score (0–64)
Fatigue	RPQ item [70]	Item score (0, 2–4)
Depressive symptoms	PHQ-9 [71]	Total score (0–27)
Anxiety-related symptoms	GAD-7 [72]	Total score (0–21)
Overall psychiatric distress	PHQ-9 [71] and GAD-7 [72]	Score of ≥10 on either scale (no/yes) [71,72]
Self-reported executive dysfunction	BRIEF-A [73]	Global Executive Composite t-score (0–100)

BRIEF-A = The Behavioral Rating of Executive Functions—Adult version, CVLT-II = California Verbal Learning Test-II, D-KEFS = Delis–Kaplan Executive Functioning Systems, GAD-7 = Generalized Anxiety Disorder 7-item, GOSE = Glasgow Outcome Scale Extended, PHQ-9 = Patient Health Questionnaire 9-item, RPQ = Rivermead Post-Concussion Symptoms Questionnaire, WAIS-IV = Weschler Adult Intelligence Scale IV.

2.4. Statistical Methods

All statistical tests were conducted in SPSS, version 26. Descriptions of patients and categorization of goals, as well as within-group changes in goal attainment from session 1 to session 8 are provided with descriptive statistics. Goal attainment per goal was not normally distributed, and Kruskal–Wallis H test was chosen to explore differences in goal attainment between domains. Distribution of GAS scores was assessed by visual inspection of QQ-plots.

To determine indicators of GAS score at session 8, two analytical approaches were performed using multiple hierarchical linear regression analyses. In the first approach, variables based on theoretical, empirical, and clinical experience ("expert model") were included in a hierarchical multiple regression analysis to compare models with or without controlling for baseline scores. Differences between the models were assessed with change in the explained variance (ΔR^2) and whether this change was significant. In the second explorative approach all variables associated ($p < 0.20$) with GAS at session 8 from univariate regression analyses were included ("explorative model"), also controlling for baseline GAS levels in a block-wise approach. The chosen explorative variables are outlined above. One factor from each domain was chosen to avoid multicollinearity. Further, multicollinearity among exploratory variables was checked using Pearson correlation coefficient (r) or Spearman's rho (ρ) of 0.7 as a cut off. The results from linear regression analyses are reported by regression coefficient (β) with 95% confidence interval (CI) and explained variance (R^2). Changes in explained variance between the steps (ΔR^2) and the significance levels are provided. Missing values of exploratory variables were 5% missing for cause of injury and 6% missing for injury severity. These data were multiple imputed under the assumption of missing at random. All available data were used to generate 15 imputed datasets. The results from each imputed dataset were combined to present single estimates.

2.5. Ethics

The study was approved by the Data Protection Office at OUH (2017/10390). The trial was registered at ClinicalTrials.gov, NCT03545594.

3. Results

3.1. Participants

Sixty participants were randomized to the intervention group. One withdrew after session 2 due to personal reasons, while the 59 remaining participants completed the intervention (session 8) and are included in the analysis. Thirty-nine (66%) had a participating family member, of whom 28 (72%) were spouses or domestic partners, 6 (15%) were parents, and 5 (13%) were other family members, such as siblings. Patient characteristics are reported in Table 2. In total, 56 (94%) participants participated in all 8 sessions, while 3 completed 7 sessions. Average length of intervention was 124 days (SD = 11.32; ~4 months).

Table 2. Patient characteristics.

Characteristics		Mean (SD)/Median (Range)/n(%)
Demographics		
Age, y		43.12 (13.61)
Gender, male		43 (73%)
Education, y		12 (10–20)
Marital status	Single	21 (36%)
	Married/domestic partner	32 (54%)
	Other (widowed, divorced, separated)	6 (10%)
Injury-related factors		
Injury severity (GCS) *		8 (3–15)
	Mild	16 (27%)
	Moderate	9 (15%)
	Severe	30 (51%)
	NA	4 (7%)
Cause of injury **	Fall	17 (29%)
	Transport-related	24 (40%)
	Violence	4 (7%)
	Other †	11 (19%)
	NA	3 (5%)
Time since injury ***, y		4 (2–23)
Work participation		
Work percentage		0 (0–100)
Work status	Works full-time	16 (27%)
	Works part-time	13 (22%)
	Disability/sick leave/retired	30 (51%)

* $n = 55$. ** $n = 56$. *** $n = 58$. †: sports- and leisure activities. GCS = Glasgow Coma Scale, SD = standard deviation, y = years.

3.2. SMART Goals

In total, 151 unique SMART goals were established and rated at session 8, with a mean of 2.61 (SD = 0.72, range: 1–4) per participant.

3.2.1. Goal Attainment

At session 8, 41 (27%) goals were scored at expected levels of goal attainment (score 0), 55 (36%) goals were scored a little better than expected (score +1) and 42 (28%) goals were scored much better than expected (+2). Only 11 (7%) goals were scored a little worse than expected (−1), and 2 (1%) goals were scored as much worse than expected (−2) at session 8.

The median overall GAS change score was 2 (range: −1.0–4.0). At session 8, 141 (93.3%) of the goals showed positive goal attainment (i.e., change scores 1–4), while 1 (0.7%) goal was with a worse goal attainment than at baseline, and 9 (6.0%) goals were scored with no change from baseline. The mean raw GAS change score per participant ($n = 59$) was 2.22 (SD = 0.91), and mean improvement per participant ranged from 0.5 to 4.0, i.e., all participants improved on at least one of their goals. The mean GAS change score at the individual level is visualized in Figure 3.

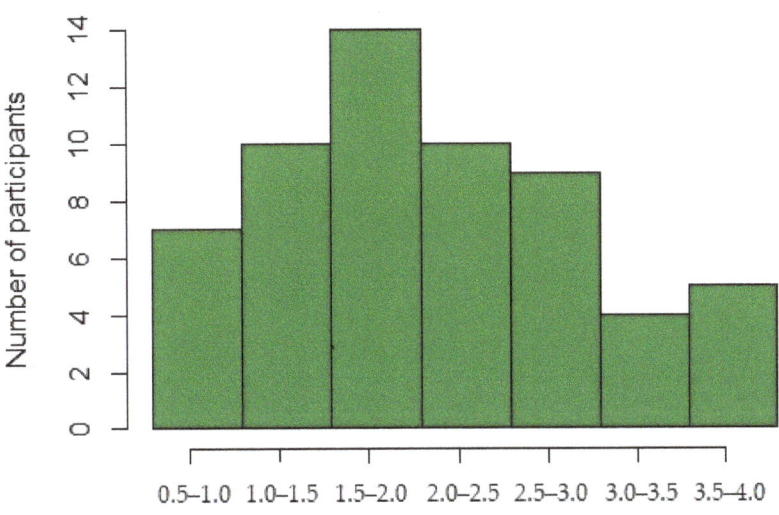

Figure 3. Mean individual change in GAS scores, across all 151 goals.

3.2.2. SMART Goal Domains and Categories

Table 3 displays the 151 SMART goals sorted by domains and sub-categories, with corresponding goal attainment. Table 3 also demonstrates that the SMART goals were classified within the same functional domains as target outcomes, confirming that goals adhered to problem areas initially reported by patients. The three most frequent SMART goal categories were related to reduced capacity and fatigue, memory difficulties, and sleep problems. Most goals were set related to physical/somatic functioning, especially regarding fatigue and sleep. Examples of such goals were "prevent episodes of fatigue >6 (VAS) during the week" and "maintain a circadian rhythm and get up at a fixed time". Within the domain of cognitive functioning most goals were related to memory and cognitive executive functioning and included goals such as "establish routines to ensure finding my belongings" and "get started on everyday tasks and stop postponing things". Goals regarding emotional functioning were most often related to anxiety and irritability and included goals such as "be less bothered by worrisome thoughts when going to bed" and "prevent and deal with episodes of irritability/anger in a calm manner". Within the social domain, goals were most frequently related to social communication difficulties and included goals such as "contribute to a more open and positive family communication" and "manage to stop losing track and veering off-topic during conversations". A Kruskal–Wallis H test was run to determine if there were differences in GAS change scores across the four goal domains, i.e., cognitive ($n = 38$), physical/somatic ($n = 53$), emotional ($n = 35$), and social ($n = 25$). Median GAS change scores were the same for all domains (2), with no significant differences between them ($\chi^2(3) = 2.674$, $p = 0.445$).

3.2.3. Indicators of Goal Attainment

The "expert model" included age, gender, injury severity, and total RPQ-score. The model showed an $R^2 = 0.128$, $F(5, 49) = 1.439$, $p = 0.227$. Controlling for baseline levels gave an R^2 change of 0.055 and a non-significant F change ($p = 0.085$).

Table 3. SMART goal categories and goal attainment at final session.

Domain/Category (number of participants)	Below Expectation n	At Expectation n	Above Expectation n	Total n
Cognitive difficulties	4 (11%)	11 (29%)	23 (60%)	38 (100%)
Attention difficulties (n = 5, 9%)	1	2	4	7
Memory difficulties (n = 15, 25%)	3	6	11	20
Language difficulties (n = 1, 2%)	0	0	1	1
Cognitive aspects of executive functioning (n = 10, 17%)	0	3	7	10
Physical/somatic difficulties	5 (9%)	13 (25%)	35 (66%)	53 (100%)
Reduced capacity and fatigue (n = 21, 36%)	2	7	13	22
Pain (n = 4, 7%)	0	0	4	4
Sleep difficulties (n = 11, 19%)	1	1	10	12
Difficulties with motor functions (n = 6, 10%)	0	5	3	8
Difficulties with dizziness and balance (n = 7, 12%)	2	0	5	7
Emotional difficulties	2 (6%)	8 (23%)	25 (71%)	35 (100%)
Emotion perception and regulation (n = 3, 5%)	0	0	3	3
Irritability (n = 9, 15%)	1	3	6	10
Anxiety (n = 9, 15%)	0	2	8	10
Depressive thoughts and feelings (n = 8, 14%)	0	2	6	8
Difficulties with coping with stress (n = 3, 5%)	1	1	1	3
Difficulties with identity, acceptance, and sense of self (n = 1, 2%)	0	0	1	1
Social function and participation	2 (8%)	9 (36%)	14 (56%)	25 (100%)
Behavioral dysregulation (n = 1, 2%)	0	0	1	1
Social communication difficulties (n = 10, 17%)	0	3	6	9
Reduced self-sufficiency (n = 4, 7%)	0	2	2	4
Reduced social participation (n = 4, 7%)	0	1	3	4
Lack of meaningful activities (n = 6, 10%)	2	3	2	7
Total	13 (8.6%)	41 (27.2%)	97 (64.2%)	151

Number of participants with goal within each category is given in the left column. Goal attainment levels at session 8 are given as "below expectation" (score −2 or −1), "at expectation" (score 0), and "above expectation" (score +1 and +2). The total number of goals per domain/category registered at each level of attainment are given in n (%).

As the model showed low predictive value, i.e., only predicted 12.8% of the total variance, univariate regression models were run to determine which explanatory variables should be included in the exploratory model. Results are presented in Table 4.

The final exploratory model of factors with a significance level <0.2 thus included gender, anxiety symptoms, self-reported executive function (BRIEF-A GEC t-score), and treatment expectation at session 3 and GAS baseline levels. This model showed R^2 of 0.322, $F (5, 52) = 4.854$, $p = 0.001$. The R^2 change was 0.116, F change significance was $p = 0.005$, i.e., the adjusted model showed complete case (Table 4), and imputed models (data not shown) showed similar results.

Table 4. Univariate regression analyses of goal attainment at final session (n = 59).

Exploratory Variables	B	95% CI	Significance	R Square	Decision
Demographic factors					
Age	0.002	−0.013 to 0.016	0.826	0.001	Discard
Gender	0.327	−0.102 to 0.757	0.133	0.039	Keep
Education (in years)	−0.042	−0.125 to 0.040	0.306	0.018	Discard
Percentage work participation (%)	0.002	−0.002 to 0.007	0.272	0.021	Discard
Injury-related factors					
GCS score	0.013	−0.034 to 0.060	0.588	0.006	Discard
Cause of injury (fall)	0.039	−0.125 to 0.204	0.633	0.004	Discard
Months since injury	0.000	−0.003 to 0.004	0.886	0.000	Discard
Functional status/symptoms at baseline					
Global functioning (GOSE)	−0.001	−0.202 to 0.201	0.994	0.000	Discard
Neuropsychology—overall impairment	−0.237	−0.623 to 0.149	0.224	0.026	Discard
Self-reported symptoms at baseline					
Post-concussion symptoms (RPQ total score)	0.004	−0.012 to 0.021	0.606	0.005	Discard
Fatigue (RPQ item)	0.047	−0.093 to 0.187	0.506	0.008	Discard
Depression (PHQ-9 total score)	−0.010	−0.045 to 0.026	0.589	0.005	Discard
Anxiety (GAD-7 total score)	−0.032	−0.078 to 0.014	0.173	0.032	*Keep*
Psychiatric symptoms (PHQ-9 and/or GAD-7 ≥ 10)	−0.072	−0.483 to 0.339	0.726	0.002	Discard
Executive dysfunction (BRIEF-A GEC t-score)	−0.023	−0.044 to −0.002	0.032	0.080	*Keep*
Intervention factors					
Treatment expectation at session 1	0.027	−0.074 to 0.127	0.595	0.005	Discard
Treatment expectation at session 3	0.125	0.019 to 0.230	0.022	0.090	*Keep*
Family member participation	0.099	−0.312 to 0.509	0.633	0.004	Discard

Italics display results at acceptable p-value (<0.20) to be carried forward. BRIEF-A = Behavioral Rating Inventory of Executive Functioning-Adult version. GAD-7 = Generalized Anxiety Disorder 7-items, GCS = Glasgow Coma Scale, GEC = Global Executive Composite, GOSE = Glasgow Outcome Scale Extended, PHQ-9 = Patient Health Questionnaire 9-item, RPQ = Rivermead Post-Concussion Questionnaire.

4. Discussion

This study aimed at describing goal attainment in patients receiving an individually tailored, home-based rehabilitation intervention and at describing goal attainment in different goal domains. We also explored indicators of goal attainment at the final session.

Goal attainment was very high. All participants had a positive total goal attainment change score, which means that all participants improved on at least one of their goals. The high levels of goal attainment found across patients with different injury severity, time since injury, current level of functioning, and different goal domains indicated that the intervention format is well suited for many individuals in the chronic phase of TBI. We believe that the high level of patient involvement in this study might have resulted in the high goal attainment seen, as suggested in the literature [74]. Additionally, setting goals and GAS has been shown to be effective in and of itself [75], which may have contributed to the results. Goals were categorized as related to either cognitive, physical/somatic, emotional, or social functioning. The level of goal attainment was equal across goal domains, which implies that the intervention was sufficiently tailored to allow participants to work effectively on a broad range of issues.

During baseline assessment in the RCT, patients and family members nominated target problem areas relating to TBI. A previously published paper [62] describes domains and categories of these problem areas. The problem areas reported at baseline were highly similar to the SMART goal areas reported in the current paper. A few problem areas reported at baseline were, however, not developed into SMART goals, i.e., visuospatial difficulties, reduced processing speed, difficulties with sensations, and difficulties with natural functions. Furthermore, some goal areas were not frequently established, such as goals related to identity difficulties and behavioral dysregulation. This may suggest that some problem areas are less easy to translate to SMART goals. If this was the result of difficulties in operationalizing abstract goal themes when applying GAS, this implies some limitation to the use of GAS. However, it might also be that abstract themes such as impaired self-awareness and identity difficulties were addressed while working on more concrete, everyday activities nominated by the patients, e.g., increased social activity.

The initial investigation of indicators of goal attainment based on theoretical, empirical, and clinical perspectives, yielded a low predictive model explaining only 12.8% of the total variance of goal attainment in this sample. As the knowledge base about predictors of goal attainment is scarce, an exploratory approach was warranted to generate new hypotheses for future work. This approach suggested that being female, having low levels of anxiety symptoms, experiencing good executive functioning as well as high rehabilitation expectations were related to positive goal attainment. This finding should be interpreted with caution as there is a risk of overestimating the association of single explanatory variables in univariate regression analyses, and future investigation is needed. Furthermore, it should be noted that although the exploratory model is significant, the explained variance is still modest (32.2%), which implies that there are factors associated with goal attainment that were not included in the current model.

The fact that both demographic factors, emotional symptoms, TBI-related deficits, and factors relating to the intervention itself may play a role in goal attainment is, however, not surprising but clinically very important. Rehabilitation is a complex, multifaceted process that involves many interacting factors, and the identification of active ingredients in rehabilitation interventions is notoriously difficult [76]. It is not surprising that individual factors may be associated with intervention outcomes. In our exploratory model, neither age, education level nor employment status predicted goal attainment. However, women displayed higher goal attainment. This finding needs replication. The literature on the influence of gender on outcome post-TBI is mixed [77]. Colantonio and colleagues [78] found that men reported larger difficulties than women in setting realistic goals, which might influence goal attainment. Other studies have suggested that women might have more intact executive functioning and better self-awareness post-TBI, but findings vary, and other authors have suggested that women show higher levels of self-awareness after

TBI [79]. Hence, we do not currently have any strong hypothesis regarding this result. The finding might even be spurious, in that gender is a proxy for a third and unknown variable. Interestingly, no injury-related factors were predictive of goal attainment. This could suggest that at the chronic stage of TBI, factors such as injury severity and time since injury do not play an important role in who benefits from every-day-oriented goal-based rehabilitation approaches. This supports the findings by Cicerone and colleagues that individuals with ongoing TBI-related difficulties should be offered support and may also benefit in the chronic stage, even years after the injury [25,26]. Additionally, self-reported executive dysfunction was shown to be detrimental to goal attainment, while performance-based cognitive impairments were not predictive of goal attainment. Thus, this only partly supports previous findings that cognitive impairment may hinder setting and achieving goals [42,43]. Despite previous findings that fatigue and emotional difficulties may be barriers to early goal-oriented rehabilitation in patients with stroke [80], only anxiety levels significantly predicted goal attainment in the current study. It may be that initial levels of fatigue and depression are a larger barrier to benefiting from rehabilitation during early recovery and are more addressable as the target of SMART goals later on. However, anxiety symptoms were shown to influence goal attainment. Anxiety levels are known to influence outcome post-TBI, although the directionality of this influence is disputed [81]. One study by Curran and colleagues [82] suggested that individuals with high levels of anxiety displayed more negative coping skills, such as worry, self-blame, and wishful thinking, and to some degree less positive coping skills such as problem solving. Whether anxiety symptoms in themselves are detrimental to goal attainment, or whether anxiety is a proxy for a variable such as coping skills is uncertain, and this finding also needs replication.

The finding that a positive expectation that the treatment could be beneficial during the third but not during the first session was predictive of goal attainment, was highly interesting. The finding may suggest that patient expectations are essential for goal attainment. However, as the wording of this question was the degree to which the participant expected that they would benefit from participating in the program, and that this belief was only predictive after participating in two or more sessions (and not at the very first session), it is likely that their response was influenced by their perceived level of therapeutic alliance. Although therapeutic alliance has received most attention in the field of psychotherapy, it has also been recognized as an important factor in brain injury rehabilitation (see [83] for a discussion). However, positive expectations might also be related to factors not measured in the current study. For example, the level of self-awareness may influence therapeutic alliance [44]. It may also be that expectations of change were influenced by the level of participant self-efficacy caused by the experienced improvement or lack thereof during the first three sessions. Self-efficacy, tenacity, and motivation have been previously shown to be predictive of goal attainment [34,41,44,45]. Future investigations should include measures of both therapeutic alliance, self-efficacy, and self-awareness in addition to change motivation to provide a clearer understanding of this interesting finding. The finding also indicated that treatment expectations should be discussed with patients early on in treatment, as this may play a role in treatment outcome. In summary, despite being exploratory, the current analyses provide hypotheses for further investigation of factors associated with goal attainment. Such investigations might be highly important to ensure a better understanding of what helps and what hinders goal attainment in rehabilitation, which again could help improve outcomes and ensure necessary tailoring of interventions.

Limitations

This work has some limitations that should be recognized. Firstly, the comparability of goal attainment across patients when delivering an individualized intervention is always uncertain, and although the intervention was manualized, the specific content was tailored to the individual patient. However, the individualized nature of the intervention is also thought to be a major strength, given the heterogeneous nature of long-term symptoms of TBI, and because it allows participants to define for themselves what areas are important for them to work on, further enhancing patient involvement. Secondly, the efficacy of this intervention has not yet been established. Although this study is based on a similar RCT, which did demonstrate significant between-group effects [55], effects have not yet been investigated in our sample pending final outcome assessments. This entails that we do not yet know whether the high level of goal attainment is accompanied by improved participation and quality of life, which are the primary outcome measures in the RCT. However, high goal attainment is an important positive finding regardless of group average changes on global outcome measures. Thirdly, the sample may not be representative of patients with TBI in general. Rather, the study included those who continue to experience TBI-related challenges in everyday life and who were motivated to participate in rehabilitation. Thus, the sample is considered representative of patients seen in specialized rehabilitation clinics. Further, GAS scoring has some limitations, i.e., there may be reliability issues in the establishment and scoring of GAS. For example, there is a risk of the development of different procedures by each therapist, and, as noted earlier, the scoring is deemed to be subjective in nature. In this study, GAS scoring was conducted by the therapists, as scoring by a blinded third party was not feasible. How to best compute GAS scores across goals and individuals is also disputed, which is the reason that GAS change scores were applied instead of t-scores, as these are controversial [84]. In addition, it is important to note that the problem categories used in the current paper were based on previous work by our research group using a data-driven approach. Different approaches could be applied that might have resulted in a somewhat different categorization of goals. There is currently no gold standard in taxonomies for goal categorization, although some suggestions have been made elsewhere [85,86]. The exploratory regression models were conducted to generate hypothesis for future research, and identified factors should not be considered as predictive of goal attainment without replication.

5. Conclusions

This study provides a transparent look at a goal-oriented approach in delivering rehabilitation interventions in the chronic phase of brain injury. Goal attainment was high, and goals were related to a broad range of problem areas typically identified in the chronic phase of TBI. Further investigation is needed to make strong conclusions regarding indicators of goal attainment, but the current study suggests that both individual, injury-related, and therapeutic factors are at play. The findings have clinical utility for therapists working with acquired brain injuries in general and other conditions where an individualized approach to treatment is warranted.

Author Contributions: Conceptualization, methodology, M.L., N.A., U.S., H.L.S., S.S., C.R.; data collection I.M.H.B., S.L.H., M.V.F., I.K.; data analysis, I.M.H.B., C.B.; writing—original draft preparation, I.M.H.B., M.L., S.L.H., M.V.F., C.R.; writing—review and editing, I.K., C.B., N.A., U.S., H.L.S., S.S.; project administration, C.R., M.L. All authors have read and agreed to the published version of the manuscript.

Funding: This research was funded by the Research Council of Norway, project number 260673/H10.

Institutional Review Board Statement: The study was conducted according to the guidelines of the Declaration of Helsinki and approved by the Data Protection Office at Oslo University Hospital (2017/10390).

Informed Consent Statement: Informed consent was obtained from all subjects involved in the study.

Data Availability Statement: Data can be viewed at secure servers at Oslo University Hospital by contacting the corresponding author.

Acknowledgments: We would like to thank participants and family members for their contribution to this study.

Conflicts of Interest: The authors declare no conflict of interest.

References

1. Tagliaferri, F.; Compagnone, C.; Korsic, M.; Servadei, F.; Kraus, J. A systematic review of brain injury epidemiology in Europe. *Acta Neurochir.* **2005**, *148*, 255–268. [CrossRef] [PubMed]
2. Peeters, W.; Brande, R.V.D.; Polinder, S.; Brazinova, A.; Steyerberg, E.W.; Lingsma, H.F.; Maas, A.I.R. Epidemiology of traumatic brain injury in Europe. *Acta Neurochir.* **2015**, *157*, 1683–1696. [CrossRef] [PubMed]
3. Peterson, A.B.; Xu, L.; Daugherty, J.; Breiding, M.J. Surveillance report of traumatic brain injury-related emergency department visits, hospitalizations, and deaths, United States, 2014. Centers for Disease Control and Prevention, U.S. Department of Health and Human Services; 2019. Available online: https://stacks.cdc.gov/view/cdc/78062 (accessed on 17 September 2021).
4. Olver, J.; Ponsford, J.L.; Curran, C.A. Outcome following traumatic brain injury: A comparison between 2 and 5 years after injury. *Brain Inj.* **1996**, *10*, 841–848. [CrossRef]
5. Brooks, J.C.; Strauss, D.J.; Shavelle, R.M.; Paculdo, D.; Hammond, F.M.; Harrison-Felix, C.L. Long-Term Disability and Survival in Traumatic Brain Injury: Results from the National Institute on Disability and Rehabilitation Research Model Systems. *Arch. Phys. Med. Rehabil.* **2013**, *94*, 2203–2209. [CrossRef] [PubMed]
6. Dikmen, S.S.; Machamer, J.; Powell, J.M.; Temkin, N.R. Outcome 3 to 5 years after moderate to severe traumatic brain injury. *Arch. Phys. Med. Rehabil.* **2003**, *84*, 1449–1457. [CrossRef]
7. Ruttan, L.; Martin, K.; Liu, A.; Colella, B.; Green, R. Long-Term Cognitive Outcome in Moderate to Severe Traumatic Brain Injury: A Meta-Analysis Examining Timed and Untimed Tests at 1 and 4.5 or More Years After Injury. *Arch. Phys. Med. Rehabil.* **2008**, *89*, S69–S76. [CrossRef] [PubMed]
8. Andelic, N.; Hammergren, N.; Bautz-Holter, E.; Sveen, U.; Brunborg, C.; Røe, C. Functional outcome and health-related quality of life 10 years after moderate-to-severe traumatic brain injury. *Acta Neurol. Scand.* **2009**, *120*, 16–23. [CrossRef]
9. Forslund, M.; Perrin, P.; Sigurdardottir, S.; Howe, E.; van Walsem, M.; Arango-Lasprilla, J.; Lu, J.; Aza, A.; Jerstad, T.; Røe, C.; et al. Health-Related Quality of Life Trajectories across 10 Years after Moderate to Severe Traumatic Brain Injury in Norway. *J. Clin. Med.* **2021**, *10*, 157. [CrossRef]
10. Miller, L. Family therapy of brain injury: Syndromes, strategies, and solutions. *Am. J. Fam. Ther.* **1993**, *21*, 111–121. [CrossRef]
11. Brickell, T.A.; French, L.; Lippa, S.M.; Lange, R.T. Burden among caregivers of service members and veterans following traumatic brain injury. *Brain Inj.* **2018**, *32*, 1541–1548. [CrossRef]
12. Saban, K.L.; Griffin, J.M.; Urban, A.; Janusek, M.A.; Pape, T.B.; Collins, E. Perceived health, caregiver burden, and quality of life in women partners providing care to Veterans with traumatic brain injury. *J. Rehabil. Res. Dev.* **2016**, *53*, 681–692. [CrossRef] [PubMed]
13. Doser, K.; Norup, A. Caregiver burden in Danish family members of patients with severe brain injury: The chronic phase. *Brain Inj.* **2016**, *30*, 334–342. [CrossRef] [PubMed]
14. Manskow, U.S.; Friborg, O.; Røe, C.; Braine, M.; Damsgard, E.; Anke, A. Patterns of change and stability in caregiver burden and life satisfaction from 1 to 2 years after severe traumatic brain injury: A Norwegian longitudinal study. *NeuroRehabilitation* **2017**, *40*, 211–222. [CrossRef]
15. Masel, B.E.; DeWitt, D.S. Traumatic Brain Injury: A Disease Process, Not an Event. *J. Neurotrauma* **2010**, *27*, 1529–1540. [CrossRef] [PubMed]
16. Corrigan, J.D.; Hammond, F.M. Traumatic Brain Injury as a Chronic Health Condition. *Arch. Phys. Med. Rehabil.* **2013**, *94*, 1199–1201. [CrossRef] [PubMed]
17. Wilson, L.; Stewart, W.; Dams-O'Connor, K.; Diaz-Arrastia, R.; Horton, L.; Menon, D.K.; Polinder, S. The chronic and evolving neurological consequences of traumatic brain injury. *Lancet Neurol.* **2017**, *16*, 813–825. [CrossRef]
18. Sigurdardottir, S.; Andelic, N.; Røe, C.; Schanke, A.-K. Trajectory of 10-Year Neurocognitive Functioning After Moderate–Severe Traumatic Brain Injury: Early Associations and Clinical Application. *J. Int. Neuropsychol. Soc.* **2020**, *26*, 654–667. [CrossRef]
19. Forslund, M.V.; Perrin, P.B.; Røe, C.; Sigurdardottir, S.; Hellstrøm, T.; Berntsen, S.A.; Lu, J.; Arango-Lasprilla, J.C.; Andelic, N. Global Outcome Trajectories up to 10 Years After Moderate to Severe Traumatic Brain Injury. *Front. Neurol.* **2019**, *10*, 219. [CrossRef]
20. Hoofien, D.; Gilboa, A.; Vakil, E.; Donovick, P.J. Traumatic brain injury (TBI) 10?20 years later: A comprehensive outcome study of psychiatric symptomatology, cognitive abilities and psychosocial functioning. *Brain Inj.* **2001**, *15*, 189–209. [CrossRef]
21. Koskinen, S. Quality of life 10 years after a very severe traumatic brain injury (TBI): The perspective of the injured and the closest relative. *Brain Inj.* **1998**, *12*, 631–648. [CrossRef]
22. Hammond, F.M.; Perkins, S.M.; Corrigan, J.D.; Nakase-Richardson, R.; Brown, A.W.; O'Neil-Pirozzi, T.M.; Zasler, N.D.; Greenwald, B.D. Functional Change from Five to Fifteen Years after Traumatic Brain Injury. *J. Neurotrauma* **2021**, *38*, 858–869. [CrossRef] [PubMed]
23. Wong, A.W.K.; Ng, S.; Dashner, J.; Baum, M.C.; Hammel, J.; Magasi, S.; Lai, J.-S.; Carlozzi, N.E.; Tulsky, D.S.; Miskovic, A.; et al. Relationships between environmental factors and participation in adults with traumatic brain injury, stroke, and spinal cord injury: A cross-sectional multi-center study. *Qual. Life Res.* **2017**, *26*, 2633–2645. [CrossRef] [PubMed]
24. Whiteneck, G.G.; Gerhart, K.A.; Cusick, C.P. Identifying Environmental Factors That Influence the Outcomes of People with Traumatic Brain Injury. *J. Head Trauma Rehabil.* **2004**, *19*, 191–204. [CrossRef] [PubMed]
25. Cicerone, K.D.; Goldin, Y.; Ganci, K.; Rosenbaum, A.; Wethe, J.V.; Langenbahn, D.M.; Malec, J.F.; Bergquist, T.F.; Kingsley, K.; Nagele, D.; et al. Evidence-Based Cognitive Rehabilitation: Systematic Review of the Literature From 2009 Through 2014. *Arch. Phys. Med. Rehabil.* **2019**, *100*, 1515–1533. [CrossRef]

26. Cicerone, K.D.; Mott, T.; Azulay, J.; Friel, J.C. Community integration and satisfaction with functioning after intensive cognitive rehabilitation for traumatic brain injury. *Arch. Phys. Med. Rehabil.* **2004**, *85*, 943–950. [CrossRef]
27. Patterson, F.; Fleming, J.; Doig, E. Group-based delivery of interventions in traumatic brain injury rehabilitation: A scoping review. *Disabil. Rehabil.* **2016**, *38*, 1961–1986. [CrossRef]
28. Evans, L.; Brewis, C. The efficacy of community-based rehabilitation programmes for adults with TBI. *Int. J. Ther. Rehabil.* **2008**, *15*, 446–458. [CrossRef]
29. Andelic, N.; Soberg, H.L.; Berntsen, S.; Sigurdardottir, S.; Roe, C. Self-Perceived Health Care Needs and Delivery of Health Care Services 5 Years After Moderate-to-Severe Traumatic Brain Injury. *PM&R* **2014**, *6*, 1013–1021. [CrossRef]
30. Andelic, N.; Røe, C.; Tenovuo, O.; Azouvi, P.; Dawes, H.; Majdan, M.; Ranta, J.; Howe, E.; Wiegers, E.; Tverdal, C.; et al. Unmet Rehabilitation Needs after Traumatic Brain Injury across Europe: Results from the CENTER-TBI Study. *J. Clin. Med.* **2021**, *10*, 1035. [CrossRef]
31. Barnes, M.P. Principles of neurological rehabilitation. *J. Neurol. Neurosurg. Psychiatry* **2003**, *74*, iv3–iv7. [CrossRef]
32. Yun, D.; Choi, J. Person-centered rehabilitation care and outcomes: A systematic literature review. *Int. J. Nurs. Stud.* **2019**, *93*, 74–83. [CrossRef] [PubMed]
33. Wilson, B.A. Neuropsychological Rehabilitation. *Annu. Rev. Clin. Psychol.* **2008**, *4*, 141–162. [CrossRef] [PubMed]
34. Rose, A.; Rosewilliam, S.; Soundy, A. Shared decision making within goal setting in rehabilitation settings: A systematic review. *Patient Educ. Couns.* **2016**, *100*, 65–75. [CrossRef] [PubMed]
35. Levack, W.M.M.; Taylor, K.; Siegert, R.J.; Dean, S.G.; McPherson, K.M.; Weatherall, M. Is goal planning in rehabilitation effective? A systematic review. *Clin. Rehabil.* **2006**, *20*, 739–755. [CrossRef]
36. Levack, W.M.M.; Weatherall, M.; Hay-Smith, E.J.C.; Dean, S.; McPherson, K.; Siegert, R. Goal setting and strategies to enhance goal pursuit for adults with acquired disability participating in rehabilitation. *Cochrane Database Syst. Rev.* **2015**, CD009727. [CrossRef]
37. Doig, E.; Fleming, J.; Kuipers, P.; Cornwell, P.; Khan, A. Goal-directed outpatient rehabilitation following TBI: A pilot study of programme effectiveness and comparison of outcomes in home and day hospital settings. *Brain Inj.* **2011**, *25*, 1114–1125. [CrossRef]
38. Powell, J.; Heslin, J.; Greenwood, R. Community based rehabilitation after severe traumatic brain injury: A randomised controlled trial. *J. Neurol. Neurosurg. Psychiatry* **2002**, *72*, 193–202. [CrossRef]
39. McClain, C. Collaborative Rehabilitation Goal Setting. *Top. Stroke Rehabil.* **2005**, *12*, 56–60. [CrossRef]
40. Wade, D.T. Goal setting in rehabilitation: An overview of what, why and how. *Clin. Rehabil.* **2009**, *23*, 291–295. [CrossRef]
41. Prescott, S.; Fleming, J.; Doig, E. Goal setting approaches and principles used in rehabilitation for people with acquired brain injury: A systematic scoping review. *Brain Inj.* **2015**, *29*, 1515–1529. [CrossRef]
42. Hersh, D.; Worrall, L.; Howe, T.; Sherratt, S.; Davidson, B. SMARTER goal setting in aphasia rehabilitation. *Aphasiology* **2012**, *26*, 220–233. [CrossRef]
43. Hart, T.; Evans, J. Self-regulation and Goal Theories in Brain Injury Rehabilitation. *J. Head Trauma Rehabil.* **2006**, *21*, 142–155. [CrossRef] [PubMed]
44. Schönberger, M.; Humle, F.; Teasdale, T.W. The development of the therapeutic working alliance, patients' awareness and their compliance during the process of brain injury rehabilitation. *Brain Inj.* **2006**, *20*, 445–454. [CrossRef] [PubMed]
45. Plant, S.; Tyson, S.; Kirk, S.; Parsons, J. What are the barriers and facilitators to goal-setting during rehabilitation for stroke and other acquired brain injuries? A systematic review and meta-synthesis. *Clin. Rehabil.* **2016**, *30*, 921–930. [CrossRef]
46. Brands, I.; Stapert, S.; Wade, D.; Van Heugten, C.; Köhler, S. Life goal attainment in the adaptation process after acquired brain injury: The influence of self-efficacy and of flexibility and tenacity in goal pursuit. *Clin. Rehabil.* **2014**, *29*, 611–622. [CrossRef]
47. Siegert, R.J.; McPherson, K.M.; Taylor, W.J. Toward a cognitive-affective model of goal-setting in rehabilitation: Is self-regulation theory a key step? *Disabil. Rehabil.* **2004**, *26*, 1175–1183. [CrossRef]
48. Playford, E.D.; Siegert, R.J.; Levack, W.; Freeman, J. Areas of consensus and controversy about goal setting in rehabilitation: A conference report. *Clin. Rehabil.* **2009**, *23*, 334–344. [CrossRef]
49. Scobbie, L.; Wyke, S.; Dixon, D. Identifying and applying psychological theory to setting and achieving rehabilitation goals. *Clin. Rehabil.* **2009**, *23*, 321–333. [CrossRef]
50. Turner-Stokes, L. Goal attainment scaling (GAS) in rehabilitation: A practical guide. *Clin. Rehabil.* **2009**, *23*, 362–370. [CrossRef]
51. Liu, C.; Mcneil, J.E.; Greenwood, R. Rehabilitation outcomes after brain injury: Disability measures or goal acheivement? *Clin. Rehabil.* **2004**, *18*, 398–404. [CrossRef]
52. Kiresuk, T.J.; Sherman, R.E. Goal attainment scaling: A general method for evaluating comprehensive community mental health programs. *Community Ment. Health J.* **1968**, *4*, 443–453. [CrossRef] [PubMed]
53. Grant, M.; Ponsford, J. Goal Attainment Scaling in brain injury rehabilitation: Strengths, limitations and recommendations for future applications. *Neuropsychol. Rehabil.* **2014**, *24*, 661–677. [CrossRef] [PubMed]
54. Hurn, J.; Kneebone, I.; Cropley, M. Goal setting as an outcome measure: A systematic review. *Clin. Rehabil.* **2006**, *20*, 756–772. [CrossRef] [PubMed]
55. Trevena-Peters, J.; McKay, A.; Ponsford, J. Activities of daily living retraining and goal attainment during posttraumatic amnesia. *Neuropsychol. Rehabil.* **2018**, *29*, 1655–1670. [CrossRef] [PubMed]

56. Behn, N.; Marshall, J.; Togher, L.; Cruice, M. Feasibility and initial efficacy of project-based treatment for people with ABI. *Int. J. Lang. Commun. Disord.* **2019**, *54*, 465–478. [CrossRef]
57. Winter, L.; Moriarty, H.J.; Robinson, K.; Piersol, C.; Vause-Earland, T.; Newhart, B.; Iacovone, D.B.; Hodgson, N.; Gitlin, L.N. Efficacy and acceptability of a home-based, family-inclusive intervention for veterans with TBI: A randomized controlled trial. *Brain Inj.* **2016**, *30*, 373–387. [CrossRef]
58. Borgen, I.M.H.; Løvstad, M.; Andelic, N.; Hauger, S.; Sigurdardottir, S.; Søberg, H.L.; Sveen, U.; Forslund, M.V.; Kleffelgård, I.; Lindstad, M.; et al. Traumatic brain injury—Needs and treatment options in the chronic phase: Study protocol for a randomized controlled community-based intervention. *Trials* **2020**, *21*, 294. [CrossRef]
59. Bovend'Eerdt, T.J.H.; Botell, R.; Wade, D. Writing SMART rehabilitation goals and achieving goal attainment scaling: A practical guide. *Clin. Rehabil.* **2009**, *23*, 352–361. [CrossRef]
60. Malec, J.F. Goal Attainment Scaling in Rehabilitation. *Neuropsychol. Rehabil.* **1999**, *9*, 253–275. [CrossRef]
61. Winter, L.; Moriarty, H.J.; Piersol, C.V.; Vause-Earland, T.; Robinson, K.; Newhart, B. Patient-and family-identified problems of traumatic brain injury: Value and utility of a target outcome approach to identifying the worst problems. *J. Patient-Cent. Res. Rev.* **2016**, *3*, 30–39. [CrossRef]
62. Borgen, I.M.H.; Kleffelgård, I.; Hauger, S.L.; Forslund, M.V.; Søberg, H.L.; Andelic, N.; Sveen, U.; Winter, L.; Løvstad, M.; Røe, C. Patient-Reported Problem Areas in Chronic Traumatic Brain Injury. *J. Head Trauma Rehabil.* **2021**, in press. [CrossRef] [PubMed]
63. Rimel, R.W.; Giordani, B.; Barth, J.T.; Jane, J.A. Moderate Head Injury: Completing the Clinical Spectrum of Brain Trauma. *Neurosurgery* **1982**, *11*, 344–351. [CrossRef]
64. Wilson, J.L.; Pettigrew, L.E.; Teasdale, G.M. Structured Interviews for the Glasgow Outcome Scale and the Extended Glasgow Outcome Scale: Guidelines for Their Use. *J. Neurotrauma* **1998**, *15*, 573–585. [CrossRef] [PubMed]
65. Wechsler, D. *Wechsler Adult Intelligence Scale*, 4th ed.; WAIS–IV; Pearson: London, UK, 2008.
66. Migliore, S.; Ghazaryan, A.; Simonelli, I.; Pasqualetti, P.; Squitieri, F.; Curcio, G.; Landi, D.; Palmieri, M.G.; Moffa, F.; Filippi, M.M.; et al. Cognitive Impairment in Relapsing-Remitting Multiple Sclerosis Patients with Very Mild Clinical Disability. *Behav. Neurol.* **2017**, *2017*, 8140962. [CrossRef] [PubMed]
67. Binder, L.M.; Iverson, G.L.; Brooks, B.L. To Err is Human: "Abnormal" Neuropsychological Scores and Variability are Common in Healthy Adults. *Arch. Clin. Neuropsychol.* **2009**, *24*, 31–46. [CrossRef]
68. Delis, D.C.; Kramer, J.H.; Kaplan, E.; Ober, B.A. *California Verbal Learning Test*, 2nd ed.; Harcourt Assessment: San Antonio, TX, USA, 2000.
69. Delis, D.C.; Kaplan, E.; Kramer, J.H. *Delis-Kaplan Executive Function System*; The Psychological Corporation: San Antonio, TX, USA, 2001.
70. King, N.S.; Crawford, S.; Wenden, F.J.; Moss, N.E.G.; Wade, D. The Rivermead Post Concussion Symptoms Questionnaire: A measure of symptoms commonly experienced after head injury and its reliability. *J. Neurol.* **1995**, *242*, 587–592. [CrossRef]
71. Kroenke, K.; Spitzer, R.L.; Williams, J.B.W. The PHQ-9: Validity of a brief depression severity measure. *J. Gen. Intern. Med.* **2001**, *16*, 606–613. [CrossRef]
72. Spitzer, R.L.; Kroenke, K.; Williams, J.B.W.; Löwe, B. A Brief Measure for Assessing Generalized Anxiety Disorder: The GAD-7. *Arch. Intern. Med.* **2006**, *166*, 1092–1097. [CrossRef]
73. Roth, R.M.; Isquith, P.K.; Gioia, G.A. *Behavior Rating Inventory of Executive Function—Adult Version (BRIEF-A)*; Psychological Assessment Resources: Lutz, FL, USA, 2005.
74. Evans, J.J. Goal setting during rehabilitation early and late after acquired brain injury. *Curr. Opin. Neurol.* **2012**, *25*, 651–655. [CrossRef]
75. Herdman, K.A.; Vandermorris, S.; Davidson, S.; Au, A.; Troyer, A.K. Comparable achievement of client-identified, self-rated goals in intervention and no-intervention groups: Reevaluating the use of Goal Attainment Scaling as an outcome measure. *Neuropsychol. Rehabil.* **2018**, *29*, 1600–1610. [CrossRef]
76. Whyte, J.; Hart, T. It's More Than a Black Box; It's a Russian Doll. *Am. J. Phys. Med. Rehabil.* **2003**, *82*, 639–652. [CrossRef] [PubMed]
77. Farace, E.; Alves, W.M. Do women fare worse: A metaanalysis of gender differences in traumatic brain injury outcome. *J. Neurosurg.* **2000**, *93*, 539–545. [CrossRef] [PubMed]
78. Colantonio, A.; Harris, J.E.; Ratcliff, G.; Chase, S.; Ellis, K. Gender differences in self reported long term outcomes following moderate to severe traumatic brain injury. *BMC Neurol.* **2010**, *10*, 1–7. [CrossRef] [PubMed]
79. Niemeier, J.P.; Perrin, P.; Holcomb, M.G.; Rolston, C.D.; Artman, L.K.; Lu, J.; Nersessova, K.S. Gender Differences in Awareness and Outcomes During Acute Traumatic Brain Injury Recovery. *J. Women's Health* **2014**, *23*, 573–580. [CrossRef] [PubMed]
80. Plant, S.; Tyson, S.F. A multicentre study of how goal-setting is practised during inpatient stroke rehabilitation. *Clin. Rehabil.* **2017**, *32*, 263–272. [CrossRef]
81. Schönberger, M.; Ponsford, J.; Gould, K.R.; Johnston, L. The Temporal Relationship Between Depression, Anxiety, and Functional Status after Traumatic Brain Injury: A Cross-lagged Analysis. *J. Int. Neuropsychol. Soc.* **2011**, *17*, 781–787. [CrossRef]
82. Curran, C.A.; Ponsford, J.L.; Crowe, S. Coping strategies and emotional outcome following traumatic brain injury: A compar-ison with orthopedic patients. *J. Head Trauma Rehab.* **2000**, *15*, 1256–1274. [CrossRef]
83. Sherer, M.; Evans, C.C.; Leverenz, J.; Stouter, J.; Irby, J.W., Jr.; Eun-Lee, J.; Yablon, S.A. Therapeutic alliance in post-acute brain injury rehabilitation: Predictors of strength of alliance and impact of alliance on outcome. *Brain Inj.* **2007**, *21*, 663–672. [CrossRef]

4. Tennant, A. Goal attainment scaling: Current methodological challenges. *Disabil. Rehabil.* **2007**, *29*, 1583–1588. [CrossRef]
5. Kuipers, P.; Foster, M.; Carlson, G.; Moy, J. Classifying client goals in community-based ABI rehabilitation: A taxonomy for profiling service delivery and conceptualizing outcomes. *Disabil. Rehabil.* **2003**, *25*, 154–162. [CrossRef]
6. Grill, E.; Lohmann, S.; Decker, J.; Müller, M.; Strobl, R.; Grill, E. The ICF forms a useful framework for classifying individual patient goals in post-acute rehabilitation. *J. Rehabil. Med.* **2011**, *43*, 151–155. [CrossRef] [PubMed]

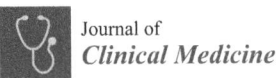

Article

Feasibility and Acceptability of a Complex Telerehabilitation Intervention for Pediatric Acquired Brain Injury: The Child in Context Intervention (CICI)

Ingvil Laberg Holthe [1,2,*], Nina Rohrer-Baumgartner [1], Edel J. Svendsen [1,3,4], Solveig Lægreid Hauger [1,2], Marit Vindal Forslund [5], Ida M. H. Borgen [2,5], Hege Prag Øra [1], Ingerid Kleffelgård [5], Anine Pernille Strand-Saugnes [6], Jens Egeland [2,7], Cecilie Røe [4,5,8], Shari L. Wade [9,10] and Marianne Løvstad [1,2]

1. Department of Research, Sunnaas Rehabilitation Hospital, 1453 Nesodden, Norway; uxronb@sunnaas.no (N.R.-B.); edel.jannecke.svendsen@sunnaas.no (E.J.S.); solveig.laegreidhauger@sunnaas.no (S.L.H.); hege.ora@sunnaas.no (H.P.Ø.); marianne.lovstad@sunnaas.no (M.L.)
2. Department of Psychology, Faculty of Social Sciences, University of Oslo, 0317 Oslo, Norway; idmbor@ous-hf.no (I.M.H.B.); jens.egeland@siv.no (J.E.)
3. Department of Nursing and Health Promotion, Oslo Metropolitan University, 0130 Oslo, Norway
4. Research Centre for Habilitation and Rehabilitation Models and Services (CHARM), Institute of Health and Society, Faculty of Medicine, University of Oslo, 0372 Oslo, Norway; cecilie.roe@medisin.uio.no
5. Department of Physical Medicine and Rehabilitation, Oslo University Hospital, 0424 Oslo, Norway; mavfor@ous-hf.no (M.V.F.); uxinff@ous-hf.no (I.K.)
6. Department of Acquired Brain Injury, Statped: Norwegian Service for Special Needs Education, 2815 Gjøvik, Norway; anine.strand-saugnes@statped.no
7. Department of Research, Vestfold Hospital Trust, 3103 Tønsberg, Norway
8. Institute of Clinical Medicine, Faculty of Medicine, University of Oslo, 0372 Oslo, Norway
9. Division of Pediatric Rehabilitation Medicine, Cincinnati Children's Hospital Medical Center, Cincinnati, OH 45229, USA; shari.wade@cchmc.org
10. Department of Pediatrics, University of Cincinnati College of Medicine, Cincinnati, OH 45267, USA
* Correspondence: ingvil.laberg.holthe@sunnaas.no

Abstract: The current study is a feasibility study of a randomized controlled trial (RCT): the Child in Context Intervention (CICI). The CICI study is an individualized, goal-oriented and home-based intervention conducted mainly through videoconference. It targets children with ongoing challenges (physical, cognitive, behavioral, social and/or psychological) after acquired brain injury (ABI) and their families at least one year post injury. The CICI feasibility study included six children aged 11–16 years with verified ABI-diagnosis, their families and their schools. The aim was to evaluate the feasibility of the intervention components, child and parent perceptions of usefulness and relevance of the intervention as well as the assessment protocol through a priori defined criteria. Overall, the families and therapists rated the intervention as feasible and acceptable, including the videoconference treatment delivery. However, the burden of assessment was too high. The SMART-goal approach was rated as useful, and goal attainment was high. The parents' ratings of acceptability of the intervention were somewhat higher than the children's. In conclusion, the CICI protocol proved feasible and acceptable to families, schools and therapists. The assessment burden was reduced, and adjustments in primary outcomes were made for the definitive RCT.

Keywords: feasibility study; goal-oriented rehabilitation; pediatric brain injury; SMART-goals; home-based rehabilitation

1. Introduction

Although children with acquired brain injury (pediatric acquired brain injury—pABI) may suffer long-lasting physical, cognitive, behavioral and social symptoms as well as disturbances in psychological adaptation [1–3], few randomized controlled trials have explored the effectiveness of complex interventions targeting these children, their families and their everyday context at home and in school. This may be due to the considerable complexity of designing and conducting such studies where one must take a range of factors into account. These include the child's age and developmental level, the heterogeneity of symptoms that may follow a pABI, family factors that may influence the ability and willingness to participate in an intervention, and the heterogeneity in factors related to the child's everyday life in the community, such as school and other areas of participation. The possible pitfalls are many. Exploring the feasibility of a complex intervention is therefore important prior to large-scale RCTs. This paper describes the investigation of the feasibility of a complex, individualized and community-based intervention targeting children with pABI and their families.

Brain damage acquired after birth can be caused by traumatic (TBI) or non-traumatic injuries such as stroke (i.e., brain hemorrhage or infarction), tumor, inflammation, infection or hypoxia. pABI may cause a wide range of disruptions in the child's developmental course [1–3]. Deficits may be persistent, leading to reduced participation in school and social life [4–6], and reduced quality of life [2,7,8]. Prior studies have identified needs for long-term follow-up after ABI; psychological support for parents, siblings and the affected child; as well as support in the return to school [9]. Interestingly, reported needs may change over time, from primarily physical concerns in the first months post injury (79%), to cognitive (47%) and socioemotional needs (68%) later on [10]. Importantly, rehabilitation needs after pABI are described as largely unmet [11].

As family needs after a pediatric brain injury are complex and heterogeneous, rehabilitation services and follow-up care should be individualized to each patient's needs. In line with this, rehabilitation should be multidisciplinary and take place within a biopsychosocial framework [12]. In addition, rehabilitation needs to be flexible, monitoring the development and goals of the patient, which may change over time [12]. A recent study mapped treatment goals set by young people with ABI to the domains in the International Classification of Functioning, Disability and Health (ICF) [13], in which 52% were related to activities and participation, and 20% to environmental factors [14]. This highlights the need to include community-based rehabilitation that is individualized and context-sensitive [14]. The complexity of pediatric ABI rehabilitation may explain the small body of evidence-based recommendations. However, existing knowledge provides evidence for family/caregiver-focused interventions and the use of technology in rehabilitation [15]. In addition, direct interventions related to cognitive functions such as attention, memory, executive function and emotional/behavioral functioning have given positive results [15]. However, a critique against the direct training approach in cognitive rehabilitation (i.e., interventions directed toward retraining the child's abilities) is that generalization to everyday functioning is often unknown or disputed [16]. Therefore, indirect approaches such as behavioral compensation and modification, environmental modification and supports, educational supports and instructional strategies are recommended, including education for parents and caregiver involvement in handling executive dysfunction [17,18]. The effects of parenting/family interventions after pABI have been explored in randomized controlled trials (RCTs) by Wade and colleagues with promising results for online problem-solving training, improving behavior problems, executive functioning, and family functioning [15,19–22]. The use of technology in rehabilitation is relatively new, but telerehabilitation has shown to be a reliable alternative to in-person meetings [23,24] with promising results in cognitive rehabilitation [25], speech and language therapy [26] and family therapy [27,28]. Recent reviews on technology-based or -assisted rehabilitation programs for children with ABI have found that in addition to the mentioned evidence for online problem-solving, there is promising evidence for training of cognitive, social and behavioral skills [15,22,29,30]. The findings are characterized by heterogeneity and small samples, but the involvement of a clinician in addition to the technology-based intervention may be of importance for a positive result [30]. Although most of this research has been conducted in the USA, some of the technology-based intervention studies presented in the literature reviews have also been performed in Europe. In addition, goal-oriented rehabilitation is considered a key ingredient in pABI rehabilitation [14,31], and goal attainment scaling can be a sensitive and meaningful way to measure rehabilitation outcomes [32]. Children's self-identified goals have been found to be as achievable as their parents' goals in a sample of children with a mean age of 9 years [33], pointing toward the importance of including the children in defining rehabilitation goals.

To our knowledge, no single intervention has included all these important perspectives simultaneously in a pABI-population. However, an intervention targeting individualized, everyday rehabilitation needs in a home setting has been carried out for the adult TBI-population in the US [34] and is currently ongoing in Norway [35]. This intervention defined individualized rehabilitation goals in collaboration with the patient and family member when available and worked on strategies to reach these goals over a period of four months. To meet the demands of holistic, person-centered and goal-oriented interventions for the pABI-population, this adult intervention was adapted to the pediatric population. In the Child in Context Intervention (CICI), the family and the child's school are included, and collaboration is established with the Norwegian Service for Special Needs Education ("Statped"). The intervention has largely been adapted to a telerehabilitation format to facilitate access to rehabilitation services, and to ease participation for families and schools.

The Medical Research Council [36] has pointed out the need to carry out feasibility studies as part of the development of complex interventions. This is especially important as the complexity of such studies is influenced not only by the intervention components, but also by contextual factors, in addition to the interactional processes occurring between the intervention components and the context [37]. In pediatric rehabilitation, one also needs to consider a range of transactional processes: between child and parent; between the child, family and school environment; and in the community and with peers, as children rely on their environment even more than adults [38]. In the CICI study, the complex interactions that may take place between children, parents, schools and the intervention components is hard to foresee before the intervention has been tried out. Some key uncertainties include whether the complex logistics of the study are feasible, whether the families are able to maintain participation in an intensive intervention (seven sessions over 4–5 months), whether recruitment is feasible, whether it will be possible to maintain a sustainable working alliance with both children and parents through the telerehabilitation format and whether the goal-oriented approach is feasible when working with an entire family that may not have the same priorities or needs. In addition, as there have been no previous studies carried out including schools in a similar rehabilitation program, it is also of importance to assess the feasibility of this intervention component. Conducting a feasibility study prior to the future definitive RCT is therefore principal in order to evaluate the intervention manual, identify possible obstacles and be able to adjust the protocol before the RCT.

Objectives

The objectives of the CICI feasibility study were to assess the feasibility of (1) the recruitment procedures and (2) the contents and structure of the intervention, including the feasibility of treatment delivery through a videoconference solution. We also wished to evaluate the acceptability of (3) the intervention for children, parents and therapists, (4) the baseline (T1) and outcome (T2) assessment methods and finally (5) the quality of treatment delivery. In order to inform the final decisions on outcome measures in the RCT, considering preliminary indications regarding the usefulness of outcome measures was also addressed.

2. Materials and Methods

This article adheres to the CONSORT extension for the Pilot and Feasibility Trials Checklist [39].

2.1. Trial Design

This feasibility trial applied a one-group pre−post design, with a baseline (T1) and a follow-up assessment immediately after the intervention period of 4-5 months (T2). The future definitive RCT will include a two-group RCT-design. For the RCT, outcome assessments will also be performed about 9 months after baseline (T3). The T3-assessment was not included in the feasibility trial to minimize time expenditure as T3 largely matches T2.

2.2. Participants and Recruitment Procedures

The inclusion criteria were (1) school-aged children (6–16 years at inclusion) with a radiologically verified diagnosis of ABI, or loss of consciousness post-insult and verified neurological symptoms in cases where radiology could not be administered; (2) time since insult at least 1 year; (3) self- or parent-reported persistent ABI-related cognitive, emotional or behavioral challenges influencing participation in everyday life related to family, friends, school or local community, assessed through a telephone interview; (4) children attending school regularly; and (5) the family is able to participate actively in a goal-oriented study for the next 4–5 months.

Exclusion criteria were (1) severe pre- or comorbid neurological or neuropsychological disorders that would confound assessment and/or outcome measurements; (2) children with brain tumors in active treatment or at great risk of relapse; (3) children with severe psychiatric illness or with injuries so severe that they were currently in institutionalized care; (4) parental severe psychiatric illness, drug abuse or indications of a history of or risk of domestic violence; and (5) not fluent in Norwegian language, although exceptions could be made for English-speaking parents who understand and read Norwegian.

Participants were identified from the medical charts at Sunnaas Rehabilitation Hospital. The families were invited to participate through written age-appropriate information for the children and information to parents. Parents and teenagers from 16 years of age provided written informed consent. A scripted telephone interview was used to screen for inclusion and exclusion criteria and willingness to participate. Eligible and consenting families performed a baseline screening (T1) at Sunnaas Rehabilitation Hospital.

After inclusion, the children's teachers and principals at their schools received written information about the study and consent form for the teachers. They were thereafter contacted by telephone by the CICI Statped collaborator.

2.3. Assessments

The outcome measures to be evaluated in the feasibility study are listed in Table 1. Neuropsychological assessment was included at baseline to provide descriptive data regarding the children with ABI and to inform the goal-setting process. Primary outcomes were post-concussive symptom burden (HBI), parenting self-efficacy (TOPSE) and quality of life (PedsQL). Questionnaires were completed at home and returned by mail.

As part of the baseline assessments, the families were asked to name the current three most challenging areas related to the child's brain injury. These were rated on a 5-point Likert scale according to how troublesome they were perceived in everyday life. Parents agreed on three areas but scaled them separately. The child was similarly asked to name and rate his or her own three most troublesome pABI-related problem areas.

2.4. Intervention

A detailed intervention manual was developed. It was based on the manual developed for an adult population by Borgen and colleagues [35] and adapted to the pediatric and family context by experienced rehabilitation therapists (authors M.L., S.L.H., I.M.H.B., M.V.F., N. R.-B., I.L.H.). In addition to descriptions of the content of each session, the manual contained general information on the study's rationale and aims as well as detailed guidance on how to establish SMART-goals and strategies, and references to evidence-based strategies and "tools" to handle different challenges. The manual also included detailed guidelines on how to manage therapy and communication through videoconference.

Table 1. Measures included in the feasibility study.

Assessment Domain	Instrument
Neuropsychological Assessment at Baseline Only	
Verbal IQ estimate	Similarities from Wechsler Intelligence Scale for Children (WISC-V) [40]
Non-verbal IQ estimate	Matrix reasoning from WISC-V
Auditory attention/verbal working memory	Digit span from WISC-V
Visuomotor processing speed	Coding from WISC-V
Verbal learning and memory	Children's Auditory Verbal Learning Test-2 (CAVLT-2) [41]
Verbal inhibition	Inhibition from the Developmental Neuropsychological Assessment (NEPSY-II) [42]
Auditory comprehension	Comprehension of instructions from NEPSY-II
Questionnaires at Baseline and Post Intervention	
Emotional, behavioral and social functioning	Strengths and Difficulties Questionnaire (SDQ) [43]
Participation: home, neighborhood, community	Child and Adolescent Scale of Participation (CASP) [44]
Quality of life	The Pediatric Quality of Life Inventory (Peds-QL) [45]
Post-concussive symptoms after ABI	Health and Behavior Inventory (HBI) [46]
Executive functioning at home and in school	Behavior Rating Inventory of Executive Function-2. ed. (BRIEF-2) [42]
Main pABI-related problem areas of daily life	Likert scale from 0 (Not at all difficult) to 4 (Very difficult)
Family functioning	Family Assessment Device (FAD) [47]
Parent self-perceived stress	Parental Stress Scale (PSS) [48]
Parenting self-efficacy	Tool to measure Parenting Self-Efficacy (TOPSE and Teen TOPSE) [49]
Unmet healthcare needs of the family	Family Needs Questionnaire Pediatric Version (FNQ-P) [50]
Parents' depression symptoms	Patient Health Questionnaire—9 item (PHQ-9) [51]
Parents' generalized anxiety symptoms	The General Anxiety Disorder—7 item (GAD-7) [52]
Acceptability of intervention, self-tailored	Acceptability Scale rated on a Likert scale from 0 (Completely disagree) to 4 (Completely agree)

The intervention included seven family sessions, four school-meetings interspersed with the family sessions (starting after the first family-session) and a one-day parent group seminar (occurring about halfway through the family sessions for all participants) over the treatment period of four to five months. Figure 1 gives an overview of the intervention components. The family sessions and the school sessions were delivered through an encrypted videoconferencing solution. The feasibility study was performed from August to December 2020. See Adaptations due to COVID-19 below.

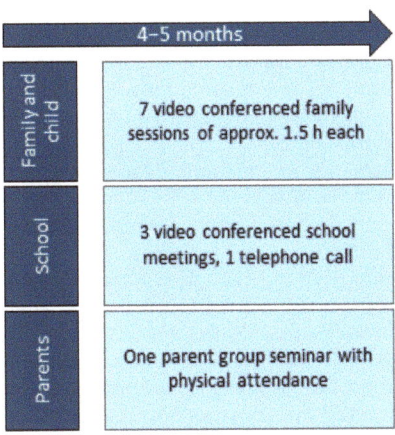

Figure 1. Overview of the intervention.

Three therapists, two clinical neuropsychologists and one experienced pediatric nurse (authors N.R.-B., I.L.H. and E.J.S., respectively) with extensive rehabilitation experience delivered the intervention. Therapists received training from the therapists of the adult community-based TBI-study [35,53] concerning the goal-oriented approach and strategies related to different commonly reported ABI-related problem areas. This was discussed in repeated meetings throughout the feasibility study. Therapists delivered nearly all the family sessions in pairs to ensure adherence to the study manual and a uniform delivery across therapists. The school sessions were performed by an experienced special education counselor from Statped (author A.P.S.-S.) in close collaboration with the three therapists. The therapists conducted the parent group seminar. Weekly meetings between the therapists, the Statped counselor and the study Principal Investigator (author M.L.) were held to discuss ongoing therapies and to ensure protocol adherence. The therapists also received training in the technical solutions of telerehabilitation as well as education on important therapeutic aspects of using this format, by a researcher with relevant experience (author H.P.Ø.), and the telerehabilitation team at Sunnaas Rehabilitation Hospital.

2.5. Content

2.5.1. Family Sessions

SMART-goals (Specific, Measurable, Achievable, Realistic/Relevant and Timed) [54] were established in collaboration between the family and the therapist in videoconference family sessions. Goal Attainment Scaling (GAS) [55] was established for each goal and recorded in the last session. To increase motivation and comprehensibility for the children, the GAS scaling was set from 1 to 5 instead of using the traditional scaling from −2 to +2, with the preferred starting point being defined as level 2 (equivalent to −1 in the standard GAS). However, in some cases where the desired behavior or action was not present at all at the points of goal-setting, the starting point was 1. A visual presentation of the goal and GAS-scaling in the form of a staircase with five steps was used to support understanding (see Figure 2 for an example). Once a goal was identified, the therapist, parent, and child identified specific strategies designed to achieve and implement the goal. The children collaborated in the goal-setting process according to their cognitive abilities and age. Strategies were based on the available evidence-based recommendations for the pediatric population [15,17,56–60] in addition to recommendations for the adult population with age-appropriate adaptations [61]. Working on and modifying strategies when needed was a main focus throughout the intervention.

Every family received a psychoeducational booklet developed for the CICI study. It was validated by the senior researchers in the project and a user consultant. The handbook consists of 12 short chapters about common challenging areas for families after a pediatric ABI, such as common brain injury symptoms, fatigue, communication in the family, stress management and psychological symptoms in children and their parents, as well as identity issues after pABI. The booklet was used primarily with the parents in relation to goals and strategies set by each family according to how comfortable and interested the parents were in reading such information.

Daily use of strategies was emphasized throughout the intervention to ease transfer to daily life activities for the families.

2.5.2. School Involvement

As the children's challenges often disrupt their educational or social settings in school, we established school-related strategies related to the families' goals. The Statped special education counselor visited the schools for observations of the child and the school context. The schools, including the child's main teacher, were invited to participate in four meetings with the research team. School strategies were established through collaboration between the CICI team, the family and the schools to ensure that the strategies were feasible and adapted to the schools' environments and resources.

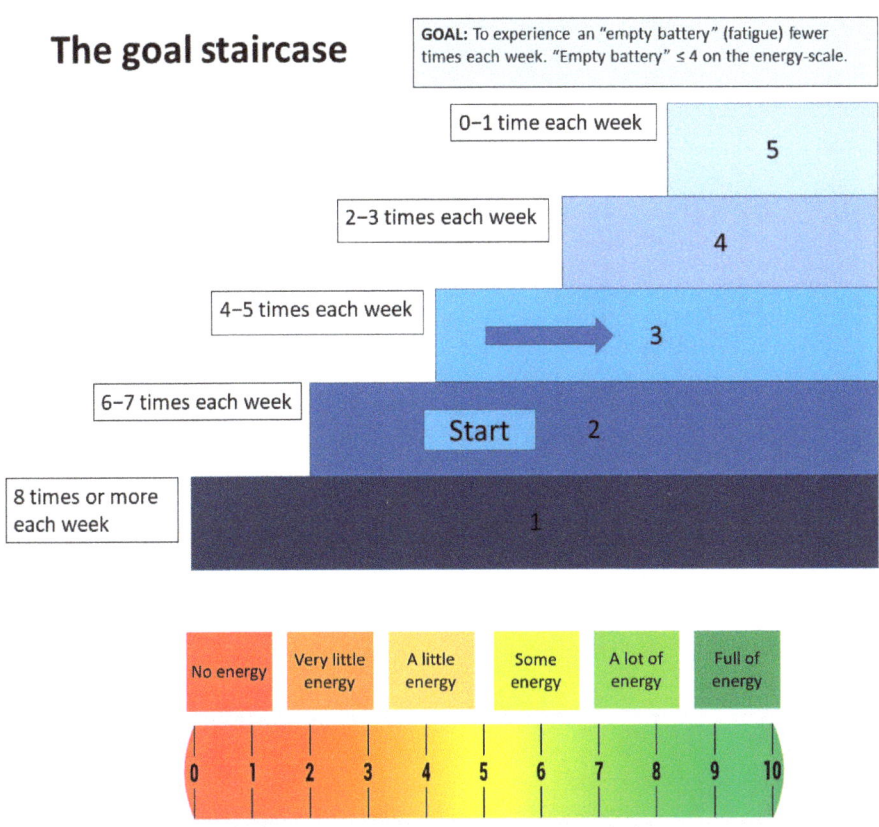

Examples of strategies to reach the goal

At home:
- Fatigue is registered morning, afternoon and evening on the energy-scale
- Maintain good routines for meals and sleep.
- Use a weekly schedule to plan the activities of the week and time for rest
- Preferably take a rest before energy level is in the red area
- Rest after school with 10–15 minutes without stimuli

At school:
- Scheduled rests at school in secluded area with minimum of stimuli
- Promote the use of earplugs to shield from noisy environment in for instance physical education, music or arts and crafts
- Information about fatigue is given to the school teachers and to classmates

Figure 2. An example of the "The goal staircase". This example shows a goal related to fatigue and how fatigue was operationalized as energy on a scale. Energy level is measured three times each day. Strategies to obtain the goal are presented in the textbox.

2.5.3. Parent Group Seminar

A one-day interactive parent group seminar focusing on family functioning and parenting challenges was held in accordance with recommendations to include caregivers in pediatric rehabilitation [62]. Topics included: parents' experiences with SMART-goals, family communication patterns, changes in family dynamics after pABI, how to care for siblings, emotional reactions in the family after pABI (e.g., guilt, grief and embarrassment), and self-care.

2.6. Telerehabilitation Delivery

A web-based encrypted videoconference solution was provided by the Norwegian Health Net (join.nhn.no, accessed on 1 February 2020), delivered by Pexip. The solution was risk assessed and approved for clinical use by Sunnaas Rehabilitation Hospital's Chief information security officer. The participants used their own computers or tablets with integrated camera, and the therapists used their work computers and external microphone speakers to enhance communication. Participants could borrow computers and microphone speakers from the project if they did not have suitable equipment. An IT consultant was available during the sessions in case of technical challenges. Guidelines for therapy through videoconference were developed and conveyed to the participants with recommendations regarding how to create a secure environment for a therapeutic conversation and how to enhance communication through videoconferencing (e.g., one speaker at a time, mute when several participants are joining the same conference, give signs to signal that you want to speak).

2.7. Adaptations Due to COVID-19

Due to the COVID-19 pandemic, there were two recruitment periods. Five families were recruited in January and February 2020. Four of these started the intervention program and had completed maximum two sessions per family, which was planned to include two home visits, in addition to the videoconference sessions and the school meetings with physical attendance. However, the study was put on hold in March 2020 due to a national Norwegian lockdown. During this time, one family that had only completed the baseline assessments withdrew. The remaining families received monthly phone calls with information on the study status. One family received psychological support approximately every other week due to high distress levels.

The study re-opened in August 2020, with some adaptations. All family sessions and school sessions were conducted through videoconference (in the original protocol at least the first and last sessions were planned as home visits), and two planned parent groups were reduced to one. Two more families were recruited. All six families started with new baseline questionnaires, interviews and a definition of the main pABI-related problem areas. Children in the two newly recruited families underwent the neuropsychological screening at baseline, but this was not repeated for the four children who were enrolled in January and February.

2.8. Procedures of Feasibility Evaluation

To evaluate the study feasibility, distinct objectives were operationalized as shown in Table 2. A more detailed description can be found in the Clinical Trials registration (NCT04186182). The custom-tailored Acceptability Scale was rated on a 5-point scale by children (21 items), parents (40 items) and therapists (33 items): Completely disagree (0), Agree a little (1), Agree moderately (2), Agree (3) and Completely agree (4).

Detailed study-specific checklists were developed in concordance with the detailed descriptions in the manual regarding the content of each session and were used to monitor protocol adherence.

Table 2. Objectives of the feasibility evaluation with predefined criteria.

Objective Assessed by	Predefined Criteria
Objective 1: Recruitment procedures	
Consent rate.	Highly feasible: More than 30% consent rate Moderately feasible: 15–29% consent rate Not feasible: Less than 15% consent rate
Duration of recruitment processes.	Highly feasible: Less than 3 h per family spent on recruitment Moderately feasible: Between 3 and 5 h Not feasible: More than 5 h
Number of participants excluded at or after the baseline assessment to reach 6 participation families.	Highly feasible: One or no families excluded at or after baseline Moderately feasible: Two families excluded at or after baseline Not feasible: More than two families excluded at or after baseline
Drop-out rate.	Highly feasible: No drop-outs Moderately feasible: One drop-out Not feasible: Two or more drop-outs
Objective 2: Contents and structure of the intervention	
Attendance rate.	Measured in % attendance
Feasibility of the SMART-goal approach by feedback from participants on three items on the Acceptability Scale concerning the importance of the goals, and how helpful the strategies were for the child and for the family.	Highly feasible: Median score over 3 ("Agree") Moderately feasible: Median score between 2 ("Agree moderately") and 3 ("Agree") Not feasible: Median score lower than 2
Feasibility of videoconference in treatment delivery as assessed by: - One question in the Acceptability Scale concerning the quality of communication through videoconference rated by the children, their parents and the therapists.	Highly feasible: Median score over 3 ("Agree") Moderately feasible: Median score between 2 ("Agree moderately") and 3 ("Agree") Not feasible: Median score lower than 2
- A technical log, where number and type of technical failures were reported by the therapists.	Highly feasible: Restart of equipment in 0–1 session per family Moderately feasible: Restart in 2–3 sessions Not feasible: Restart in more than 4 sessions per family
Objective 3: Acceptability for the children, parents and therapists	
Working alliance in the intervention was measured by child and parent ratings on six items concerning the relation with the therapist; the experience of being heard, taken seriously and given information; and whether they would recommend the study to others. In addition, working alliance was rated by the therapists on five items concerning the experienced quality of relationship with the families.	Highly feasible: Median score over 3 ("Agree") Moderately feasible: Median score between 2 ("Agree moderately") and 3 ("Agree") Not feasible: Median score lower than 2
Usefulness of the intervention was rated on six items on the Acceptability Scale for the children and nine items for the parents, concerning the helpfulness of the intervention, the knowledge transfer to other situations and whether one learned something new. In addition, the therapists rated their experience of the usefulness of the intervention for the families on seven items concerning helpfulness of the intervention, importance of the goals, usefulness of the parent group seminar and awareness of and openness toward the child's challenges.	Highly feasible: Median score over 3 ("Agree") Moderately feasible: Median score between 2 ("Agree moderately") and 3 ("Agree") Not feasible: Median score lower than 2
Objective 4: Methods of assessment at baseline and T2	
Burden of assessment was rated on the Acceptability Scale by four children, and parents rated items concerning whether the child was comfortable being tested and expressing his/her symptoms and opinions through the questionnaires, understood the questionnaires, and was fatigued by the assessments. Parents also rated two items concerning the number of questionnaires and the relevance of the topics in the questionnaires.	Highly feasible: Median score over 3 ("Agree") Moderately feasible: Median score between 2 ("Agree moderately") and 3 ("Agree") Not feasible: Median score lower than 2
Duration of the baseline assessment.	Highly feasible: Less than 3 h Moderately feasible: 3 to 4 h Not feasible: More than 4 h
Objective 5: Quality of treatment delivery	
Protocol adherence by study-specific checklists monitoring discrepancies between actual intervention delivery and the CICI manual.	Highly feasible: Less than 15% deviation Moderately feasible: 16–25% deviation Not feasible: More than 25% deviation

3. Results

For protection of privacy, the families are presented in variable order throughout the results section.

3.1. Participants

The feasibility trial was carried out with six families, corresponding to 9.4% of the planned total sample size of the RCT (64 families after attrition). This is adequate according to the recommendations for optimal sample size in clinical pilot studies [63,64].

The children were three girls and three boys between 11 and 16 years old at baseline (median 13 years). Time since injury ranged between one and 13 years (median 5.5 years). The injuries were TBI (2), anoxia (2) and brain hemorrhage (2). The mother and father of each child participated, constituting 12 parents in total. All children had siblings and all parents lived together. The majority of the parents had completed 14–16 years of education (seven parents), three parents had 17 years or more and two had 11–13 years of education. Eight parents worked fulltime, while one couple received 50% compensational social support from governmental welfare systems related to their child's problems due to brain injury. Two parents were on 50 and 100% sick leave. All schools agreed to participate. Four children were in regular schools with some (e.g., structured time-outs, extended time on tests) or no adaptations to their injury-related symptoms; one child attended a private school and had a comprehensive special educational service; and one attended a special educational class. The neuropsychological screening indicated that the range of cognitive functioning overall varied between typical for their age and impaired. See Table 3 for details.

Table 3. Neuropsychological functioning and main pABI-related problem areas.

Family	Neuropsychological Functioning	Parents' Identified Problem Areas	Child's Identified Problem Areas
1	Within normal range	Fatigue, emotion regulation, study technique	Fatigue, study skills
2	Impaired memory and verbal reasoning (≤-2 sd). Slightly impaired processing speed, working memory and visual reasoning (≤-1 sd).	Fatigue, cognitive gap to peers, worry for child's emotional health	Fatigue
3	Executive dysfunction and impaired processing speed (≤-3 sd), impaired working memory (-2 sd), reduced memory functions and verbal reasoning (≤-1.3 sd).	Social challenges, headache, fatigue	Social challenges, headache
4	Reduced working memory (-1.3 sd)	Parenting a child with ABI, child's social insecurity, pain	Pain, sleep, fatigue
5	Overall, severely reduced neurocognitive functioning with all scores in the impaired range (between -1.3 to -3 sd, with all but 2 tests ≤-2 sd)	Parental exhaustion tied to challenges in getting adequate help for child, child's social isolation	Losing track in conversations with peers, not able to follow activities and changes in the same tempo as peers
6	Executive dysfunction (≤-2.3 sd), impaired processing speed (-2 sd) and reduced visual reasoning (-1.3 sd)	Social challenges; physical challenges such as balance, coordination and strength; lack of independence in getting around	Getting around independently

Identification of Main pABI-Related Problem Areas

The three most challenging areas related to the child's brain injury are shown in Table 3. The most commonly identified pABI problem area was fatigue, reported by three parents and three children. In addition to reporting the child's symptoms as challenging, the parents also reported problem areas related to parenting, worries and communication with the health care system. Overall, it was difficult for some of the children to report their most challenging areas. The therapists put initial effort into getting to know and build trust with the child. The phrasing of the question was adapted to the child's developmental level and cognitive functioning. When needed, the child was also reminded of the troubles he/she had reported in the questionnaires. Some children still had difficulties with this task, probably due to cognitive deficits such as an underdeveloped ability to generalize and to maintain a meta-perspective on their own level of functioning. Moreover, some children expressed that they did not wish to talk about their difficulties. For ethical reasons, therapists did not push children to define problem areas when they were clearly struggling with the task. The children thus reported fewer challenging areas than their parents. The parents had no trouble reporting three challenging areas in their everyday life related to the child's injury. The parents of each child agreed on three areas, although they sometimes initially had different opinions on what to choose. The parents often had different opinions regarding how challenging the areas were and therefore scaled them separately.

3.2. Objective 1: Recruitment Procedures

Seventeen families were screened for inclusion and twelve were deemed eligible. Of these, seven families (60%) were willing to participate (see Figure 3). The reasons for declining participation were not experiencing challenges that the family currently needed help with ($n = 2$) and not having enough time ($n = 3$). The recruitment rate was deemed highly feasible according to the predefined criteria, as we had set the a priori level of highly feasible to 30%, and we included 60% of the families we approached. Given that the existing literature indicates that at least 30% of these families experience unmet needs [9,11,65], we would expect an inclusion rate in the same range or higher when recruiting from a rehabilitation hospital. Time spent on recruitment for each family was also deemed feasible (less than 3 h per family). None were excluded after baseline, indicating that the screening process was satisfactory. One family withdrew before starting the intervention during the COVID-19 lockdown, due to having second thoughts on whether the intervention would help their child. All families that started the intervention completed it. In total, the recruitment procedures were highly feasible.

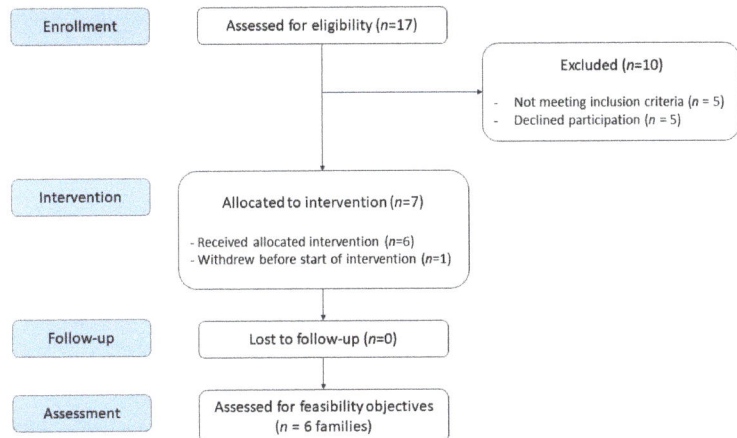

Figure 3. Illustration of the recruitment process.

3.3. Objective 2: Contents and Structure of the Intervention
3.3.1. Attendance

Members from all six families completed the family sessions (100% family attendance), and all families were represented in the parent seminar. Due to illness, one parent neither completed the second half of the intervention nor the T2 assessment. However, the child and the other parent completed as planned. All four school meetings were conducted for all participants (100% school attendance), and four families participated in at least one school meeting. The rest of the meetings that parents did not attend were forgotten by the parents. On average, the family sessions lasted 98 min including breaks. The children attended parts of all the sessions, according to what topic was being discussed and the child's concentration and willingness to participate. All families received extra telephone follow-ups related to their goals and strategies in addition to the procedures described in the manual (with a total duration of 20 to 150 min per family). For two families, telephone contact was also made to other collaborators: physiotherapist (20 min), school nurse (20 min) and the special educational service (45 min) for one family, and two phone calls to the child's assistant for the other family (40 min). Overall, the high attendance rates indicate that the intervention implementation was feasible.

3.3.2. Evaluation of the SMART-Goal and GAS Approach

All families set SMART-goals that were related to some or all of the main problem areas they reported at baseline (Table 3). For two families, new areas to work on became evident during the intervention. Five families defined three goals and one family defined five, providing a total of 20 goals. Of these, six goals had their starting point at GAS 1, whereas the rest started at GAS 2. The most frequent topic was fatigue, which was the focus of at least one goal in five families. Increased independence in everyday life was a topic for two children, including leaving the house on his/her own in the morning, keeping track of appointments, taking the bus and starting to ride a bike again. Two worked on goals to reduce pain and two had goals regarding social functioning. Two families worked toward parental mental health goals, and two families had goals regarding family communication and learning how to talk about the injury with others. One family aimed to apply a problem-solving technique and one set a goal related to the child's study skills.

The children's participation in the goal-setting process varied according to their abilities and motivation. For instance, the youngest child (11 years) would participate in setting the goal and name already existing good strategies to obtain the goal (for instance, rest after school). The child would also participate in discussing new possible strategies to ensure ownership and collaboration (for instance, how the child would be comfortable resting at school). Due to short attention span, strategies related to the parents' actions would be discussed when the child took a break (for instance, encouraging the child to name the level of experienced fatigue three times a day on an "energy-scale" and taking notes of the different activities the child had endured that day). In contrast, one of the teenagers was cognitively able to participate in larger parts of the sessions, the goal-setting processes and discussions on strategies. During the family sessions, all children were encouraged to share their experiences in working with the strategies since the last session and to state their opinions on whether the strategies were helpful and feasible for them. The strategies were adapted and/or new strategies were established as needed. To a large extent, the strategies were external, which means adapting the environment or facilitating the establishment of new skills. One example is parents who trained their child to use a smart-watch by using principles of errorless learning [66], where the parents gradually offered less help as the child gained confidence and skills. Implementation of the strategies in everyday life was highlighted throughout the intervention by basing the strategies on the individual family's everyday life routines and resources and through encouraging daily use of the strategies.

The families attained all their goals but one (in family B). For 14 of the 20 goals, goal achievement was beyond the expected level on the GAS. Figure 4 shows goal attainment scaling per goal for each family. None of the goals showed negative GAS change.

3.3.3. Responses to the SMART-Goal Approach

Both parents and children perceived the SMART-goals as highly relevant, with all but one score ranging from 3 (agree) to 4 (completely agree) on the corresponding item on the Acceptability Scale. See Table 4 for the individual ratings. All children confirmed the importance of the goals and were pleased to achieve the skill, but some of them found working on the skills and spending time in meetings instead of being at school or with friends tiresome. The parents reported that the strategies to achieve the goals had helped their children, with four families responding with 4 (completely agree) on this item and two families scoring 3 (agree). Overall, the SMART-goal and GAS-methodology was deemed highly feasible.

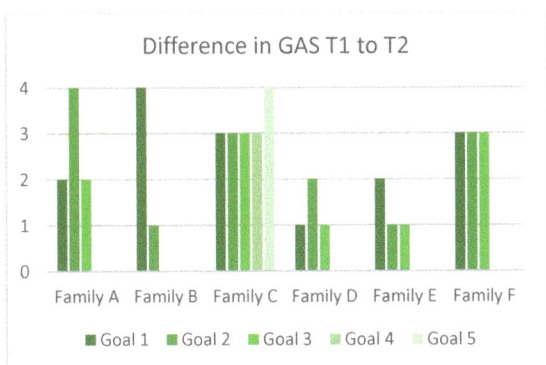

Figure 4. Goal attainment scaling on each goal per family, measured by the GAS change from T1 to T2. A positive number means that the goal was achieved. For family B, one goal had no progress on the GAS and is not visible in the figure.

Table 4. Working alliance, usefulness and evaluation of SMART-goals and strategies, scale from 0 ("Completely disagree") to 4 ("Completely agree").

Participant	Relevance of SMART-Goals	Helpful Strategies for the Child [1]	Satisfaction with Video-conference in Treatment	Working Alliance	Usefulness
Child	4	-	3	4	3.5
Mother	4	4	4	4	4
Father	4	4	4	4	4
Child	3	-	3	1.5	2
Mother	4	3	3	4	3
Father	3	3	3	4	3
Child	4	-	3	0.5	2
Mother	4	4	4	4	4
Father	4	4	3	4	4
Child	2	-	3	3	1
Mother	*	*	*	*	*
Father	3	3	3	4	3.5
Child	4	-	3	4	4
Mother	4	4	3	4	4
Father	4	4	4	4	3.5
Child	3	-	3	3	3
Mother	3	4	3	4	3
Father	3	4	3	4	3

* Indicates missing data. [1] Parent rated

3.3.4. The Use of Videoconferences in Treatment Delivery

Overall, the technical solutions worked very well. All families but one had excellent internet connection, and every family owned equipment suitable for videoconferences (PC or tablet). Support was provided to the family with slow internet connection, and solutions were found to enhance the quality of the videoconferences. External microphone speakers were sent to the families to optimize the sound. There were only a few incidents of needing to restart the equipment (less than one session per family) throughout all of the 40 videoconferences. According to the predefined criteria, the technical solutions were highly feasible.

The satisfaction with the use of videoconference in the intervention (see Table 4) was rated as high by both parents and children (median score 3 for both). The therapists rated the use of videoconferences in the intervention as good overall (median 3) and also experienced it as highly feasible to set goals and strategies and to implement the intervention with the family (median score 4). However, the therapists rated it as challenging to maintain good communication with the children through videoconference, with most ratings at the lower end of the scale on the question framed "communication was good with the child". The therapists' ratings varied from 0 to 4, with the lowest rating being in regard to a child with very severe cognitive deficit. Overall, the use of videoconference was evaluated as an acceptable approach for treatment delivery, but with a special focus on involving the children.

3.4. Objective 3: Acceptability for the Children, Parents and Therapists

3.4.1. Working Alliance in the Intervention

The parents' ratings of working alliance were high (median score of 4, all scores either 3 or 4), whereas the children showed more variation, but with median scores at the high end of the scale (median 3, range 0.5 to 4). See Table 4. Two of the children rated the working alliance as low (1.5 and 0.5). These were one teenager who expressed that he in general did not want to focus on the brain injury, and also that he was not happy that the therapists and his parents talked about his challenges in his absence. The younger child was reluctant to participate in the last sessions, although the goals were achieved.

The therapists' ratings of working alliance were high with regards to feeling welcome to contact the family and the general tone of communication (median 5 for both), but two questions concerning relation and communication with the child had more variable responses, similar to the children's own ratings (median 3, range 1–5). The therapists rated the collaboration with the schools as good (median 4.5, range 3–5).

3.4.2. Usefulness of the Intervention

The parents rated the intervention as highly useful (median 4, range 3 to 4). The children's ratings showed large variations also for usefulness, ranging from 1 to 4 with a median of 3. The variability between the children was similar to the responses on the questions related to working alliance (see Table 4), with yet another teenager rating the usefulness as low. The parents rated the CICI handbook as very useful (median score 4). Some parents reported that they read the entire booklet several times during the intervention, whereas others mainly used the booklet during psychoeducation in sessions. The parent group seminar was rated as overall very useful (median score 5).

The therapists rated their experience of the usefulness of the intervention for the families as high (median 5, range 2–5). Only 1/77 responses was a 2, which was due to the fact that the therapist considered that a child with very severe cognitive deficit had not gained an increased understanding of his/her symptoms due to the intervention. The remaining items were scored within a range of 3–5.

Parents of two of the children who gave low ratings of working alliance and usefulness specifically commented that the child was tired and in a bad mood when filling out the Acceptability Scale, which in their opinion had influenced response validity. Overall, working alliance and usefulness were judged as highly feasible according to the predefined criteria for both parents and children, although with notable variation in responses among and regarding the children.

3.5. Objective 4: Methods of Assessment at Baseline and T2

3.5.1. Burden of Assessments

Regarding the burden of assessments, all children reported that they understood the questionnaires and all but one reported that it was good to be able to report on how they were doing through the questionnaires. However, three children were very fatigued from the assessments, as reported by both children and parents. In addition, three children experienced the neuropsychological assessment as very burdensome. Four of the 11 parents reported that their child had trouble understanding the questionnaires. Two parents reported that there were too many questionnaires, while the remaining parents reported that they did not find the number of questionnaires too burdensome. All parents but one agreed that the topics of the questionnaires were relevant.

The duration of the baseline assessment was on average more than 4 h per family, equivalent to "not feasible" on our predetermined criteria. In addition, we experienced challenges in collecting questionnaires from both parents and children at T2. In summary, the assessments were considered too lengthy and too much of a burden especially for children, but also for the parents.

3.5.2. Outcome Measures

The feasibility of the outcome measures was assessed with the aim of informing the final decisions regarding primary and secondary outcomes in the RCT. The results of the questionnaires were explored, but no group-average-based statistical analyses of change were performed. The individual scores for selected questionnaires are presented. Group mean and median scores are not presented as the main aim of a feasibility trial is to assess the intervention protocol, not the outcomes. Furthermore, the small sample does not render statistical group analysis useful.

When inspecting the planned primary outcomes (post-concussive symptom burden (HBI)), parenting self-efficacy (TOPSE) and the child's quality of life (PedsQL), there appeared to be low correspondence between parent- and child-ratings. The results of the HBI displayed a lower symptom burden post intervention for all participants on the somatic subscale, and for 10 of 17 respondents on the cognitive subscale (see Figure 5). The TOPSE (parenting self-efficacy) showed improvement (higher scores) for eight of the eleven responding parents after the intervention, with the largest positive changes in fathers (see Figure 6). The PedsQL, however, showed a less consistent pattern of change post intervention, with improvements reported by three of six children and eight of the eleven parents (see Figure 7). All parents but one mother and one father rated their family needs (FNQ-P) as met to a larger degree after the intervention. Emotional distress in parents varied, with more depressive symptoms at T2 for six of ten parents (PHQ-9), and more anxiety symptoms in four of nine parents (GAD-7). However, only one parent scored above the clinical cut-off post intervention, and one mother who reported moderate symptoms pre intervention was below the cut-off post intervention. The emotional symptom burden was thus in the low range for all parents but one at T2.

3.6. Objective 5: Quality of Treatment Delivery

In total, there were only small deviations from the study protocol, with a mean adherence of 95.6%. The 4.4% deviations resulted mainly from the fact that the psychoeducational CICI handbook was used less than expected in the individual sessions. The quality of treatment delivery was deemed highly feasible according to the predefined criteria.

3.7. Harms

There were no reported harms or unintended effects.

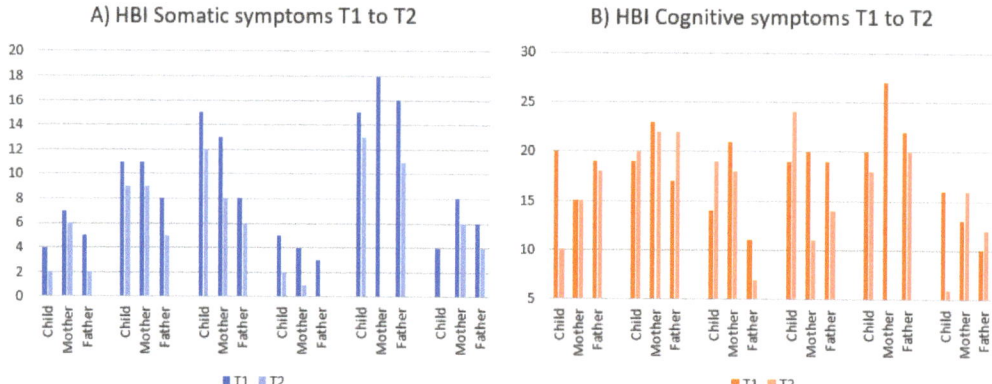

Figure 5. Ratings on the (**A**) somatic and (**B**) cognitive sub-scales of the HBI at T1 and T2 for each family. Lower scores imply lower symptom burden.

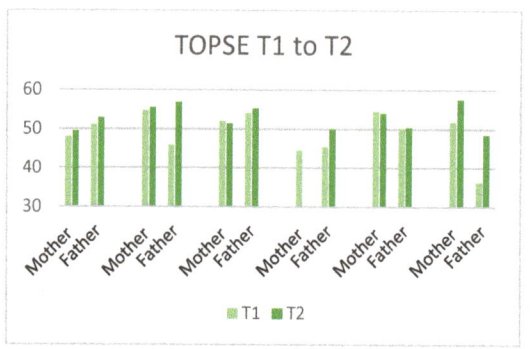

Figure 6. Ratings on the TOPSE each family at T1 and T2. Higher scores imply higher parenting self-efficacy.

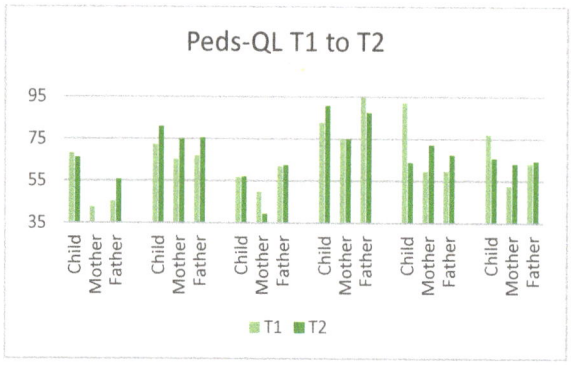

Figure 7. Ratings on the PEDS-QL for each family at T1 and T2. Higher scores imply higher reported quality of life.

4. Discussion

Although the intervention was found to be feasible overall, valuable information was obtained on issues that needed to be considered before the future definitive RCT.

4.1. Contents and Structure of the Intervention

Recruitment rates were high in this feasibility study, as 60% of the eligible families were willing to participate. Of the declining families, two did not report challenges which they needed help with, and three did not have the time to participate in an extensive rehabilitation program at this point. The participating families were recruited from Sunnaas Rehabilitation Hospital, where children with specialized rehabilitation needs are referred to after acute care. In the future definitive RCT, patients will also be recruited from the acute hospital of the South-Eastern Health Region and from the national special education service, providing a population with a broader spectrum of severity and possibly different long-term needs. The RCT-recruitment will thus include less severe injuries. Furthermore, the relation that the recruited families had to Sunnaas Rehabilitation Hospital may have influenced their willingness to participate in this study. The fact that we recruited participants from a rehabilitation hospital may indicate a selection bias toward participants with severe injuries and therefore a high level of unmet needs. The final inclusion rate in the future RCT remains to be established but may be expected to be somewhat lower.

Attendance rates were very high. However, the attendance of parents in the school meetings was lower than expected, which was interpreted as too many meetings during the intervention. It was, however, not crucial that the parents attended all school meetings. The CICI therapists made sure that important information was shared between the families and schools, and emphasis was put on establishing means of communication before the intervention ended. The high attendance rate of the schools showed that it was feasible to include schools in the intervention. In the future definitive RCT, parents will be offered to attend school meetings to the extent that they find useful and manageable. Contact with local health care providers was established for two of the six participants. Interestingly, most of the participants did not receive help from local health care providers, confirming the high incidence of unmet needs in areas of, for instance, fatigue, cognitive rehabilitation and issues related to increased independence in everyday life. In this respect, the CICI provided services that the families would not have received elsewhere.

Defining the three main pABI-related problem areas of daily life worked well for the parents, but it became apparent that parents of the same child did not always experience the same problem areas or experience the problems as equally challenging. In addition to being able to scale the pABI-related problem areas separately, parents will also have the opportunity to define separate areas in the future definitive RCT, to avoid important areas being overlooked. Some of the children struggled with this task, and clinical consideration will be taken in the future RCT, as was done in the feasibility trial, by accepting a lower number of problem areas from the children when necessary.

Overall, the satisfaction with the SMART-goal approach was high in parents and children. Interestingly, the SMART-goals were obtained and perceived as useful also for the children who responded with low ratings of working alliance and usefulness of the intervention. This finding may reflect that children have poorer abilities of abstract thinking and generalizing than adults. It may reflect a common challenge in all therapy with children: children rarely seek help by themselves, they have a less developed insight into their challenges, they are less motivated to change, and they often have a different understanding of their problems and how to solve them than their parents [67]. This influences children's motivation to take part in treatment. In addition, children with brain injuries have varying degrees of awareness of their deficits, further adding to reluctance to participate in treatment.

Goal attainment was high. Although there was some variation in goal attainment (Figure 4), all but one of 20 goals reached at least the expected level of achievement. The variation in goal attainment might depend on the complexity of the goal. High goal attainment (highest level of GAS) was achieved for less complex skills such as learning to ride a bike, whereas goals related to more complex skills, e.g., communication and mental health, showed progress as expected. The high goal attainment showed that it was possible to achieve positive change in symptom areas that are common after pABI, such as fatigue, independence in everyday life, pain and problem solving. The SMART-goal approach was thus a feasible and appreciated method for working with a broad range of problems. Whether the intervention as a whole will have a significant effect remains to be established in the definitive RCT.

4.2. Acceptability

The families responded well to the use of videoconference in treatment delivery, and the technical solutions were satisfactory. The therapists found that using videoconferences worked surprisingly well for building trust and for treatment with the parents, but it was more challenging to establish a high-quality communication with the child. In line with this, the perceived working alliance and usefulness of the intervention was higher for parents than for the children, but with large variation among the participating children. Some of the children tended to disappear from the video meetings when they lost concentration. Some of them did not want to talk much in the sessions, which made it difficult for the therapists to engage them. This was experienced as especially challenging in communication with the teenagers, who seemed more reluctant to focus on the brain injury than the younger participants. Unfortunately, this feasibility study did not succeed in recruiting the youngest children (from age 6 to 11).

Building a relationship with a child is facilitated by establishing joint attention and engaging in joint activities, which is challenging in videoconferences. Maintaining the child's attention is often facilitated by eye contact and by the therapist's ability to adjust conversational strategies to the child's needs, which may be more difficult to achieve through videoconferences. In addition, building alliances with children in therapy is complicated by the fact that therapists also need to establish an alliance and negotiate goals with caregivers as well [68]. Thus, general aspects concerning the treatment of children were seen that may not have been directly related to the intervention being videoconference-based, although videoconference may have amplified them. On a positive note, research on treatment effects and alliance in therapy with children and families has found that the alliance with parents influences treatment outcomes more than the alliance with the child [69]. The therapists in this intervention rated communication with the parents through videoconference as good. However, they rated it as more challenging to maintain good communication with the children, even with the children who rated their own satisfaction with the intervention as high. The fact that therapists may rate the satisfaction with the telerehabilitation lower than the participants has been found in other studies [70] and may be influenced by the complex therapeutic tasks. In a telerehabilitation environment, therapists face several tasks simultaneously: preserving therapeutic alliance, delivering therapy and dealing with technical difficulties, which demands multitasking beyond face-to-face delivery. Participants, however, tend to display a higher technology failure tolerance than the therapists [71]. These factors may have influenced the therapists' experience of the telerehabilitation communication with the children, where expectations from the experienced therapists were high beforehand.

For the future definitive RCT, some of the intervention material will be further developed to engage the child in conversations and to establish a sense of ownership to the intervention. Although most children and parents reported gains through the intervention and appreciated the accessibility that video sessions provided, a videoconference-based-intervention may be particularly challenging for some children. The children's participation in the sessions and ability to generalize and reflect on their experience will necessarily vary according to factors such as the child's age, state of mind, cognitive difficulties, level of fatigue and personality, as well as the child's relationship to and interaction with their parents and the therapeutic alliance. In addition, the children's state of mind at the time of completing the Acceptability Scale seemed to influence how they responded, possibly influencing the validity of their responses. The intervention was conducted during the COVID-19 pandemic, and the children's ratings may also have been influenced by both frustrations related to the lack of normal activities in their lives, and perhaps a low motivation for videoconferenced activities at a time where school was mostly conducted through this medium for the teenagers.

Due to the COVID-19 pandemic, conducting an intervention through videoconference enabled the provision of health care services that would not otherwise have been possible. In Norway, most families have grown accustomed to using videoconference as a medium of communication, as both school and work have been carried out through digital media during lockdown for a large part of the population. As such, the pandemic has changed the prerequisites for a telerehabilitation intervention, making it more available.

4.3. Methods of Assessment at Baseline and Post Treatment

The baseline assessment protocol was too lengthy and burdensome for children and parents. Adaptations will thus be made for the future RCT. Firstly, the neuropsychological screening on baseline will be reduced to only two subtests of abstract thinking (Matrix and Similarities from WISC-V). The reduction in neuropsychological measures was deemed appropriate as the main focus of the intervention is on everyday challenges, regardless of cognitive profile. Secondly, reducing the number of questionnaires for children and parents was also necessary. As CICI is an individualized intervention, it is challenging to define one common outcome at the group level. After careful considerations, we decided to include outcome measures that target areas that are commonly experienced as challenging after pABI [9,14], and which we also expect will be targeted in the intervention. Furthermore, we wished to include broader domains such as quality of life and participation. Given the family focus, it was important to also include measures that would capture parent factors such as parent mental health and parenting self-efficacy, as well as family function. The feasibility study provided important information on the selected assessment methods which, together with a thorough literature review, was used to inform the final decisions on assessment and outcome methods in the future definitive RCT. Three questionnaires (CASP, PSS and SDQ) were excluded as they were judged to have significant overlap with other questionnaires, appeared to not be very sensitive to change, and/or were judged to contribute with less important information for the study purpose. This feasibility trial also aided in the determination of what should be primary outcome measures in the future definitive RCT. Due to correction of the alpha level according to multiple primary outcomes, a maximum of two primary outcomes was decided to ensure adequate statistical power with a feasible sample size. The large variability and possible low validity in the children's responses led to the decision to use parent ratings as primary outcomes, which is common in family interventions and interventions including children with brain injury [72–75]. To be able to capture changes in symptom severity in the child as well as important parent factors [49], changes in parent-reported brain injury symptom severity (HBI) and parenting self-efficacy (TOPSE) were thus chosen as primary outcome measures. The final CICI protocol with all changes resulting from the feasibility study is described in detail in a published CICI protocol article [76].

Regarding the questionnaire results, the positive feedback on the Acceptability Scale appeared to be captured in some of the measures, such as reduced brain injury symptoms reported by parents (HBI), lower levels of executive deficit (BRIEF), improved quality of life (PedsQL), higher parenting self-efficacy (TOPSE) and fewer unmet family needs (FNQ-p). Although some parents reported more emotional symptoms after the intervention, only one had symptoms equivalent to moderate depression. The elevated symptoms might reflect a more accurate rating of emotional state at T2, as the therapeutic alliance results in more openness from the parents. On the other hand, parents face long-term challenges that are likely to not be fully overcome in a 4–5-month intervention. Particular interest should be devoted to this issue in the future RCT, as we should be cautious about the risk of parents feeling overwhelmed at the prospect of again being left to deal with their problems on their own.

4.4. Limitations

The low number of participants in this study constitutes a limitation regarding generalizability of the results, especially concerning the results of the outcome measures. However, the main purpose of this study was to assess feasibility and not to investigate statistical effects. The participating children had different types of injuries and a large span in time since injury, which was considered a strength, while the restricted variation in age should be considered a limitation. In addition, the parents' educational level was high and all parents were married, which reduces the generalizability of the findings.

5. Conclusions

The findings from the CICI feasibility study indicate high intervention feasibility and acceptability, particularly for the parents. As the use of external strategies in cognitive rehabilitation of children with ABI tends to be the most reliable approach, it was considered acceptable and to a certain degree expected that the alliance and communication with the parents was superior to that of the children. The focus on SMART-goals was perceived as useful by all participants, and including schools in the intervention proved beneficial. The telerehabilitation format seems acceptable, although some concerns regarding the engagement of children need to be monitored. The number of neuropsychological tests and questionnaires was reduced, and new primary outcome measures were defined as parent-reported brain injury symptom severity (HBI) and enhanced parenting self-efficacy (TOPSE). Except for this, no major adjustments to the protocol were made (see protocol article by Rohrer-Baumgartner et al. (2022) REF).

Author Contributions: Conceptualization and methodology: I.L.H., N.R.-B., M.L., E.J.S., S.L.H., M.V.F., I.M.H.B., H.P.Ø., I.K., A.P.S.-S., J.E., C.R. and S.L.W.; recruitment, intervention and data collection: I.L.H., N.R-B., E.J.S. and A.P.S.-S.; project management: M.L.; data analysis: I.L.H., N.R.-B. and M.L.; writing—original draft preparation: I.L.H., N.R.-B. and M.L.; writing—review and editing: I.L.H., N.R.-B., M.L., E.J.S., S.L.H., M.V.F., I.M.H.B., H.P.Ø., I.K., A.P.S.-S., J.E., C.R. and S.L.W. All authors have read and agreed to the published version of the manuscript.

Funding: This research was funded by The Norwegian Research Council, grant number 288172.

Institutional Review Board Statement: The study was conducted according to the guidelines of the Declaration of Helsinki and approved by the Data Protection Office at Sunnaas Rehabilitation Hospital (approval number: REK 2019/1283, Trial registration: ClinicalTrials.gov (accessed on 1 January 2020) Identifier: NCT04186182).

Informed Consent Statement: Informed consent was obtained from all subjects involved in the study who were 16 years of age or older. Children under the age of 16 received age-appropriate information about the study before participating.

Data Availability Statement: The data presented in this study are not publicly available due to protection of privacy.

Acknowledgments: We would like to thank all participants for their contribution to this study.

Conflicts of Interest: The authors declare no conflict of interest.

References

1. Anderson, V.; Brown, S.; Newitt, H.; Hoile, H. Long-term outcome from childhood traumatic brain injury: Intellectual ability, personality, and quality of life. *Neuropsychology* **2011**, *25*, 176–184. [CrossRef] [PubMed]
2. Babikian, T.; Asarnow, R. Neurocognitive outcomes and recovery after pediatric TBI: Meta-analytic review of the literature. *Neuropsychology* **2009**, *23*, 283–296. [CrossRef] [PubMed]
3. Babikian, T.; Merkley, T.; Savage, R.C.; Giza, C.C.; Levin, H. Chronic Aspects of Pediatric Traumatic Brain Injury: Review of the Literature. *J. Neurotrauma* **2015**, *32*, 1849–1860. [CrossRef] [PubMed]
4. Câmara-Costa, H.; Francillette, L.; Opatowski, M.; Toure, H.; Brugel, D.; Laurent-Vannier, A.; Meyer, P.G.; Dellatolas, G.; Watier, L.; Chevignard, M. Participation seven years after severe childhood traumatic brain injury. *Disabil. Rehabil.* **2019**, *42*, 2402–2411. [CrossRef] [PubMed]

5. Law, M.; Anaby, D.; DeMatteo, C.; Hanna, S. Participation patterns of children with acquired brain injury. *Brain Inj.* **2011**, *25*, 587–595. [CrossRef]
6. Rivara, F.P.; Ennis, S.K.; Mangione-Smith, R.; MacKenzie, E.J.; Jaffe, K.M. Quality of Care Indicators for the Rehabilitation of Children with Traumatic Brain Injury. *Arch. Phys. Med. Rehabil.* **2012**, *93*, 381–385.e9. [CrossRef]
7. Di Battista, A.; Soo, C.; Catroppa, C.; Anderson, V. Quality of Life in Children and Adolescents Post-TBI: A Systematic Review and Meta-Analysis. *J. Neurotrauma* **2012**, *29*, 1717–1727. [CrossRef]
8. Rosema, S.; Crowe, L.; Anderson, V. Social Function in Children and Adolescents after Traumatic Brain Injury: A Systematic Review 1989–2011. *J. Neurotrauma* **2012**, *29*, 1277–1291. [CrossRef]
9. Keetley, R.; Radford, K.; Manning, J. A scoping review of the needs of children and young people with acquired brain injuries and their families. *Brain Inj.* **2019**, *33*, 1117–1128. [CrossRef]
10. Keenan, H.T.; Clark, A.E.; Holubkov, R.; Ewing-Cobbs, L. Changing Healthcare and School Needs in the First Year After Traumatic Brain Injury. *J. Head Trauma Rehabil.* **2020**, *35*, E67–E77. [CrossRef]
11. Jones, S.; Davis, N.; Tyson, S.F. A scoping review of the needs of children and other family members after a child's traumatic injury. *Clin. Rehabil.* **2018**, *32*, 501–511. [CrossRef] [PubMed]
12. Wade, D.T. What is rehabilitation? An empirical investigation leading to an evidence-based description. *Clin. Rehabil.* **2020**, *34*, 571–583. [CrossRef] [PubMed]
13. World Health Organization. *International Classification of Functioning, Disability, and Health: Children & Youth Version: ICF-CY*; World Health Organization: Geneva, Switzerland, 2007.
14. McCarron, R.H.; Watson, S.; Gracey, F. What do Kids with Acquired Brain Injury Want? Mapping Neuropsychological Rehabilitation Goals to the International Classification of Functioning, Disability and Health. *J. Int. Neuropsychol. Soc.* **2019**, *25*, 403–412. [CrossRef] [PubMed]
15. Laatsch, L.; Dodd, J.; Brown, T.; Ciccia, A.; Connor, F.; Davis, K.; Doherty, M.; Linden, M.; Locascio, G.; Lundine, J.; et al. Evidence-based systematic review of cognitive rehabilitation, emotional, and family treatment studies for children with acquired brain injury literature: From 2006 to 2017. *Neuropsychol. Rehabil.* **2020**, *30*, 130–161. [CrossRef]
16. Catroppa, C.; Anderson, V. Traumatic brain injury in childhood: Rehabilitation considerations. *Dev. Neurorehabil.* **2009**, *12*, 53–61. [CrossRef]
17. Catroppa, C.; Soo, C.; Crowe, L.; Woods, D.; Anderson, V. Evidence-based approaches to the management of cognitive and behavioral impairments following pediatric brain injury. *Future Neurol.* **2012**, *7*, 719–731. [CrossRef]
18. Chavez-Arana, C.; Catroppa, C.; Carranza-Escárcega, E.; Godfrey, C.; Yáñez-Téllez, G.; Corona, P.; De León, M.A.; Anderson, V. A Systematic Review of Interventions for Hot and Cold Executive Functions in Children and Adolescents with Acquired Brain Injury. *J. Pediatr. Psychol.* **2018**, *43*, 928–942. [CrossRef]
19. Wade, S.L.; Fisher, A.P.; Kaizar, E.E.; Yeates, K.O.; Taylor, H.G.; Zhang, N. Recovery Trajectories of Child and Family Outcomes Following Online Family Problem-Solving Therapy for Children and Adolescents after Traumatic Brain Injury. *J. Int. Neuropsychol. Soc.* **2019**, *25*, 941–949. [CrossRef]
20. Wade, S.L.; Kaizar, E.E.; Narad, M.; Zang, H.; Kurowski, B.G.; Yeates, K.O.; Taylor, H.G.; Zhang, N. Online Family Problem-solving Treatment for Pediatric Traumatic Brain Injury. *Pediatrics* **2018**, *142*, e20180422. [CrossRef]
21. Zhang, N.; Kaizar, E.E.; Narad, M.E.; Kurowski, B.G.; Yeates, K.O.; Taylor, H.G.; Wade, S.L. Examination of Injury, Host, and Social-Environmental Moderators of Online Family Problem Solving Treatment Efficacy for Pediatric Traumatic Brain Injury Using an Individual Participant Data Meta-Analytic Approach. *J. Neurotrauma* **2019**, *36*, 1147–1155. [CrossRef]
22. Wade, S.L.; Narad, M.E.; Shultz, E.L.; Kurowski, B.G.; Miley, A.E.; Aguilar, J.M.; Adlam, A.-L.R. Technology-assisted rehabilitation interventions following pediatric brain injury. *J. Neurosurg. Sci.* **2018**, *62*, 187–202. [CrossRef] [PubMed]
23. Subbarao, B.S.; Stokke, J.; Martin, S.J. Telerehabilitation in Acquired Brain Injury. *Phys. Med. Rehabil. Clin. N. Am.* **2021**, *32*, 223–238. [CrossRef] [PubMed]
24. Wade, S.L.; Raj, S.P.; Moscato, E.L.; Narad, M.E. Clinician perspectives delivering telehealth interventions to children/families impacted by pediatric traumatic brain injury. *Rehabil. Psychol.* **2019**, *64*, 298–306. [CrossRef] [PubMed]
25. Solana, J.; Caceres, C.; Garcia-Molina, A.; Opisso, E.; Roig, T.; Tormos, J.M.; Gomez, E.J. Improving Brain Injury Cognitive Rehabilitation by Personalized Telerehabilitation Services: Guttmann Neuropersonal Trainer. *IEEE J. Biomed. Health Inform.* **2015**, *19*, 124–131. [CrossRef] [PubMed]
26. Øra, H.P.; Kirmess, M.; Brady, M.C.; Partee, I.; Hognestad, R.B.; Johannessen, B.B.; Thommessen, B.; Becker, F. The effect of augmented speech-language therapy delivered by telerehabilitation on poststroke aphasia—A pilot randomized controlled trial. *Clin. Rehabil.* **2020**, *34*, 369–381. [CrossRef] [PubMed]
27. McLean, S.A.; Booth, A.T.; Schnabel, A.; Wright, B.J.; Painter, F.L.; McIntosh, J.E. Exploring the Efficacy of Telehealth for Family Therapy Through Systematic, Meta-analytic, and Qualitative Evidence. *Clin. Child Fam. Psychol. Rev.* **2021**, *24*, 244–266. [CrossRef]
28. Owen, R.R.; Woodward, E.N.; Drummond, K.L.; Deen, T.L.; Oliver, K.A.; Petersen, N.J.; Meit, S.S.; Fortney, J.C.; Kirchner, J.E. Using implementation facilitation to implement primary care mental health integration via clinical video telehealth in rural clinics: Protocol for a hybrid type 2 cluster randomized stepped-wedge design. *Implement. Sci.* **2019**, *14*, 33. [CrossRef]
29. Corti, C.; Oldrati, V.; Oprandi, M.C.; Ferrari, E.; Poggi, G.; Borgatti, R.; Urgesi, C.; Bardoni, A. Remote Technology-Based Training Programs for Children with Acquired Brain Injury: A Systematic Review and a Meta-Analytic Exploration. *Behav. Neurol.* **2019**, *2019*, 1346987. [CrossRef]

30. Linden, M.; Hawley, C.; Blackwood, B.; Evans, J.; Anderson, V. Technological aids for the rehabilitation of memory and executive functioning in children and adolescents with acquired brain injury. *Cochrane Database Syst. Rev.* **2016**, *7*, 11020. [CrossRef]
31. Kelly, G.; Dunford, C.; Forsyth, R.; Kavcic, A. Using child- and family-centred goal setting as an outcome measure in residential rehabilitation for children and youth with acquired brain injuries: The challenge of predicting expected levels of achievement. *Child Care Health Dev.* **2019**, *45*, 286–291. [CrossRef]
32. Krasny-Pacini, A.; Hiebel, J.; Pauly, F.; Godon, S.; Chevignard, M. Goal Attainment Scaling in rehabilitation: A literature-based update. *Ann. Phys. Rehabil. Med.* **2013**, *56*, 212–230. [CrossRef] [PubMed]
33. Vroland-Nordstrand, K.; Eliasson, A.-C.; Jacobsson, H.; Johansson, U.; Krumlinde-Sundholm, L. Can children identify and achieve goals for intervention? A randomized trial comparing two goal-setting approaches. *Dev. Med. Child Neurol.* **2016**, *58*, 589–596. [CrossRef] [PubMed]
34. Winter, L.; Moriarty, H.J.; Robinson, K.; Piersol, C.; Vause-Earland, T.; Newhart, B.; Iacovone, D.B.; Hodgson, N.; Gitlin, L.N. Efficacy and acceptability of a home-based, family-inclusive intervention for veterans with TBI: A randomized controlled trial. *Brain Inj.* **2016**, *30*, 373–387. [CrossRef] [PubMed]
35. Borgen, I.M.H.; Løvstad, M.; Andelic, N.; Hauger, S.; Sigurdardottir, S.; Søberg, H.L.; Sveen, U.; Forslund, M.V.; Kleffelgård, I.; Lindstad, M.Ø.; et al. Traumatic brain injury—Needs and treatment options in the chronic phase: Study protocol for a randomized controlled community-based intervention. *Trials* **2020**, *21*, 294. [CrossRef] [PubMed]
36. Skivington, K.; Matthews, L.; Simpson, S.; Craig, P.; Baird, J.; Blazeby, J.; Boyd, K.; Craig, N.; French, D.; McIntosh, E.; et al. A new framework for developing and evaluating complex interventions: Update of Medical Research Council guidance. *BMJ* **2021**, *374*, n2061. [CrossRef]
37. Moore, G.; Audrey, S.; Barker, M.; Bond, L.; Bonell, C.; Cooper, C.; Hardeman, W.; Moore, L.; O'Cathain, A.; Tinati, T.; et al. Process evaluation in complex public health intervention studies: The need for guidance. *J. Epidemiol. Community Health* **2014**, *68*, 101–102. [CrossRef]
38. King, G.; Imms, C.; Stewart, D.; Freeman, M.; Nguyen, T. A transactional framework for pediatric rehabilitation: Shifting the focus to situated contexts, transactional processes, and adaptive developmental outcomes. *Disabil. Rehabil.* **2018**, *40*, 1829–1841. [CrossRef]
39. Eldridge, S.M.; Chan, C.L.; Campbell, M.J.; Bond, C.M.; Hopewell, S.; Thabane, L.; Lancaster, G.A.; PAFS Consensus Group. CONSORT 2010 statement: Extension to randomised pilot and feasibility trials. *Pilot Feasibility Stud.* **2016**, *2*, 64. [CrossRef]
40. Wechsler, D. *Wechler Intelligence Scale for Children*, 5th ed.; NCS Pearson: San Antonio, TX, USA, 2014.
41. Talley, J.L. *Children's Auditory Verbal Learning Test-2*; Psychological Assessment Resources: Lutz, FL, USA, 1992.
42. Korkman, M.; Kirk, U.; Kemp, S. *NEPSY-II*, 2nd ed.; Harcourt Assessment: San Antonio, TX, USA, 2007.
43. Goodman, R. The extended version of the Strengths and Difficulties Questionnaire as a guide to child psychiatric caseness and consequent burden. *J. Child Psychol. Psychiatry* **1999**, *40*, 791–799. [CrossRef]
44. Bedell, G. Further validation of the Child and Adolescent Scale of Participation (CASP). *Dev. Neurorehabil.* **2009**, *12*, 342–351. [CrossRef]
45. Varni, J.W.; Seid, M.; Kurtin, P.S. PedsQL™ 4.0: Reliability and validity of the pediatric quality of Life Inventory™ Version 4.0 generic core scales in healthy and patient populations. *Med. Care* **2001**, *39*, 800–812. [CrossRef] [PubMed]
46. Ayr, L.K.; Yeates, K.O.; Taylor, H.G.; Browne, M. Dimensions of postconcussive symptoms in children with mild traumatic brain injuries. *J. Int. Neuropsychol. Soc.* **2009**, *15*, 19–30. [CrossRef] [PubMed]
47. Epstein, N.B.; Baldwin, L.M.; Bishop, D.S. The McMaster Family Assessment Device. *J. Marital Fam. Ther.* **1983**, *9*, 171–180. [CrossRef]
48. Berry, J.O.; Jones, W.H. The Parental Stress Scale: Initial Psychometric Evidence. *J. Soc. Pers. Relatsh.* **1995**, *12*, 463–472. [CrossRef]
49. Kendall, S.; Bloomfield, L. Developing and validating a tool to measure parenting self-efficacy. *J. Adv. Nurs.* **2005**, *51*, 174–181. [CrossRef]
50. Gan, C.; Wright, F.V. Development of the family needs questionnaire—Pediatric version [FNQ-P]—Phase I. *Brain Inj.* **2019**, *33*, 623–632. [CrossRef] [PubMed]
51. Kroenke, K.; Spitzer, R.L.; Williams, J.B.W. The PHQ-9—Validity of a brief depression severity measure. *J. Gen. Intern. Med.* **2001**, *16*, 606–613. [CrossRef] [PubMed]
52. Spitzer, R.L.; Kroenke, K.; Williams, J.B.W.; Löwe, B. A brief measure for assessing generalized anxiety disorder—The GAD-7. *Arch. Intern. Med.* **2006**, *166*, 1092–1097. [CrossRef]
53. Borgen, I.M.H.; Hauger, S.L.; Forslund, M.V.; Kleffelgård, I.; Brunborg, C.; Andelic, N.; Sveen, U.; Søberg, H.L.; Sigurdardottir, S.; Røe, C.; et al. Goal Attainment in an Individually Tailored and Home-Based Intervention in the Chronic Phase after Traumatic Brain Injury. *J. Clin. Med.* **2022**, *11*, 958. [CrossRef]
54. Bovend'Eerdt, T.J.H.; Botell, R.E.; Wade, D. Writing SMART rehabilitation goals and achieving goal attainment scaling: A practical guide. *Clin. Rehabil.* **2009**, *23*, 352–361. [CrossRef]
55. Malec, J.F. Goal Attainment Scaling in Rehabilitation. *Neuropsychol. Rehabil.* **1999**, *9*, 253–275. [CrossRef]
56. Catroppa, C.; Anderson, V.; Beauchamp, M.; Yeates, K. *New Frontiers in Pediatric Traumatic Brain Injury: An Evidence Base for Clinical Practice*; Routledge: New York, NY, USA, 2016.
57. Schrieff-Elson, L.E.; Thomas, K.G.F.; Rohlwink, U.K. Pediatric Traumatic Brain Injury: Outcomes and Rehabilitation. In *Textbook of Pediatric Neurosurgery*; Di Rocco, C., Pang, D., Rutka, J., Eds.; Springer: Cham, Switzerland, 2017.

58. Limond, J.; Leeke, R. Practitioner Review: Cognitive rehabilitation for children with acquired brain injury. *J. Child Psychol. Psychiatry* **2005**, *46*, 339–352. [CrossRef] [PubMed]
59. Laatsch, L.; Harrington, D.; Hotz, G.; Marcantuono, J.; Mozzoni, M.P.; Walsh, V.; Hersey, K.P. An Evidence-based Review of Cognitive and Behavioral Rehabilitation Treatment Studies in Children with Acquired Brain Injury. *J. Head Trauma Rehabil.* **2007**, *22*, 248–256. [CrossRef] [PubMed]
60. Resch, C.; Rosema, S.; Hurks, P.; de Kloet, A.; Van Heugten, C. Searching for effective components of cognitive rehabilitation for children and adolescents with acquired brain injury: A systematic review. *Brain Inj.* **2018**, *32*, 679–692. [CrossRef]
61. Sohlberg, M.M. Cognitive Rehabilitation Manual: Translating Evidence-Based Recommendations into Practice. *Arch. Clin. Neuropsychol.* **2012**, *27*, 931–932. [CrossRef]
62. Crowe, L.M.; Catroppa, C.; Anderson, V. Sequelae in children: Developmental consequences. In *Handbook of Clinical Neurology*; Elsevier: Amsterdam, The Netherlands, 2015; Volume 128, pp. 661–677.
63. Stallard, N. Optimal sample sizes for phase II clinical trials and pilot studies. *Stat. Med.* **2012**, *31*, 1031–1042. [CrossRef]
64. Billingham, S.A.; Whitehead, A.L.; Julious, S.A. An audit of sample sizes for pilot and feasibility trials being undertaken in the United Kingdom registered in the United Kingdom Clinical Research Network database. *BMC Med. Res. Methodol.* **2013**, *13*, 104. [CrossRef]
65. Slomine, B.S.; McCarthy, M.L.; Ding, R.; MacKenzie, E.J.; Jaffe, K.M.; Aitken, M.E.; Durbin, D.R.; Christensen, J.R.; Dorsch, A.M.; Paidas, C.N.; et al. Health Care Utilization and Needs After Pediatric Traumatic Brain Injury. *Pediatrics* **2006**, *117*, e663–e674. [CrossRef]
66. Baddeley, A.; Wilson, B.A. When implicit learning fails: Amnesia and the problem of error elimination. *Neuropsychologia* **1994**, *32*, 53–68. [CrossRef]
67. DiGiuseppe, R.; Linscott, J.; Jilton, R. Developing the therapeutic alliance in child—Adolescent psychotherapy. *Appl. Prev. Psychol.* **1996**, *5*, 85–100. [CrossRef]
68. Fjermestad, K. Therapeutic alliance in cognitive behavioural therapy for children and adolescents. *Tidsskr. Nor. Psykologforen.* **2011**, *48*, 12–15.
69. McLeod, B.D.; Weisz, J.R. The Therapy Process Observational Coding System-Alliance Scale: Measure Characteristics and Prediction of Outcome in Usual Clinical Practice. *J. Consult. Clin. Psychol.* **2005**, *73*, 323–333. [CrossRef] [PubMed]
70. Øra, H.P.; Kirmess, M.; Brady, M.C.; Sørli, H.; Becker, F. Technical Features, Feasibility, and Acceptability of Augmented Telerehabilitation in Post-stroke Aphasia—Experiences from a Randomized Controlled Trial. *Front. Neurol.* **2020**, *11*, 671. [CrossRef] [PubMed]
71. Keck, C.S.; Doarn, C. Telehealth Technology Applications in Speech-Language Pathology. *Telemed. e-Health* **2014**, *20*, 653–659. [CrossRef]
72. Antonini, T.N.; Raj, S.P.; Oberjohn, K.S.; Cassedy, A.; Makoroff, K.L.; Fouladi, M.; Wade, S.L. A Pilot Randomized Trial of an Online Parenting Skills Program for Pediatric Traumatic Brain Injury: Improvements in Parenting and Child Behavior. *Behav. Ther.* **2014**, *45*, 455–468. [CrossRef]
73. Wade, S.L.; Taylor, H.G.; Cassedy, A.; Zhang, N.; Kirkwood, M.W.; Brown, T.M.; Stancin, T. Long-Term Behavioral Outcomes after a Randomized, Clinical Trial of Counselor-Assisted Problem Solving for Adolescents with Complicated Mild-to-Severe Traumatic Brain Injury. *J. Neurotrauma* **2015**, *32*, 967–975. [CrossRef]
74. Hypher, R.E.; Brandt, A.E.; Risnes, K.; Rø, T.B.; Skovlund, E.; Andersson, S.; Finnanger, T.G.; Stubberud, J. Paediatric goal management training in patients with acquired brain injury: Study protocol for a randomised controlled trial. *BMJ Open* **2019**, *9*, e029273. [CrossRef]
75. Wade, S.L.; Cassedy, A.E.; Shultz, E.L.; Zang, H.; Zhang, N.; Kirkwood, M.W.; Stancin, T.; Yeates, K.; Taylor, H.G. Randomized Clinical Trial of Online Parent Training for Behavior Problems After Early Brain Injury. *J. Am. Acad. Child Adolesc. Psychiatry* **2017**, *56*, 930–939.e2. [CrossRef]
76. Rohrer-Baumgartner, N.; Holthe, I.L.; Svendsen, E.J.; Røe, C.; Egeland, J.; Borgen, I.M.H.; Hauger, S.L.; Forslund, M.V.; Brunborg, C.; Prag Øra, H.; et al. Rehabilitation for children with chronic acquired brain injury in the Child in Context Intervention (CICI) study: Study protocol for a randomized controlled trial. *Trials* **2022**, *23*, 169. [CrossRef]

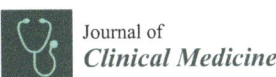

Article

Evaluating a Novel Treatment Adapting a Cognitive Behaviour Therapy Approach for Sexuality Problems after Traumatic Brain Injury: A Single Case Design with Nonconcurrent Multiple Baselines

Elinor E. Fraser [1,2,*], Marina G. Downing [1,2], Kerrie Haines [1], Linda Bennett [1], John Olver [3] and Jennie L. Ponsford [1,2]

[1] Turner Institute for Brain and Mental Health, School of Psychological Sciences, Monash University, Clayton, VIC 3800, Australia; marina.downing@monash.edu (M.G.D.); kehaines@bigpond.net.au (K.H.); linda@lindabennettpsychology.com.au (L.B.); jennie.ponsford@monash.edu (J.L.P.)
[2] Monash-Epworth Rehabilitation Research Centre, Epworth Healthcare, Richmond, VIC 3121, Australia
[3] Rehabilitation Medicine, Epworth HealthCare, Richmond, VIC 3121, Australia; john.olver@epworth.org.au
* Correspondence: elinor.fraser@monash.edu

Abstract: There has been little progress in development of evidence-based interventions to improve sexuality outcomes for individuals with traumatic brain injury (TBI). This study aimed to evaluate the preliminary efficacy of an individualised intervention using a cognitive behaviour therapy (CBT) framework to treat sexuality problems after TBI. A nonconcurrent multiple baseline single-case design with 8-week follow-up and randomisation to multiple baseline lengths (3, 4, or 6 weeks) was repeated across nine participants (five female) with complicated mild–severe TBI (mean age = 46.44 years (SD = 12.67), mean post-traumatic amnesia = 29.14 days (SD = 29.76), mean time post-injury = 6.56 years (median = 2.50 years, SD = 10.11)). Treatment comprised eight weekly, individual sessions, combining behavioural, cognitive, and educational strategies to address diverse sexuality problems. Clinical psychologists adopted a flexible, patient-centred, and goal-orientated approach whilst following a treatment guide and accommodating TBI-related impairments. Target behaviour was subjective ratings of satisfaction with sexuality, measured three times weekly. Secondary outcomes included measures of sexuality, mood, self-esteem, and participation. Goal attainment scaling (GAS) was used to measure personally meaningful goals. Preliminary support was shown for intervention effectiveness, with most cases demonstrating sustained improvements in subjective sexuality satisfaction and GAS goal attainment. Based on the current findings, larger clinical trials are warranted.

Keywords: Sexuality; cognitive behaviour therapy; traumatic brain injury; Rehabilitation

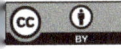

1. Introduction

Sexuality is a healthy and natural part of living. It is much more than sexual activity and behaviour, encompassing identity, self-esteem, body image, attitudes, motivation, pleasure, and relationships [1,2]. Sexuality is influenced by several sociocultural processes and invariably changes in its meaning and importance across a lifetime [3]. After traumatic brain injury (TBI), a substantial proportion of individuals experience difficulties with sexuality, with prevalence rates generally ranging from 36–54% [4–7]. The majority report global reductions in sexual arousal and orgasm, perceived importance of sexuality, and frequency of sexual behaviour (i.e., hyposexuality) [6,8,9] In most cases, there is an immediate decrease in sexuality post-TBI with only a small degree of improvement shown across the first year of recovery [10]. Increased sexual arousal and inappropriate sexual behaviour (i.e., hypersexuality) is thought to occur in a smaller proportion of individuals [11]. Hypersexuality, connected to the early post-TBI phase of recovery, is often reversible, whilst persistent hypersexuality is generally underpinned by disinhibition in brain function [12,13].

The biopsychosocial model conceptualises the complex and multifactorial nature of TBI-related sexuality changes as a culmination of biological and medical, psychological and neuropsychological, and social and relationship factors [14]. Neurophysiological mechanisms underpinning sexuality problems may include damage to neuroanatomical regions, altered neurotransmission, and disrupted hormonal regulation [15–17]. Although there is agreement that neuroendocrine dysfunction may contribute to post-TBI sexuality changes, including decreased libido, impotence, fertility issues, and irregular menstrual cycles [15,18,19], studies investigating the diagnosis and prognosis of neuroendocrine deficiencies and their implications for sexuality outcomes following TBI are lacking [20]. Although the association between older age and reduced sexuality post-injury has been highlighted in previous research [6,10,21–23], the onset of hyposexuality problems following TBI does not appear to be strongly linked to injury severity or time post-injury [6,21,22,24]. With regards to psychological factors, there is strong evidence supporting the role of depression in the onset and maintenance of sexuality problems after TBI [9,22,23]. Self-esteem, anxiety, and antidepressant medication may also be associated with sexuality changes [6,21,22], although it is unclear to what extent concomitant depression also contributes to these associations. Adults with TBI may show increased distractibility, as well as impaired behavioural control, communication, and egocentricity, all of which have the potential to affect one's capacity to engage in intimate relationships and relate to others [14,15]. Two studies have highlighted an association between decreased social participation and reduced sexuality [23,25], whilst role changes, loss of emotional intimacy, and uninjured partners emotional reactions to the cognitive behavioural changes are likely to pose challenges to sexual readjustment within relationships [26].

Several models and recommendations have been put forth for the management of sexuality problems after TBI. Extant literature advocates for the PLISSIT model [27] as one approach that may be used to address sexual health and wellbeing across TBI healthcare settings [14,28–30]. The acronym PLISSIT classifies four levels of intervention: permission to discuss sexuality, provision of limited information, specific suggestions regarding the individual's sexual problem, and intensive therapy with a qualified healthcare professional. Taylor and Davis [31] later published the extended PLISSIT (Ex-PLISSIT) model which proposes that all levels begin with explicit giving of permission. In previous TBI sexuality research, more emphasis has been placed on addressing the first two levels through the development and evaluation of handouts, booklets, and information resources [32–38]. As a result, there is little information on interventions for persistent and complex post-TBI sexuality problems at the Specific Suggestions and Intensive Therapy levels. Although previous research has offered broad and nonspecific recommendations for the use of counselling, individual and group psychotherapy, sex therapy, pharmacology, and cognitive and behavioural therapy to address sexuality problems after TBI [5,17,29,32,39–41], only a handful of descriptive case reports [41–43] and single case studies [44,45] have been completed. Studies have generally focused on treating male sexual dysfunction through the application of standard medical and sex therapy treatments [44,45]. Small sample sizes and a narrow focus on male sexual dysfunction, in addition to an absence of standardised treatment manuals and limited description of how treatment was modified to accommodate TBI-related sequelae, are also relevant limitations of previous research.

To meet the comprehensive and holistic needs of the TBI population, adopting a flexible, integrative, patient-centred, sex-positive, and biopsychosocial approach that emphasises individuals' strengths rather than limitations is necessary [46,47]. Cognitive behaviour therapy (CBT) is a widely researched, time-limited psychotherapeutic approach that has been shown to be efficacious in the treatment of a wide range of disorders, including TBI-related depression and anxiety [48–50] and sleep and fatigue [51,52]. The utility of CBT as a therapeutic option for sexuality disturbances in non-TBI populations is strongly endorsed in the literature [53]. The therapeutic framework proposes that cognitions (thoughts), emotions (feelings), and behaviours all contribute to personal functioning and changes in one domain can lead to changes in others [54]. A mainstay of the CBT approach includes challenging distorted thinking (e.g., negative thoughts related to one's sexual appeal) and maladaptive behaviours (e.g., avoidance of intimate contact) to achieve more balanced and affirming self-talk and behaviour [55]. Indeed, therapists play an active role in guiding therapeutic interactions and topics of discussion. Relevant to the TBI cohort, the CBT approach acknowledges the multifactorial nature of sexuality and the need to go beyond treating the physiological basis of sexual dysfunction and address psychological and social factors that contribute to sexual wellbeing. Such an intervention can be accessed by adult TBI survivors regardless of sex, gender, sexual orientation, marital status, or type of sexuality issue. Furthermore, CBT includes a significant educational component and can be adapted to accommodate TBI-related cognitive impairment to enhance individuals' ability to take in and recall information, understand concepts, and remember to complete homework [50–52]. Common strategies include greater structure, using more behavioural techniques when cognition is impaired, implementing new skills in vivo, simplifying complex concepts, summarising and repetition of information, pictorial representations of concepts, handouts, external memory aids (e.g., use of a logbook or diary), and provision of organisational support, as well as pre-emptive rest breaks to maintain energy levels [56].

To the best of our knowledge, no study has designed a novel, individualised intervention using a CBT framework tailored to address TBI-related sexuality problems and evaluated its efficacy. The current study aimed to (1) describe a novel, individualised CBT-based intervention in adult TBI survivors with persistent post-injury sexuality problems, (2) use a single case methodology to explore the efficacy of this intervention in improving subjective satisfaction with sexuality, and (3) explore whether this intervention results in improvements in depression, anxiety, self-esteem, social participation, or participants' attainment of individualised goals.

2. Materials and Methods

2.1. Study Design

The study used a nonconcurrent, multiple baselines, AB single-case experimental design (SCED) with follow-up (i.e., baseline; treatment; follow-up) repeated across nine participants to explore the effectiveness of an eight-session, individualised CBT intervention on the primary outcome measure of subjective satisfaction with sexuality. Prior to commencing treatment, participants were randomly assigned to baseline durations of 3, 4, or 6 weeks. Experimental control is demonstrated by using the multiple baseline design, which controls for threats to internal validity (e.g., maturation, history) [57,58], whilst the randomisation enhances scientific rigour [59]. The baseline phase was immediately followed by an eight-week treatment phase, before a final eight-week follow-up phase. The Risk of Bias in N of 1 Trials scale (RoBiNT) [60] and the Single-Case Reporting guideline In Behavioural Interventions (SCRIBE) [61] were followed to ensure methodological quality in design and reporting (see Supplementary Table S1 for scoring).

2.2. Participants

Participants were five women and four men recruited via two mechanisms: (1) community advertising to clinicians treating individuals with TBI, and (2) through an established research project that involves collection of follow up outcome data across individuals' recovery after TBI. Figure 1 shows the flow of participants throughout the study. Informed written consent was obtained from all participants. No financial compensation was provided to the study participants, although participants received treatment free of charge. Inclusion criteria were as follows: (a) aged 18 to 65 years, (b) had sustained complicated mild to very severe TBI, (b) greater than three months post injury, (c) self-reported sexuality disturbance. The following exclusion criteria were used: (a) presence of other neurological disorder, (b) history of psychotic disorder, (c) current alcohol or drug abuse, and (d) insufficient English language or cognitive ability to complete questionnaires or therapy tasks, and (e) sexual dysfunction prior to TBI. Ethical approval for the study was granted by relevant ethics committees. Demographic, injury, and cognitive variables for participants are displayed in Table 1.

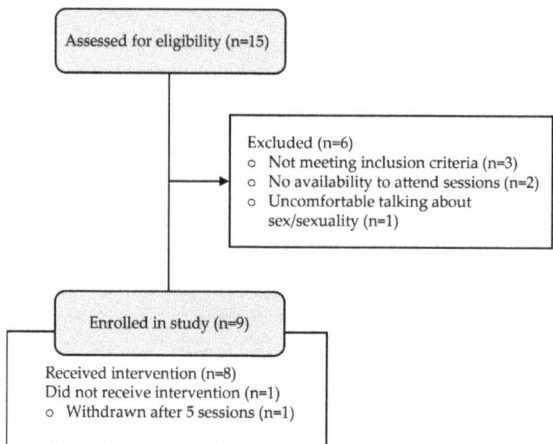

Figure 1. Recruitment and flow of participants throughout the study.

2.3. Intervention

A detailed treatment guide was developed though an iterative process characterised by a comprehensive review of scientific and grey literature and publicly available information sourced from media, books, expert opinions, and web pages together with discussions and idea generation among a small working group of healthcare practitioners (neuropsychologists, psychologists, doctors) and researchers with expertise in this field. The contents of the treatment guide were organised into 12 modules with accompanying handouts. The overarching aims of CBT were to (1) foster shifts in cognition and/or behaviour that allow individuals/couples to feel more in control of their sexuality, (2) improve satisfaction with sexuality in the individual with TBI, and (3) help individuals with TBI accept and manage changes in sexuality. A medical review was incorporated into the treatment design to aid therapists/clients understanding of the problem and to help differentiate between organic and psychogenic causes and contributing factors.

The intervention consisted of eight 60-min sessions delivered weekly and one booster session completed approximately two months later. The intervention was delivered by two clinical psychologists, KH and LB, licensed to treat clients with CBT and experienced in working with adults with TBI. Therapists had between 13 and 25-years of clinical experience. During periods of non-pandemic related lockdowns, participants had the choice of attending sessions via teleconference (videocall) or in person at the clinicians' respective private practices. For couples, the intervention was offered to both the participant and their partner.

It was the working group's intention that the treatment guide be used in a flexible manner. The first treatment session focused on engaging the participant, initiating rapport building, and undertaking a comprehensive assessment and history taking (module 1). The assessment and formulation process followed a biopsychosocial method of classifying predisposing, precipitating, maintaining, and protective factors. The provision of psychoeducation together with goal setting and ongoing rapport building are key features of session 2 that can be built upon and revisited across the duration of treatment. To increase participant engagement, generating the clinical formulation and defining specific goals was intended to be a collaborative process.

Table 1. Demographic, injury, and cognitive characteristics of the participants.

Variables	AA	BB	CC	DD	EE	FF	GG	HH *	II *
Demographic data									
Age (years)	49	31	64	47	63	56	33	33	41
Sex	Male	Female	Male	Female	Male	Female	Female	Male	Female
Education (years)	12	18	14	12	12	15	16	14	18
Preinjury relationship	Single	De-facto	Married	Married	Married	De-facto	De-facto	De-facto	Married
Baseline relationship	Single	Single	Married	Married	Married	Single	Single	De-facto	Married
Injury characteristics									
Cause of TBI	Bicycle Accident	MVA	Work-related injury	MVA	MVA	MVA	MVA	Fall	Pedestrian struck by car
PTA duration (days)	70	16	21	1	0.5	20	8	68	23
Worst GCS score	3	15	8	[b]	15	14	3	3	13
Time since injury (years)	33	6	6	5	2	3	1	1	0.90
CT brain imaging	Petecchial haemorrhages in frontal and paraventricular regions	Frontal contusion, subarachnoid haemorrhage, contrecoup injury with contusion in the orbitofrontal region	NAD	Fractured occipital lobe, epidural haematoma, subarachnoid haemorrhage, pneumocephalus, thrombosis of transverse sigmoid sinus and jugular vein	Interhemispheric subarachnoid haemorrhage	NAD	Fractured parietal and temporal bones, contusion and intracerebral haemorrhage in temporal region, extra-axial haemorrhage	Fractured occipital lobe, subfalcine herniation, inferior frontal contusion, grey and white matter loss, haemorrhage	Left subdural haematoma, contusions in right frontal and temporal regions, fractured left temporal bone
Cognitive performance									
Digit Symbol Coding Test z-score	−1.33	0.00	−1.00	−1.00	−1.67	0.00	NA	NA	0.67
RAVLT Verbal Learning Trials 1–5 Sum z-score	−1.52	−0.92	−0.70	0.22	−0.96	1.53	NA	−2.12	0.22
Trail Making Test Part-B z-score	−0.67	−0.67	−1.00	−0.67	−1.00	0.00	NA	NA	1.33
Estimated Premorbid Intellectual Functioning (NART Standard Score)	103	104	105	113	115	117	NA	NA	100

TBI, traumatic brain injury; MVA, motor vehicle accident; PTA, post traumatic amnesia; GCS, Glasgow Coma Scale; CT, computed tomography; NAD, no abnormality detected; NA, not applicable—no formal testing was able to be undertaken; DSCT, digit symbol coding test; RAVLT, Rey Auditory Verbal Learning Test; NART, National Adult Reading Test. [b] Blank cells represent missing data. * Completed the intervention with their partner.

For sessions 3–7, therapists were encouraged to apply clinical judgement in identifying, selecting, and modifying the delivery of modules to suit the needs of the client, taking into consideration their presenting problem, clinical formulation, and goals. Hence, the content of each session and the overall number of modules delivered was expected to vary according to the individual/couple. As a tangible representation of each module, the purpose of the accompanying handouts was to provide structure to the treatment, as well as aid communication and delivery of information between the therapist and client. Handouts were used not only in the context of building psychoeducation but also the exploration of cognitive and behavioural strategies.

The purpose of Session 8 was consolidation of treatment content, skills, and strategies. Functional goals were reviewed as a marker of treatment progress, whilst relapse prevention was explored in the context of supporting maintenance of treatment gains. When delivering the treatment, clinical psychologists implemented several strategies to support engagement in sessions and retention of information. Key strategies included educational scaffolding, visual handouts, written summaries, repetition, and simplification of concepts. The degree to which strategies were applied, however, varied between individuals according to their needs. The treatment structure as it related to sessions and delivery of modules and accompanying handouts is displayed in Table 2.

Table 2. Treatment structure and modules.

Session	Module	Objective
1–2	Module 1: Assessment and Formulation	Work closely with the individual/couple to develop a shared understanding of the problem and collaboratively set treatment goals.
	Module 2: Psychoeducation and Goals	Explore the individual's/couple's understanding of sexuality and provide psychoeducation surrounding sexuality, TBI, and overall health and wellbeing.
3–7	Module 3: Self-esteem and Body Image	Explore self-esteem or body image and identify and adjust biased expectations, negative self-evaluations, and rules and assumptions
	Module 4: Understanding Arousal	Define desire and arousal, explore dimensions of touch, identify brakes and accelerators
	Module 5: Reframing thoughts	Explore links between thoughts, emotions, and behaviours. Employ cognitive restructuring techniques that allow the individual/couple to feel in control of their sexuality.
	Module 6: Communication	Understand expressive and receptive listening skills using modelling and in-session coaching.
	Module 7: Relaxation	Teach mindfulness, breathing, and progressive muscle relaxation techniques to enhance sexual experiences
	Module 8: Psychosexual Skill Exercises	Practise exercises targeted to the individual's/couple's sexual problem.
	Module 9: Social Skills	Establish relevant techniques to increase positive and rewarding social behaviours and decrease negative social behaviour.
	Module 10: Sleep and Fatigue Management	Identify practical strategies to improve sleep and manage physical and mental fatigue.
	Module 11: Medical Review	Assess neurological/medical basis to sexuality problem.
8	Module 12: Relapse Prevention	Summarise skills and content learned throughout treatment and generate plan for managing setbacks.

TBI, traumatic brain injury.

2.4. Measures

2.4.1. Measures of Participant Baseline Characteristics

The National Adult Reading Test (NART) [62] was used as an estimate of premorbid intellectual ability in the current study. New learning and memory were assessed using the total words recalled in trials 1–5 on the Rey Auditory Verbal Learning Test [63], whilst executive function and speed of information processing were measured using the total time taken to complete the Trail Making Test Part B [64] and digit symbol-coding test [65], respectively. The Fatigue Severity Scale (FSS) [66] together with the pain and independence subscales of the Traumatic Brain Injury-Quality of Life (TBI-QOL) [67] were also administered (See supplementary Table S2 for scores).

2.4.2. Primary Outcome Measure

For the purposes of this study, the authors developed a rating scale to measure participants' subjective satisfaction with their sexuality [68]. Participants were asked to rate the following question 'How satisfied are you with your current sexuality?' on a 7-point Likert scale ranging from 'extremely unsatisfied' to 'extremely satisfied'.

2.4.3. Secondary Outcome Measures

Several secondary measures were used to provide converging evidence for treatment effectiveness. The Brain Injury Questionnaire of Sexuality (BIQS) [69] is a 15-item, self-report questionnaire comprising three subscales measuring sexual functioning, relationship quality and self-esteem, and mood. Respondents are required to compare aspects of their sexuality with preinjury status on a 5-point Likert scale ranging from "greatly decreased" to "greatly increased". Total sexuality scores between 14 and 44 are classified as decreased from pre-injury levels, the same for scores of 45, and increased from pre-injury levels for scores between 46 and 75.

The Hospital Anxiety and Depression Scale (HADS) [70] was used as a reliable 14-item measure of anxiety and depression symptoms. Higher scores on the HADS subscales reflect higher levels of depression and anxiety. The Rosenberg self-esteem scale (RSES) [71] was utilised as a 10-item measure of self-esteem. On this measure, higher scores reflect better self-esteem, with scores less than 15 suggestive of low self-esteem. As a reliable and valid measure of social participation after TBI, the Participation Assessment with Recombined Tools-Objective (PART-O) [72] comprises 17 items across three subscales measuring productivity, social relations, and 'out and about' (e.g., going to the movies). The averaged total score was used as an indication of overall social participation, with higher scores indicative of greater social participation.

Goal attainment scaling (GAS) [73] was used to set individualised goals, allowing for measurement of personally meaningful progress [60]. Possible outcomes were defined according to a standard five-point symmetrical scale (-2 a lot less than expected; -1 less than expected; 0 at expectation; +1 more than expected; +2 a lot more than expected). Level of goal attainment was assessed at post-intervention and follow-up timepoints. GAS goals were initially set at -1 to allow for measurement of deterioration [74].

2.5. Treatment Integrity

Treatment sessions were audio recorded for assessment of treatment integrity. Specifically designed treatment integrity monitoring forms were developed to measure, (1) overall adherence to elements common in a CBT approach, (2) adherence to the chosen module(s) used in the session, and (3) therapist competency in module delivery [52]. The three domains were rated on an 8-point Likert scale ranging from 'unacceptable' to 'excellent'. Two randomly selected recordings per participant were chosen for evaluation by an independent practitioner with 21 years of professional clinical psychology experience.

2.6. Procedure

Data were collected between March 2021 and March 2022. Participants were provided with information about the research project and screened for eligibility via telephone. Participants who met eligibility criteria were scheduled for an initial baseline assessment. Participants were then randomly allocated to a baseline monitoring phase of 3, 4, or 6 weeks. The target behaviour (i.e., subjective satisfaction with sexuality) was assessed three times per week via a text message reminder system. Ratings were recorded online across all three study phases (baseline, intervention, follow-up) to provide a continuous measure of rate of change. Secondary outcome measures assessing sexuality, depression and anxiety, self-esteem, and social participation were collected prior to the intervention (conclusion of the baseline period), at the conclusion of the intervention, and eight weeks post conclusion of the intervention. The majority completed secondary measures on the online platform Qualtrics™ (Qualtrics, Provo, UT, USA) to minimise bias in data collection. They were otherwise collected by a researcher independent of the therapist. Goal attainment scaling goals were set in collaboration with the therapist and reassessed at two timepoints (at the conclusion of the intervention and eight weeks post conclusion of the intervention).

Participants received eight one-hour therapy sessions with clinical psychologists KH or LB either face to face or via teleconference (videocall). After cessation of therapy, a 30–45-min semi-structured interview was administered by the first author to evaluate the usefulness of the intervention, to identify its strengths and limitations and ascertain whether the participant would recommend it to others in the future.

2.7. Data Analysis

Descriptive statistics were generated for all variables of interest. For cognitive measures, raw scores were converted to standardised z-scores using age- and education-based normative data. Primary outcome sexuality satisfaction ratings were displayed graphically using Graphpad Prism (Version 8) and evaluated using visual analysis in line with established guidelines proposed by Lane and Gast [75], incorporating both within and between phase analysis. The SCDA plugin for R [76] was used to fit a linear trend to data using the split middle method [59,77]. Stability was defined as 80% of data points being within an envelope of ±25% of the phase median. When evidence for a functional effect was present, we proceeded to estimate the effect sizes using statistical analysis.

Statistical analyses used the Tau-U statistic, which is a nonparametric index of the percentage of the data that do not overlap minus the percentage of the data that overlap between phases [78]. Tau-U is a distribution-free non-parametric technique, with an index well-suited for small datasets and is useful in aggregating data across phases to provide an overall effect size [78]. Baseline correction was applied when Tau-U values for baseline exceeded 0.20 and the trend occurred in the same direction as the aims of the intervention (i.e., when baseline displayed a trend to improving sexuality satisfaction) [79]. Tau-U values below 0.2 were considered small, 0.2–0.6 medium, 0.6–0.8 large, and greater than 0.8 large to very large [80]. Analysis was conducted using the online calculator at http://www.singlecaseresearch.org/calculators/tau-u (accessed on 15 January 2022).

Informal comparisons were made between pre-treatment, post-treatment, and follow-up secondary outcome measures. Functional change on participants' individual GAS goals were descriptively explored with any change considered to constitute clinical significance [81]. Independently collected semi-structured interview data related to participants' experience of the intervention were also qualitatively examined, although they will be reported in later publications.

3. Results

3.1. Case Description

Nine community dwelling adults with a diagnosis of TBI were recruited into the study (five female, four male). Participants varied in age (31–64 years), severity of injury as measured by PTA duration (<1–70 days), and time since injury (0.90–33 years), and most displayed impairment on at least one measure of cognition. Five participants were receiving psychological intervention for other issues, unrelated to sexuality, at the time of study participation. The majority completed the treatment via teleconference (videocall), with only one participant (AA) attending sessions in person. Participant DD withdrew during the treatment phase due to extenuating circumstances that meant they did not have the time or capacity to continue with the study. All other participants completed the study in its entirety. No adverse events were recorded for any participant across the duration of the study.

With regards to presenting problems in the current sample, all participants presented with sexuality issues consistent with reduced sexuality, or hyposexuality, regardless of age, sex, marital status, or time post injury. Individuals endorsed reductions in sexual desire and arousal and ability to climax (AA, BB, CC, DD, EE, FF, GG, HH, II), self-esteem (DD, HH), body image (BB, DD, II), and communication (FF, GG, II). Of the four males, three (AA, CC, EE) presented with erectile dysfunction, and for those who had partners, there was a consistent reduction in frequency of, and satisfaction with, sexual intimacy within the relationship (CC, DD, EE, HH, II). Despite overlap in the nature of participants' sexuality complaints, establishing the probable aetiological basis of the individual's issue through comprehensive assessment and formulation was a crucial first step of the intervention. For two participants (AA, FF), this also involved undergoing medical review to clarify the relative contributions of injury-related, neurological, and/or biological factors.

Given the diversity in presenting problems, it was of the utmost importance that treatment planning and delivery were individualised and tailored. To illustrate how this was implemented in this study, it can be helpful to briefly describe and compare cases with similar characteristics. CC and EE were both males in their 60's and married, and both reported a loss of intimacy in their relationship related to the post-injury onset of erectile dysfunction. For CC, treatment involved increasing his awareness of factors related to erectile dysfunction and trialling psychosexual skill exercises. By the final session, CC was able to successfully obtain an erection. On the other hand, EE's erectile dysfunction was a direct result of damage sustained to his pelvis and genital area in the accident. As a result, treatment focused on expanding EE's understanding of sexuality and masculinity and working on ways in which EE could facilitate emotional closeness and connectedness' with his wife outside of sexual intercourse. Single and actively dating, AA was the third participant who presented with erectile dysfunction. In this case, low self-esteem, high levels of performance anxiety, and lifestyle factors (weight, alcohol, smoking) were key contributing factors. Among other things, the therapist worked with AA on defining his personal strengths, recognising that sexual intercourse is only one part of sexuality, and specifying what has facilitated and inhibited desire and arousal for AA in the past. Cognitive impairment combined with unrealistic treatment expectations, however, limited his ability to engage in CBT techniques aimed at modifying thoughts, challenging unrealistic standards regarding sexual function, and engaging in behavioural experiments.

For female participants, there was equal variability in factors contributing to reduced sexual drive, desire, and arousal. FF experienced changes in sensations, which meant she was unable to tolerate touch. Trialling remedial massage in a non-intimate context was one behavioural experiment that FF and the therapist subsequently worked on. Negative body image formed part of the clinical formulation for three participants' (BB, DD, and II), although treatment needed to be tailored to address other relevant factors including anticipatory anxiety to chronic fatigue relapses (BB), high levels of self-blame (DD) and irritability and anger outbursts (II).

Only two participants, II and HH, completed the treatment with their partner. The latter was a unique case in that HH's partner had taken on a carer's role in his recovery, and at one-year post-injury, it was his partner who was reporting low sexual desire and arousal, whilst HH himself struggled with low self-esteem and difficulties communicating his sexual needs. In this case, a core facet of the treatment was delineating intimacy and sexuality from sexual intercourse and enhancing the couple's comfort and communication on the topic. Overall, the case descriptions offer insight into the complexities of the presentations and treatment of sexuality after TBI, highlighting the need to adopt a flexible and individualised approach predicated on comprehensive assessment and formulation.

3.2. Treatment Adherence and Integrity

Completed by a clinical psychologist, integrity monitoring of the delivery of the treatment indicated 'acceptable' to 'excellent' ratings for overall delivery (mean 5.76 [range 4.5–7.5]), adherence (mean 6.24 [range 4.5–8]), and competency (mean 5.55 [range 4–7]). An overview of each participant's target behaviour (sexuality satisfaction, with improvements reflected by higher scores) is presented in text and in Figure 2.

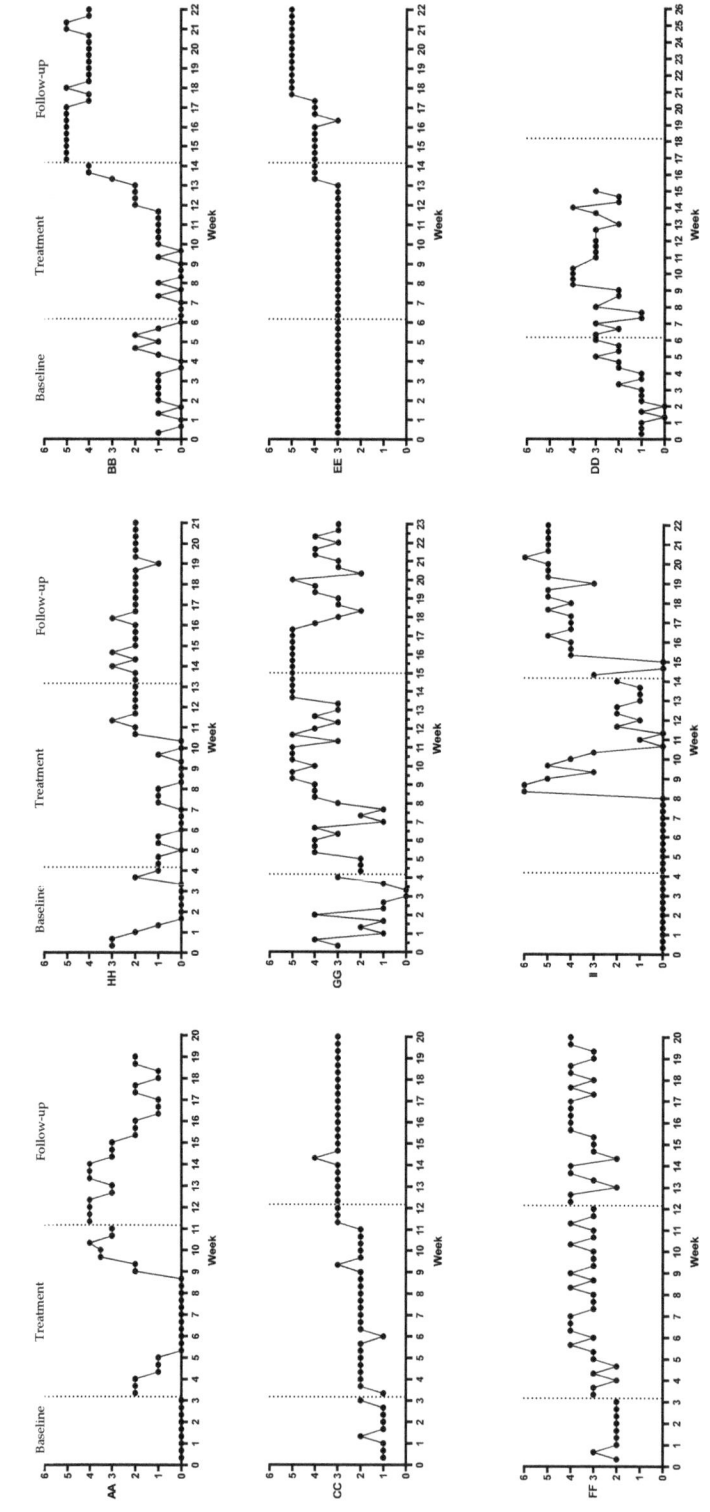

Figure 2. Participants' self-reported subjective sexuality satisfaction across baseline, intervention, and follow up phases.

3.3. Self-Reported Subjective Sexuality Satisfaction

The application of the stability envelope suggested stability of baseline phase for participants AA, EE, FF, and II. Participants GG and HH demonstrated decreasing baseline trend, whilst participants BB, CC, and DD showed increasing baseline trend. For the latter participants, a visual trend correction using the split middle method was applied. Participants AA, CC, FF, GG, HH, and II showed an increasing trend in the therapeutic direction following the introduction of the intervention. Therapeutic gains were maintained between treatment and follow-up phases for participants CC, FF, HH, and II, whilst a decreasing trend was shown in follow-up phase data for participants AA and GG. Although participant BB and EE showed no significant trend change in sexuality satisfaction during the treatment phase, an increasing trend was shown during the follow-up phase suggestive of the delayed onset of therapeutic gains following the delivery of the intervention.

With respect to the between phase change, the introduction of treatment was associated with a median level increase in subjective sexuality satisfaction for participants AA, CC, FF, GG, and II. Participant HH demonstrated a marginal between phase increase in sexuality satisfaction, whilst the introduction of the intervention was associated with a delayed median level change in sexuality satisfaction for participants BB and EE, occurring during the follow-up phase of the study.

Tau-U analysis was used to determine statistically significant changes in subjective satisfaction with sexuality between baseline and treatment phases and treatment and follow-up phases. Sexuality satisfaction significantly increased between the baseline and treatment phases for participants AA, CC, FF, GG, and II. Tau-U analyses further demonstrated statistically significant increases in subjective sexuality satisfaction between treatment and follow-up phases for participants AA, BB, CC, EE, HH, and II (See Table 3).

Table 3. Tau-U planned comparison for self-reported ratings of sexuality satisfaction.

Participant	Baseline Corrected	Baseline vs. Treatment	p Value	Treatment vs. Follow-up	p Value
AA	No	0.54 *	0.018	0.54 **	0.001
BB	No	0.13	0.461	0.96 **	0.001
CC	No	0.74 **	0.001	0.86 **	0.001
DD	b	b	b	b	b
EE	No	0.22	0.211	0.89 **	0.001
FF	No	0.84 **	0.001	0.29	0.084
GG	No	0.69 **	0.001	0.02	0.923
HH	No	0.01	0.980	0.68 **	0.001
II	No	0.53 *	0.008	0.65 **	0.001

* Significance at $p < 0.05$; ** Significance at $p \leq 0.001$. b Blank cells represent missing data due to participant withdrawal.

3.4. Secondary Outcome Measures

Descriptive analyses of the BIQS, HADS-A, HADS-D, RSES, and PART-O revealed variable results (see Table 4). On the BIQS, all participants' pre-treatment total sexuality scores were classified as decreased from pre-injury sexuality status. All participants displayed increased sexuality scores at post-treatment. The participants who commenced treatment with elevated symptoms of anxiety (AA, FF, GG) and depression (FF, GG) recorded no meaningful change on the HADS at post-treatment. With regards to self-esteem, however, those who were classified as having low self-esteem at pre-treatment (AA and HH) demonstrated significantly improved self-esteem at post-treatment, which was maintained at follow-up. Social participation measured by the PART-O was considered a more distal secondary outcome measure and did not show any convincing change between pre-treatment, post-treatment, and follow-up measurements.

Table 4. Participants' pre-treatment, post-treatment, and follow-up raw scores for secondary outcome questionnaire measures.

Participant	BIQS			HADS-A			HADS-D			RSES			PART-O		
	Pre	Post	Follow-up	Pre	Post	Follow-up	Pre	Post	Follow-up	Pre	Post	Follow-up	Pre	Post	Follow-up
AA	29	44	39	9	8	5	1	2	8	15	18	16	1.78	1.95	1.98
BB	34	49	46	4	1	1	2	2	3	28	30	30	1.38	1.68	1.66
CC	26	35	41	2	1	1	3	0	1	20	20	22	2.11	1.61	2.04
DD	21	b	b	10	b	b	11	b	b	9	b	b	2.42	b	b
EE	22	50	28	0	1	1	2	3	3	21	26	26	0.84	1.25	1.30
FF	29	33	24	14	11	12	10	8	10	21	22	23	1.48	1.21	1.42
GG	22	39	34	13	8	13	13	9	8	17	18	11	1.35	1.46	1.51
HH	37	40	41	6	5	5	7	10	9	10	15	17	1.79	1.79	1.90
II	19	25	20	5	4	3	2	0	0	18	19	20	2.84	2.94	3.03

BIQS; Brain Injury Questionnaire of Sexuality; HADS-A, anxiety subscale from the Hospital Anxiety and Depression Scale; HADS-D, depression subscale from the Hospital Anxiety and Depression Scale; RSES, Rosenberg Self-Esteem Scale; PART-O, Participation Assessment with Recombined Tools-Objective. Note: Data represents participants' raw scores for each measure. [b] Blank cells represent missing data due to participant withdrawal.

All participants reported improvement in at least one goal area following treatment, which was generally maintained, and even showed improvement for participants BB, EE, HH, and II when rated at the conclusion of the eight-week follow-up period. Although participant AA reported the attainment of goals following the intervention, this change was not maintained for two of the goals at follow-up (see Table 5).

Table 5. Description and attainment of participant GAS goals.

Participant	Goals	Pre-Treatment	Post-Treatment	Follow-up
AA	1. To work towards having an emotionally connected/supportive relationship with a female	−1	0	−1
	2. To work on erectile dysfunction	−1	+1	0
	3. To learn how to communicate clearly and honestly before engaging in sexual activity	−1	0	−1
BB	1. To feel better about body image	−1	+2	+2
	2. To not feel anxious about experiencing chronic fatigue syndrome relapses	−1	+1	+2
CC	1. To be physically intimate with partner	−1	0	0
	2. To work on erectile dysfunction	−1	0	0
DD	1. To be physically intimate with partner	−1	b	b
	2. To improve self-esteem	−1	b	b
EE	1. To increase understanding of sexuality and TBI	−1	+2	+2
	2. To explore pain management options	−1	+1	+2
	3. To explore masculinity in the context of pre- vs. post-injury self	−1	+2	+2
FF	1. To be confident to put self out there	−1	−1	0
	2. To feel more in touch with body	−1	0	0
GG	1. To improve desire/motivation/sex drive	−1	+1	+2
	2. To work on communication and reduce emotionally closing off	−1	+1	+1
HH	1. To improve sexual relationship with partner	−1	+2	+2
	2. To feel better about sexuality	−1	+1	+1
	3. To improve self-esteem	−1	+1	+1
	4. To reduce the need for partner to take on a care-taking role	−1	+1	+1
	5. To increase understanding of sexuality and TBI	−1	+2	+2
	6. To know more about partner's sexuality	−1	+2	+2
II	1. To increase knowledge of how TBI has impacted sexuality	−1	+2	+2
	2. To improve management of fatigue	−1	+1	+2
	3. To create more opportunities for intimacy behaviours	−1	+1	+1
	4. To develop more effective communication skills	−1	+2	+2

GAS, goal attainment scaling; TBI, traumatic brain injury. [b] Blank cells represent missing data due to participant withdrawal.

4. Discussion

This study served to evaluate the preliminary efficacy of a novel intervention using a CBT framework that aimed to improve individuals' satisfaction with sexuality following TBI. Hyposexuality problems identified in this study included erectile dysfunction, reduced sex drive and orgasm, negative changes in self-esteem and body image, loss of relationship intimacy, and difficulty establishing new intimate partnerships. Five participants showed treatment response in the therapeutic direction following the introduction of the intervention, whilst an additional three participants demonstrated delayed treatment response. Gains in sexuality satisfaction were generally maintained at two months following the completion of treatment. The finding that participants varied in their response to treatment was not unexpected given the individualised nature of the intervention. Signals of efficacy were also identified on secondary outcome measures of sexuality, functional goal attainment, and self-esteem. The intervention demonstrated good feasibility and adequate treatment adherence. Although the findings are encouraging, it is of note that only three participants recorded feeling 'satisfied' with their sexuality on the primary outcome measure at post-treatment and four at follow-up timepoints. Furthermore, one participant demonstrated the limited maintenance of treatment gains on the primary outcome measure and functional goals. Factors that may have contributed to this included the participants' expectation that the treatment would resolve all physical sexual issues, as well as ongoing pandemic-related lockdowns that prevented socialisation and dating.

The comparison of results with previous research is limited by the lack of studies that have previously reported on the treatment of persistent or complex post-TBI sexuality problems, with none having taken a CBT approach but rather delivered standard sex therapy and medical techniques [44,45]. Certainly, the current findings align with recommendations regarding the need for evidence-based interventions to be accessible and available at the Intensive Therapy level of the PLISSIT/Ex-PLISSIT model [14]. The proposition that intensive therapy may be offered at any stage of recovery is supported by the current research [31]. Indeed, the primary barrier to implementing intensive therapy is the lack of evidence regarding what specific techniques and tools are efficacious in ameliorating persistent post-TBI sexuality disturbances and how treatments should be tailored to suit the needs of individuals and couples following TBI [7,17]. The case descriptions outlined in this research demonstrate the complexity and nuance that needs to be considered in sexuality assessment and treatment after TBI. The continued development of interventions that are purposefully designed to meet the needs of individuals and couples following TBI is necessary to facilitate the clinical implementation of structured approaches to sexuality management, such as the PLISSIT/Ex-PLISSIT model.

4.1. Clinical Implications and Future Research

This study offers provisional support for the development of an evidence-based adapted CBT therapeutic intervention for people experiencing persistent and complex sexuality difficulties after TBI. The findings have important clinical implications for the treatment of sexuality in a TBI population. Given the heterogeneous nature of TBI, any one or combination of factors may lead to sexuality changes after TBI. Medical issues, TBI sequelae, pain, chronicity of TBI, profile of cognitive impairment, marital status, length of relationship, age, and lifestyle factors were all intricately interwoven with the sexuality problems addressed in this study. As such, adopting a holistic, flexible, and patient-centred approach is necessary to ensure tailored treatment planning and delivery.

Beyond consideration of the multifactorial aetiology of sexuality changes after TBI, there are implications associated with using a CBT framework delivered by a clinical psychologist that are worth highlighting. Specifically, it is important to note that in cases where there has been permanent alteration in an individual's physiological sexual response, an eight-week CBT intervention is unlikely to improve physical sexual function. At best, treatment will help to facilitate the emotional acceptance of the primary dysfunction, a greater understanding of sexuality, and ways to facilitate intimacy in ways other than sexual intercourse. Furthermore, there are cases where sexuality changes may directly reflect injury-related physical limitations, such as pain, increased or decreased sensitivity, and muscle weakness or spasticity, which influence body positioning and movement. In these instances, a psychological-based intervention characterised by eight sessions with a clinical psychologist may not be beneficial, rather a different discipline, such as physiotherapy or occupational therapy, may be better placed to address the issues. Indeed, there is a strong consensus that interdisciplinary sexuality service delivery is required to meet the needs of the TBI population [17,29,30].

Although further studies are required, this research provides a model for how sexuality changes may be addressed in this clinical population. Future studies evaluating sexuality treatment for individuals with TBI may benefit from larger or targeted sampling, which may allow for the evaluation of the extent to which the nature of the presenting sexuality issues or factors, such as cognitive impairment, cultural background, age, sex, gender, sexual orientation, marital status, duration of time post-injury, and other biopsychosocial variables influence responses to treatment. Increasing understanding of the potential impact of such variables will assist the design and implementation of interventions and further increase clinicians' awareness of factors to consider when addressing TBI-related sexuality changes. Additional research is needed to identify the optimal number and length of sessions and support the development and dissemination of the treatment guide and associated resources. Finally, there is a need for greater recognition and inclusion of participants with diverse gender and sexuality backgrounds, including those who identify as LGBTIQ+, in future research.

4.2. Limitations

There are several limitations to this study. First, the small number of participants included in this study limits the interpretation of the results. Participants had also undergone rehabilitation in the context of a no-fault accident compensation system, which may limit the generalisability of study findings to individuals with TBI who have not received rehabilitation. In addition to the sample consisting of white cisgender, heterosexual participants, it is worth noting the lack of recruited participants aged between 18 and 30 years, which may represent a unique period in the life cycle for sexual health and wellbeing. The results may also not extrapolate to individuals with TBI from non-Western countries or cultural backgrounds, especially those with more conservative attitudes towards sexuality. Although the diversity in sexuality problems highlighted in the current research is likely indicative of that seen in the community, the lack of uniformity prevents comparisons between individuals in terms of level and rate of improvement. Furthermore, it is unclear which components of the intervention influenced therapy response, given that an individualised approach was adopted, and a variety of therapeutic techniques were utilised. Importantly, however, the single-case experimental design did allow for the evaluation of a tailored intervention in a heterogeneous group of adults with TBI at an individual level. Other limitations, such as the lack of participants and therapist blinding and potential measurement error, also apply. GAS ratings may be subject to Rater bias as they were completed by non-blinded participants in cooperation with therapists and, therefore, should be interpreted cautiously. The authors acknowledge that the primary outcome measure was not psychometrically validated, however, there were no other validated measures that would be considered appropriate to use in this specific study. Indeed, there continues to be a lack of precision in TBI sexuality measurement, evidenced by the variability in measures utilised in the few treatment studies completed to date [44,45]. Another limitation to this intervention is the lack of involvement from occupational therapists and physiotherapists in the assessment, as well as treatment planning and delivery process. Finally, a longer follow-up (e.g., 6 to 12 months) would have been valuable to see whether improvements on outcome measures were maintained in the longer term.

5. Conclusions

To the best of our knowledge, this is the first published account of a preliminary empirical evaluation of a novel intervention adapting a CBT approach to treat sexuality problems after TBI. The findings make a unique contribution to the sexuality and TBI literature and confirm that using a CBT framework to treat TBI-related sexuality difficulties may represent a promising therapeutic avenue. As a rigorous, albeit small-scale, sexuality intervention study of individuals with TBI, this research provides preliminary evidence of efficacy and feasibility and thus is relevant to stakeholders in research, policy, and clinical practice.

Supplementary Materials: The following supporting information can be downloaded at: https://www.mdpi.com/article/10.3390/jcm11123525/s1, Supplementary Table S1: The Risk of Bias in N of 1 Trials scale. Supplementary Table S2: Participants' fatigue, pain interference, and independence baseline raw scores.

Author Contributions: Conceptualisation, E.E.F., M.G.D. and J.L.P.; methodology, E.E.F., M.G.D. and J.L.P.; formal analysis, E.E.F.; validation, M.G.D. and J.L.P.; investigation, E.E.F., K.H., L.B. and J.O.; writing—original draft preparation, E.E.F.; writing—review and editing, M.G.D., J.L.P., K.H., L.B. and J.O.; supervision, M.G.D. and J.L.P. All authors have read and agreed to the published version of the manuscript.

Funding: This research was funded by the Summer Foundation, the Epworth Medical Foundation, the Transport Accident Commission, and a National Health and Medical Research Council (NHMRC) Investigator Grant (APP1174473).

Institutional Review Board Statement: The study was conducted in accordance with the Declaration of Helsinki and approved by the Institutional Review Board (or Ethics Committee) of Monash University, Project ID No. 26148 (16 November 2020).

Informed Consent Statement: Informed consent was obtained from all participants involved in the study.

Data Availability Statement: The data presented in this study are available on request from the corresponding author. The data are not publicly available due to ethical restrictions.

Acknowledgments: The authors would like to acknowledge and sincerely thank all participants for their involvement in this research as well as our independent auditor, Tiffany Reichert, for completing the integrity monitoring.

Conflicts of Interest: The authors declare no conflict of interest. The funders had no role in the design of the study; in the collection, analyses, or interpretation of data; in the writing of the manuscript, or in the decision to publish the results.

References

1. Moreno, J.; Gan, C.; Zasler, N.D. Neurosexuality: A transdisciplinary approach to sexuality in neurorehabilitation. *NeuroRehabilitation* **2017**, *41*, 255–259. [CrossRef] [PubMed]
2. Verschuren, J.E.; Enzlin, P.; Dijkstra, P.U.; Geertzen, J.H.; Dekker, R. Chronic disease and sexuality: A generic conceptual framework. *J. Sex Res.* **2010**, *47*, 153–170. [CrossRef] [PubMed]
3. World Health Organisation. *Developing Sexual Health Programmes: A Framework for Action*; World Health Organization: Geneva, Switzerland, 2010; pp. 3–6.
4. Robert, H.; Pichon, B.; Haddad, R. Sexual dysfunctions after traumatic brain injury: Systematic review of the literature. *Prog. En Urol. J. De L'association Fr. D'urologie Et De La Soc. Fr. D'urologie* **2019**, *29*, 529–543. [CrossRef]
5. Hentzen, C.; Musco, S.; Amarenco, G.; Del Popolo, G.; Panicker, J.N. Approach and management to patients with neurological disorders reporting sexual dysfunction. *Lancet Neurol.* **2022**, *21*, 551–562. [CrossRef]
6. Ponsford, J. Sexual changes associated with traumatic brain injury. *Neuropsychol. Rehabil.* **2003**, *13*, 275–289. [CrossRef]
7. Turner, D.; Schöttle, D.; Krueger, R.; Briken, P. Sexual behavior and its correlates after traumatic brain injury. *Curr. Opin. Psychiatry* **2015**, *28*, 180–187. [CrossRef]
8. Sander, A.; Maestas, K.; Pappadis, M.; Sherer, M.; Hammond, F.; Hanks, R.; NIDRR Traumatic Brain Injury Model Systems Module Project on Sexuality After TBI. Sexual functioning 1 year after traumatic brain injury: Findings from a prospective traumatic brain injury model systems collaborative study. *Arch. Phys. Med. Rehabil.* **2012**, *93*, 1331–1337. [CrossRef]
9. Hibbard, M.; Gordon, W.; Flanagan, S.; Haddad, L.; Labinsky, E. Sexual dysfunction after traumatic brain injury. *NeuroRehabilitation* **2000**, *15*, 107–120. [CrossRef]
10. Hanks, R.; Sander, A.; Millis, S.; Hammond, F.; Maestas, K. Changes in Sexual Functioning From 6 to 12 Months Following Traumatic Brain Injury. *J. Head Trauma Rehabil.* **2013**, *28*, 179–185. [CrossRef]
11. Simpson, G.K.; Baguley, I.J. Prevalence, correlates, mechanisms, and treatment of sexual health problems after traumatic brain injury: A scoping review. *Crit. Rev. Phys. Rehabil. Med.* **2012**, *24*, 1–34. [CrossRef]
12. Britton, K.R. Case study: Medroxyprogesterone in the treatment of aggressive hypersexual behaviour in traumatic brain injury. *Brain Inj.* **1998**, *12*, 703–707. [CrossRef] [PubMed]
13. Komisaruk, B.R.; Del Cerro, M.C.R. Human sexual behavior related to pathology and activity of the brain. *Handb. Clin. Neurol.* **2015**, *130*, 109–119. [CrossRef] [PubMed]
14. Moreno, J.; Arango-Lasprilla, J.; Gan, C.; McKerral, M. Sexuality after traumatic brain injury: A critical review. *NeuroRehabilitation* **2013**, *32*, 69–85. [CrossRef]

15. Aloni, R.; Katz, S. A review of the effect of traumatic brain injury on the human sexual response. *Brain Inj.* **1999**, *13*, 269–280. [CrossRef] [PubMed]
16. Horn, L.J.; Zasler, N.D. Neuroanatomy and neurophysiology of sexual function. *J. Head Trauma Rehabil.* **1990**, *5*, 1–13. [CrossRef]
17. Latella, D.; Maggio, M.G.; De Luca, R.; Maresca, G.; Piazzitta, D.; Sciarrone, F.; Carioti, L.; Manuli, A.; Bramanti, P.; Calabro, R.S. Changes in sexual functioning following traumatic brain injury: An overview on a neglected issue. *J. Clin. Neurosci.* **2018**, *58*, 1–6. [CrossRef] [PubMed]
18. Elliot, M.L.; Biever, L.S. Head injury and sexual dysfunction. *Brain Inj.* **1996**, *10*, 703–718. [CrossRef]
19. Wilkinson, C.W.; Pagulayan, K.F.; Petrie, E.C.; Mayer, C.L.; Colasurdo, E.A.; Shofer, J.B.; Hart, K.L.; Hoff, D.; Tarabochia, M.A.; Peskind, E.R. High prevalence of chronic pituitary and target-organ hormone abnormalities after blast-related mild traumatic brain injury. *Front. Neurol.* **2012**, *3*, 11. [CrossRef]
20. Rothman, M.S.; Arciniegas, D.B.; Filley, C.M.; Wierman, M.E. The neuroendocrine effects of traumatic brain injury. *J. Neuropsychiatry Clin. Neurosci.* **2007**, *19*, 363–372. [CrossRef]
21. Downing, M.; Stolwyk, R.; Ponsford, J. Sexual changes in individuals with traumatic brain injury: A control comparison. *J. Head Trauma Rehabil.* **2013**, *28*, 171–178. [CrossRef]
22. Ponsford, J.; Downing, M.G.; Stolwyk, R. Factors associated with sexuality following traumatic brain injury. *J. Head Trauma Rehabil.* **2013**, *28*, 195–201. [CrossRef]
23. Fraser, E.E.; Downing, M.G.; Ponsford, J.L. Understanding the multidimensional nature of sexuality after traumatic brain injury. *Arch. Phys. Med. Rehabil.* **2020**, *101*, 2080–2086. [CrossRef] [PubMed]
24. Kreuter, M.; Dahllöf, A.; Gudjonsson, G.; Sullivan, M.; Siösteen, A. Sexual adjustment and its predictors after traumatic brain injury. *Brain Inj.* **1998**, *15*, 349–368. [CrossRef] [PubMed]
25. Sander, A.; Maestas, K.; Nick, T.; Pappadis, M.; Hammond, F.; Hanks, R.; Ripley, D. Predictors of sexual functioning and satisfaction 1 year following traumatic brain injury: A TBI model systems multicenter study. *J. Head Trauma Rehabil.* **2013**, *28*, 186–194. [CrossRef] [PubMed]
26. Gill, C.; Sander, A.; Robins, N.; Mazzei, D.; Struchen, M. Exploring experiences of intimacy from the viewpoint of individuals with traumatic brain injury and their partners. *J. Head Trauma Rehabil.* **2011**, *26*, 56–68. [CrossRef]
27. Annon, J.S. The PLISSIT model: A proposed conceptual scheme for the behavioral treatment of sexual problems. *J. Sex Educ. Ther.* **1976**, *2*, 1–15. [CrossRef]
28. Simpson, G. Addressing the sexual concerns of persons with traumatic brain injury in rehabilitation settings: A framework for action. *Brain Impair.* **2001**, *2*, 97–108. [CrossRef]
29. Marier-Deschênes, P.; Lamontagne, M.; Gagnon, M.; Moreno, J. Talking about sexuality in the context of rehabilitation following traumatic brain injury: An integrative review of operational aspects. *Sex. Disabil.* **2019**, *37*, 297–314. [CrossRef]
30. Dyer, K.; Das Nair, R. Talking about sex after traumatic brain injury: Perceptions and experiences of multidisciplinary rehabilitation professionals. *Disabil. Rehabil.* **2014**, *36*, 1431–1438. [CrossRef]
31. Taylor, B.; Davis, S. The extended PLISSIT model for addressing the sexual wellbeing of individuals with an acquired disability or chronic illness. *Sex. Disabil.* **2007**, *25*, 135–139. [CrossRef]
32. Aloni, R.; Katz, S. *Sexual Difficulties after Traumatic Brain Injury and Ways to Deal with It*; Charles C Thomas Publisher: Springfield, IL, USA, 2003.
33. Marier-Deschênes, P.; Gagnon, M.-P.; Lamontagne, M.-E. Co-creation of a post-traumatic brain injury sexuality information toolkit: A patient-oriented project. *Disabil. Rehabil.* **2021**, *43*, 2045–2054. [CrossRef] [PubMed]
34. Marier-Deschênes, P.; Gagnon, M.-P.; Déry, J.; Lamontagne, M.-E. Traumatic Brain Injury and Sexuality: User Experience Study of an Information Toolkit. *J. Particip. Med.* **2020**, *12*, e14874. [CrossRef] [PubMed]
35. Simpson, G. *You and Me: An Educational Program about Sex and Sexuality after a Traumatic Brain Injury*; Brain Injury Rehabilitation Unit, South Western Sydney Area Health Service: Sydney, Australia, 1999.
36. Simpson, G. *You and Me: A Guide to Sex and Sexuality after Traumatic Brain Injury*, 2nd ed.; Brain Injury Rehabilitation Unit, South Western Sydney Area Health Service: Sydney, Australia, 2003.
37. Simpson, G.; Long, E. An evaluation of sex education and information resources and their provision to adults with traumatic brain injury. *J. Head Trauma Rehabil.* **2004**, *19*, 413–428. [CrossRef] [PubMed]
38. Khajeei, D.; Smith, D.; Kachur, B.; Abdul, N. Sexuality Re-education Program Logic Model for People with Traumatic Brain Injury (TBI): Synthesis via Scoping Literature Review. *Sex. Disabil.* **2019**, *37*, 41–61. [CrossRef]
39. Blackerby, W. A treatment model for sexuality disturbance following brain injury. *J. Head Trauma Rehabil.* **1990**, *5*, 73–82. [CrossRef]
40. Bélanger, D. Traumatic brain injury and sexual rehabilitation. *Sexologies* **2009**, *18*, 83–85. [CrossRef]
41. Dombrowski, L.K.; Petrick, J.D.; Strauss, D. Rehabilitation treatment of sexuality issues due to acquired brain injury. *Rehabil. Psychol.* **2000**, *45*, 299–309. [CrossRef]
42. Aloni, R.; Keren, O.; Katz, S. Sex therapy surrogate partners for individuals with very limited functional ability following traumatic brain injury. *Sex. Disabil.* **2007**, *25*, 125–134. [CrossRef]
43. Medlar, T.M. Sexual counseling and traumatic brain injury. *Sex. Disabil.* **1993**, *11*, 57–71. [CrossRef]
44. Simpson, G.; Mccann, B.; Lowy, M. Treatment of premature ejaculation after traumatic brain injury. *Brain Inj.* **2003**, *17*, 723–729. [CrossRef]

45. Simpson, G.K.; McCann, B.; Lowy, M. Treating male sexual dysfunction after traumatic brain injury: Two case reports. *NeuroRehabilitation* **2016**, *38*, 281–289. [CrossRef] [PubMed]
46. Eisenberg, N.W.; Andreski, S.-R.; Mona, L.R. Sexuality and physical disability: A disability-affirmative approach to assessment and intervention within health care. *Curr. Sex. Health Rep.* **2015**, *7*, 19–29. [CrossRef]
47. Nimbi, F.M.; Galizia, R.; Rossi, R.; Limoncin, E.; Ciocca, G.; Fontanesi, L.; Jannini, E.A.; Simonelli, C.; Tambelli, R. The Biopsychosocial model and the Sex-Positive approach: An integrative perspective for sexology and general health care. *Sex. Res. Soc. Policy* **2021**, 1–15. [CrossRef]
48. Little, A.; Byrne, C.; Coetzer, R. The effectiveness of cognitive behaviour therapy for reducing anxiety symptoms following traumatic brain injury: A meta-analysis and systematic review. *NeuroRehabilitation* **2021**, *48*, 67–82. [CrossRef]
49. Hsieh, M.-Y.; Ponsford, J.; Wong, D.; Schönberger, M.; Taffe, J.; Mckay, A. Motivational interviewing and cognitive behaviour therapy for anxiety following traumatic brain injury: A pilot randomised controlled trial. *Neuropsychol. Rehabil.* **2012**, *22*, 585–608. [CrossRef]
50. Ponsford, J.; Lee, N.K.; Wong, D.; McKay, A.; Haines, K.; Alway, Y.; Downing, M.; Furtado, C.; O'Donnell, M.L. Efficacy of motivational interviewing and cognitive behavioral therapy for anxiety and depression symptoms following traumatic brain injury. *Psychol. Med.* **2016**, *46*, 1079–1090. [CrossRef]
51. Nguyen, S.; McKay, A.; Wong, D.; Rajaratnam, S.M.; Spitz, G.; Williams, G.; Mansfield, D.; Ponsford, J.L. Cognitive behavior therapy to treat sleep disturbance and fatigue after traumatic brain injury: A pilot randomized controlled trial. *Arch. Phys. Med. Rehabil.* **2017**, *98*, 1508–1517.e2. [CrossRef] [PubMed]
52. Ymer, L.; McKay, A.; Wong, D.; Frencham, K.; Grima, N.; Tran, J.; Nguyen, S.; Junge, M.; Murray, J.; Spitz, G. Cognitive behavioural therapy versus health education for sleep disturbance and fatigue after acquired brain injury: A pilot randomised trial. *Ann. Phys. Rehabil. Med.* **2021**, *64*, 101560. [CrossRef]
53. Avasthi, A.; Grover, S.; Rao, T.S. Clinical practice guidelines for management of sexual dysfunction. *Indian J. Psychiatry* **2017**, *59*, 91–115. [CrossRef]
54. Metz, M.E.; Epstein, N.B.; McCarthy, B. *Cognitive-Behavioral Therapy for Sexual Dysfunction*; Routledge: New York, NY, USA, 2017.
55. Frühauf, S.; Gerger, H.; Schmidt, H.M.; Munder, T.; Barth, J. Efficacy of psychological interventions for sexual dysfunction: A systematic review and meta-analysis. *Arch. Sex. Behav.* **2013**, *42*, 915–933. [CrossRef]
56. Gallagher, M.; McLeod, H.J.; McMillan, T.M. A systematic review of recommended modifications of CBT for people with cognitive impairments following brain injury. *Neuropsychol. Rehabil.* **2019**, *29*, 1–21. [CrossRef] [PubMed]
57. Nikles, J.; Tate, R.L.; Mitchell, G.; Perdices, M.; McGree, J.M.; Freeman, C.; Jacob, S.; Taing, M.W.; Sterling, M. Personalised treatments for acute whiplash injuries: A pilot study of nested N-of-1 trials in a multiple baseline single-case experimental design. *Contemp. Clin. Trials Commun.* **2019**, *16*, 100480. [CrossRef] [PubMed]
58. Tate, R.L.; Perdices, M. *Single-Case Experimental Designs for Clinical Research and Neurorehabilitation Settings: Planning, Conduct, Analysis and Reporting*; Routledge: London, UK, 2019.
59. Kratochwill, T.R.; Levin, J.R. Enhancing the scientific credibility of single-case intervention research: Randomization to the rescue. In *Single-Case Intervention Research: Methodological and Statistical Advances*, Kratochwill, T.R., Levin, J.R., Eds.; American Psychological Association: Washington, DC, USA, 2014; pp. 53–89.
60. Tate, R.L.; Perdices, M.; Rosenkoetter, U.; Wakim, D.; Godbee, K.; Togher, L.; McDonald, S. Revision of a method quality rating scale for single-case experimental designs and n-of-1 trials: The 15-item Risk of Bias in N-of-1 Trials (RoBiNT) Scale. *Neuropsychol. Rehabil.* **2013**, *23*, 619–638. [CrossRef] [PubMed]
61. Tate, R.L.; Perdices, M.; Rosenkoetter, U.; Shadish, W.; Vohra, S.; Barlow, D.H.; Horner, R.; Kazdin, A.; Kratochwill, T.; McDonald, S. The single-case reporting guideline in behavioural interventions (SCRIBE) 2016 statement. *Phys. Ther.* **2016**, *96*, e1–e10. [CrossRef] [PubMed]
62. Nelson, H.E. *National Adult Reading Test (NART): For the Assessment of Premorbid Intelligence in Patients with Dementia: Test Manual*; NFER-Nelson Publishing Co: Berkshire, UK, 1982.
63. Schmidt, M. *Rey Auditory Verbal Learning Test (RAVLT): A Handbook*; Western Psychological Services: Los Angeles, CA, USA, 1996.
64. Reitan, R. *Trail Making Test: Manual for Administration and Scoring*; Reitan Neuropsychology Laboratory: Tucson, AZ, USA, 1992.
65. Wechsler, D. *WAIS-III Wechsler Adult Intelligence Scale-Third Edition*; The Psychological Corporation: San Antonio, TX, USA, 1997.
66. Krupp, L.B.; LaRocca, N.G.; Muir-Nash, J.; Steinberg, A.D. The fatigue severity scale: Application to patients with multiple sclerosis and systemic lupus erythematosus. *Arch. Neurol.* **1989**, *46*, 1121–1123. [CrossRef]
67. Tulsky, D.S.; Kisala, P.A.; Victorson, D.; Carlozzi, N.; Bushnik, T.; Sherer, M.; Choi, S.W.; Heinemann, A.W.; Chiaravalloti, N.; Sander, A.M. TBI-QOL: Development and calibration of item banks to measure patient reported outcomes following traumatic brain injury. *J. Head Trauma Rehabil.* **2016**, *31*, 40–51. [CrossRef]
68. Krasny-Pacini, A.; Evans, J. Single-case experimental designs to assess intervention effectiveness in rehabilitation: A practical guide. *Ann. Phys. Rehabil. Med.* **2018**, *61*, 164–179. [CrossRef] [PubMed]
69. Stolwyk, R.J.; Downing, M.G.; Taffe, J.; Kreutzer, J.S.; Zasler, N.D.; Ponsford, J.L. Assessment of sexuality following traumatic brain injury: Validation of the Brain Injury Questionnaire of Sexuality. *J. Head Trauma Rehabil.* **2013**, *28*, 164–170. [CrossRef]
70. Snaith, R.; Zigmund, A. *Hospital Anxiety and Depression Scale*; NFER-Nelson Publishing Co: Berkshire, UK, 1994.
71. Rosenberg, M. *Society and the Adolescent Self Image*; Princeton University Press: Princeton, NJ, USA, 1965.

72. Bogner, J.; Bellon, K.; Kolakowsky-Hayner, S.A.; Whiteneck, G. Participation assessment with recombined tools–objective (PART-O). *J. Head Trauma Rehabil.* **2013**, *28*, 337–339. [CrossRef]
73. Kiresuk, T.J.; Sherman, R.E. Goal attainment scaling: A general method for evaluating comprehensive community mental health programs. *Community Ment. Health J.* **1968**, *4*, 443–453. [CrossRef]
74. Turner-Stokes, L. Goal attainment scaling (GAS) in rehabilitation: A practical guide. *Clin. Rehabil.* **2009**, *23*, 362–370. [CrossRef]
75. Lane, J.D.; Gast, D.L. Visual analysis in single case experimental design studies: Brief review and guidelines. *Neuropsychol. Rehabil.* **2014**, *24*, 445–463. [CrossRef] [PubMed]
76. Bulté, I.; Onghena, P. The single-case data analysis package: Analysing single-case experiments with R software. *J. Mod. Appl. Stat. Methods* **2013**, *12*, 450–478. [CrossRef]
77. Manolov, R. R Syntax: Projection of Baseline Trend with Construction of Envelope. Available online: https://dl.dropboxusercontent.com/s/5z9p5362bwlbj7d/ProjectTrend.R2014 (accessed on 1 January 2022).
78. Parker, R.I.; Vannest, K.J.; Davis, J.L. Non-overlap analysis for single-case research. In *Single-Case Intervention Research: Methodological and Statistical Advances*, Kratochwill, T.R., Levin, J.R., Eds.; American Psychological Association: Washington, DC, USA, 2014; pp. 127–151.
79. Vannest, K.J.; Ninci, J. Evaluating intervention effects in single-case research designs. *J. Couns. Dev.* **2015**, *93*, 403–411. [CrossRef]
80. Vannest, K.J.; Peltier, C.; Haas, A. Results reporting in single case experiments and single case meta-analysis. *Res. Dev. Disabil.* **2018**, *79*, 10–18. [CrossRef] [PubMed]
81. Perdices, M. How do you know whether your patient is getting better (or worse)? A user's guide. *Brain Impair.* **2005**, *6*, 219–226. [CrossRef]

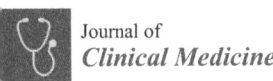

Article

Neurological Music Therapy Rebuilds Structural Connectome after Traumatic Brain Injury: Secondary Analysis from a Randomized Controlled Trial

Aleksi J. Sihvonen [1,2,3,*], Sini-Tuuli Siponkoski [1,2], Noelia Martínez-Molina [1,2], Sari Laitinen [2,4], Milla Holma [5], Mirja Ahlfors [6], Linda Kuusela [7,8], Johanna Pekkola [8], Sanna Koskinen [9] and Teppo Särkämö [1,2]

1. Cognitive Brain Research Unit, Department of Psychology and Logopedics, Faculty of Medicine, University of Helsinki, 00014 Helsinki, Finland
2. Centre of Excellence in Music, Mind, Body and Brain, University of Jyväskylä & University of Helsinki, 00014 Helsinki, Finland
3. School of Health and Rehabilitation Sciences, Queensland Aphasia Research Centre and UQ Centre for Clinical Research, The University of Queensland, Brisbane, QLD 4029, Australia
4. Espoo Hospital, 02740 Espoo, Finland
5. Independent Researcher, 00550 Helsinki, Finland
6. Independent Researcher, 02330 Espoo, Finland
7. Department of Physics, University of Helsinki, 00014 Helsinki, Finland
8. HUS Medical Imaging Center, Department of Radiology, Helsinki Central University Hospital and University of Helsinki, 00014 Helsinki, Finland
9. Clinical Neuropsychology Research Group, Department of Psychology and Logopedics, Faculty of Medicine, University of Helsinki, 00014 Helsinki, Finland
* Correspondence: aleksi.sihvonen@helsinki.fi

Abstract: Background: Traumatic brain injury (TBI) is a common and devastating neurological condition, associated often with poor functional outcome and deficits in executive function. Due to the neuropathology of TBI, neuroimaging plays a crucial role in its assessment, and while diffusion MRI has been proposed as a sensitive biomarker, longitudinal studies evaluating treatment-related diffusion MRI changes are scarce. Recent evidence suggests that neurological music therapy can improve executive functions in patients with TBI and that these effects are underpinned by neuroplasticity changes in the brain. However, studies evaluating music therapy induced structural connectome changes in patients with TBI are lacking. Design: Single-blind crossover (AB/BA) randomized controlled trial (NCT01956136). Objective: Here, we report secondary outcomes of the trial and set out to assess the effect of neurological music therapy on structural white matter connectome changes and their association with improved execute function in patients with TBI. Methods: Using an AB/BA design, 25 patients with moderate or severe TBI were randomized to receive a 3-month neurological music therapy intervention either during the first (AB, $n = 16$) or second (BA, $n = 9$) half of a 6-month follow-up period. Neuropsychological testing and diffusion MRI scans were performed at baseline and at the 3-month and 6-month stage. Findings: Compared to the control group, the music therapy group increased quantitative anisotropy (QA) in the right dorsal pathways (arcuate fasciculus, superior longitudinal fasciculus) and in the corpus callosum and the right frontal aslant tract, thalamic radiation and corticostriatal tracts. The mean increased QA in this network of results correlated with improved executive function. Conclusions: This study shows that music therapy can induce structural white matter neuroplasticity in the post-TBI brain that underpins improved executive function.

Keywords: music therapy; traumatic brain injury; TBI; executive function; rehabilitation; structural connectivity; connectometry; DTI

1. Introduction

Traumatic brain injury (TBI) is a common and devastating neurological disorder, affecting over 50 million people each year worldwide [1], with often poor long-term outcomes [2].

The primary neuropathology associated with TBI is structural white matter damage, that is, axonal injury, established already half a century ago by the seminal post-mortem studies [3,4]. In TBI, the white matter damage disrupts effective neural communication and impairs neural networks that link brain structure to function, typically causing deficits in cognitive, social, and emotional functioning [5–7]. Among the most common, persistent, and disabling aspects of cognitive impairment following TBI is executive dysfunction [8], which is often caused by diffuse axonal injury (DAI) resulting in widespread connectivity deficits in the brain [9,10].

Due to the neuropathology of TBI, neuroimaging plays a crucial role in its assessment. In the acute setting, MRI scans are used to guide appropriate management by detecting brain injuries that require neurosurgical interventions or further monitoring. However, routinely acquired MRI might not reveal findings even in patients with symptoms due to the DAI mechanism [11,12]. Therefore, advanced neuroimaging techniques reflecting white matter structures such as diffusion tensor imaging (DTI) have been under active research in TBI. Studies have shown that TBI patients have structural connectivity deficits in multiple white matter tracts, most commonly in long coursing and commissural fibres that are most vulnerable to injury in TBI [12–14]. After the initial injury, the degeneration of white matter tracts persists for years [15,16] and is associated with poor long-term functional and cognitive outcomes in TBI [16,17].

While DTI has been used to improve the diagnostics and classification system of TBI, very little research has thus far been carried out in determining treatment-induced white matter neuroplasticity changes in TBI. Given the dynamic nature of DAI, intervention studies charting the possible discontinued deterioration or recovery of white matter injury over time would be of great interest. Ultimately, this information would help to target clinical interventions for rehabilitation. A recent animal study suggests that cognitive TBI treatments can induce white matter plasticity [18], but to our best knowledge, studies on treatment-induced structural white matter neuroplasticity in TBI patients have not been published.

Cognitive therapies have emerged as efficient treatments to restore cognitive functions and improve functional outcomes in TBI [19,20]. In cognitive neurological rehabilitation, music has emerged as a viable and applicable tool during the past decades, partly owing to its capacity to engage widespread neural networks across bilateral cortical and subcortical areas [21]. Research findings in stroke patients suggest that music-based interventions engage an array of cognitive functions, resulting in cognitive improvement [22,23] and structural and functional neuroplasticity changes [24,25] in the damaged brain. In our recent randomized controlled trial (RCT) on patients with moderate-to-severe TBI, we found that a 3-month neurological music therapy (NMT) intervention enhanced executive function and increased structural grey matter neuroplasticity in prefrontal areas [26] as well as normalized or enhanced functional connectivity in the brain, especially in frontal and parietal regions [27]. Given the extent of the brain regions and pathways stimulated by music, it is possible that NMT may induce also more widespread structural connectivity changes in TBI, but this has not been studied previously.

Here, using longitudinal diffusion MRI (dMRI) data from our previous RCT [26,27], we set out to determine as a secondary outcome of the trial NMT-induced structural white matter connectivity changes and their association with improved executive function in a sample of 25 TBI patients with a 6-month follow-up. To do this, we carried out white matter connectometry analysis utilizing quantitative anisotropy (QA), which has been shown to be superior to conventional single-tensor based or tract-based analysis [28]. Connectometry analysis utilizes permutation testing to identify group differences in white matter tracts across the whole brain and has been used in neurological patients, for example, to uncover white matter tracts subserving word production [29] and verb retrieval [30] in post-stroke aphasia. Based on our previous findings of increased grey matter volume and functional connectivity, which were most evident in right prefrontal areas, after the NMT [26,27], we hypothesized that it would induce structural connectivity changes especially in the right frontal and dorsal pathways.

2. Materials and Methods

2.1. Subjects and Study Design

Forty TBI patients from the Helsinki and Uusimaa Region of Finland were recruited through the Brain Injury Clinic of the Helsinki University Central Hospital (HUCH), Validia Rehabilitation Helsinki, and the Department of Neurology of the Lohja Hospital during 2014–2017 to this RCT (NCT01956136). The inclusion criteria were: (1) diagnosed TBI according to the International Statistical Classification of Diseases and Related Health Problems, 10th revision (ICD-10), fulfilling the criteria of at least moderate severity (Glasgow Coma Scale [GCS] score: ≤ 12 and/or loss of consciousness >30 min and/or post-traumatic amnesia [PTA] ≥ 24 h and positive findings on CT/MRI); (2) time since injury ≤ 24 months at the time of recruitment; (3) cognitive symptoms caused by TBI (attention, executive function, memory); (4) no previous neurological or severe psychiatric illnesses or substance abuse; (5) age 16–60 years; (6) native Finnish speaking or bilingual with sufficient communication skills in Finnish; (7) living in the Helsinki-Uusimaa area; and (8) understanding the purpose of the study and being able to give an informed consent. Patients with GCS score 9–12 and/or loss of consciousness 30 min–24 h and/or PTA 1–7 days and abnormal structural imaging on CT/MRI were defined as having a moderate TBI, and patients with GCS score 1–9 and/or loss of consciousness >24 h and/or PTA > 7 days and abnormal structural imaging on CT/MRI were defined as having a severe TBI [31]. Both the extended Glasgow Outcome Scale (GOSE) [32] and the Neurological Outcome Scale for Traumatic Brain Injury (NOS-TBI) [33] were administered to obtain information of the overall symptoms and current functional outcome after TBI. The trial was conducted according to the Declaration of Helsinki and was consistent with good clinical practice and the applicable regulatory requirements. The trial protocol was approved by the Coordinating Ethics Committee of the Hospital District of Helsinki and Uusimaa (reference number 338/13/03/00/2012) and all participants signed an informed consent.

The study was a single-blind crossover RCT with a 6-month follow-up period. During 2014–2017, 4994 patients with TBI were screened for eligibility, 190 met the inclusion criteria, and 40 were randomized to the AB (n = 20) and BA (n = 20) groups. The randomization was stratified for lesion laterality and performed using a random number generator by a person not involved in patient recruitment or assessments. To ensure steady allocation to both groups across the trial, the randomization was done in batches of two consecutive patients. After the baseline measurements at time point 1 (TP1), which included MRI scans and neuropsychological assessments, the AB group received NMT in addition to standard care for the first 3 months, whereas the BA group received only standard care. At the 3-month crossover point (TP2), follow-up measurements using the same outcome measures were carried out. After this, the BA group received NMT and standard care for 3 months and the AB group received only standard care. At the 6-month completion point (TP3), the measurements were carried out once again. All assessments were carried out by research personnel blinded to the patients' group allocation. Due to the nature of the intervention, patients were not blinded. Standard care comprised any physical therapy, occupational therapy, speech therapy or neuropsychological rehabilitation which the patients received in public (or private) healthcare during the study period. There were no statistically significant differences between the AB and BA groups in the amount of received standard care [26].

Out of the 40 randomized patients, 1 participant dropped out before the TP1 measurements, 2 participants dropped out before TP2, and another 3 participants dropped out before TP3. The dropouts were mainly due to lack of energy and motivation. All dropouts (n = 6) occurred in the BA group, which was likely linked to the long waiting period before the intervention. Of these, five took place before the onset of the intervention. Of the remaining 34 patients, 1 was excluded from the analyses due to intensive self-implemented piano training, which was not part of the trial protocol, and 8 were excluded from the analyses due to lack of MRI data owing to contraindications or technical difficulties during the scanning. Finally, 25 patients (AB: $n = 16$, BA: $n = 9$) completed the MRI acquisition in the three time points and were included in the present study. The flowchart of the included patients with TBI is shown in Figure 1.

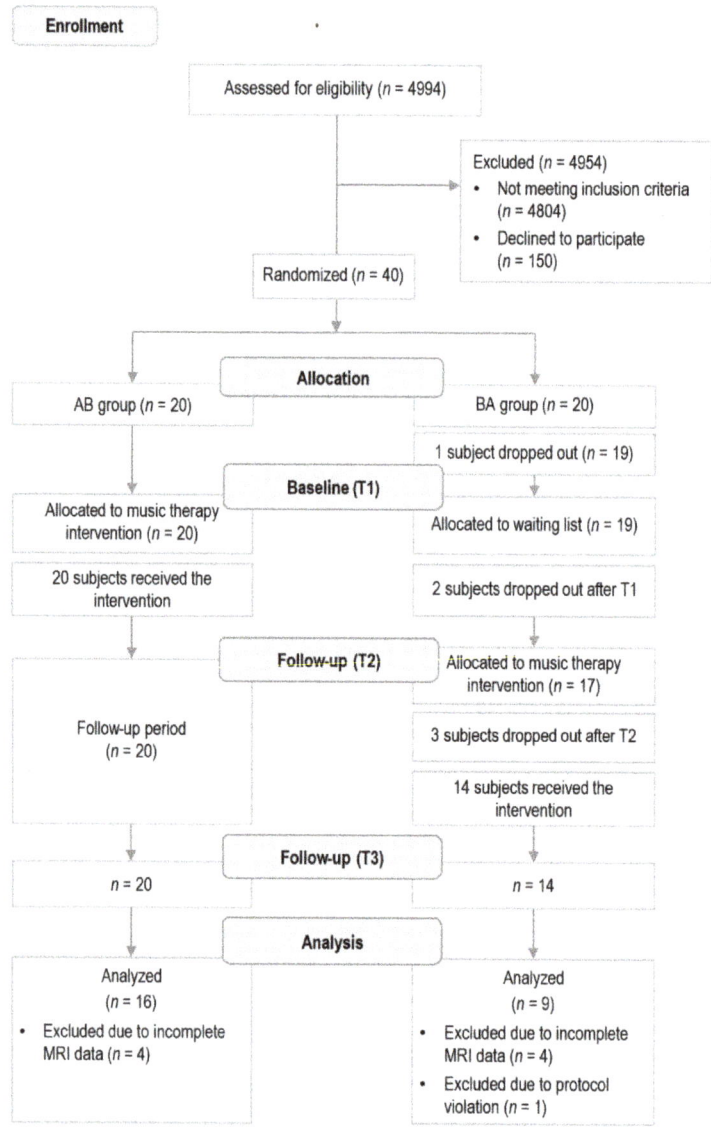

Figure 1. Flow diagram outlining the trial.

2.2. Intervention

The NMT intervention is described in detail in our previous publication [26]. Briefly, it consisted of 20 individual therapy sessions (2 times/week, 60 min/session) held by a trained music therapist at Validia Rehabilitation Helsinki. No previous musical experience was required to participate in the NMT. The focus of the NMT was on active musical production using different instruments (drums, piano) in three training modules involving (i) rhythmical training (playing sequences of musical rhythms and coordinated bimanual movements on a djembe drum and on own body), (ii) structured cognitive-motor training (playing musical exercises on a drum set with varying levels of movement elements and composition of drum pads), and (iii) assisted music playing (learning to play own favourite songs on the piano with the help of figure notes). All modules also included musical improvisation to facilitate more creative and interactive musical expression The difficulty level of the exercises was initially adjusted and then increased in a stepwise manner within and across the NMT sessions, to meet the skill level and progression of the patient.

2.3. Neuropsychological Assessment

The primary behavioural outcome measure was change in performance on the Frontal Assessment Battery (FAB) [34]. Assessing global executive function and being applicable across all severity levels of TBI, the FAB measures different aspects of frontal lobe functions and consists of six subtests exploring conceptualization (similarities subtest), mental flexibility (lexical fluency), motor programming (Luria's fist-edge-palm test), sensitivity to interference (conflicting instructions), inhibitory control (go-no go task) and environmental autonomy (prehension behaviour). The FAB total percent score (percentage correct) formed the composite score of executive function.

2.4. MRI Data Acquisition and Reconstruction

All patients were scanned on a 3T Philips Achieva MRI scanner (Philips Medical Systems) with a standard 8-channel head matrix coil at the HUS Helsinki Medical Imaging Center at HUCH. The MRI protocol comprised high-resolution T1-weighted anatomical images and whole-brain diffusion-weighted imaging (DWI) data (TR = 11,106 ms, TE = 60 ms, acquisition matrix = 112 × 112, 70 axial slices, voxel size = 2.0 × 2.0 × 2.0 mm^3) with one non-diffusion weighted volume and 32 diffusion weighted volumes (b = 1000 s/mm^2).

The DWI data were reconstructed in the Montreal Neurological Institute (MNI) space using q-space diffeomorphic reconstruction (QSDR) [35] that allows the construction of spin distribution functions (SDFs) [36]. The b-table was checked by an automatic quality control routine to ensure its accuracy [37]. Normalization was carried out using the anisotropy map of each participant and a diffusion sampling length ratio of 1.25 was used. The data output was resampled to 2 mm isotropic resolution. Quality of the normalization was inspected using the R^2 values denoting goodness-of-fit between the participant's anisotropy map and template as well as inspecting the anatomical localisation of each participant's forceps major and minor to confirm the normalization quality [29]. The restricted diffusion was quantified using restricted diffusion imaging [38] and QA was extracted as the local connectome fingerprint [39] and used in the connectometry analysis. QA-based tractography has been shown to outperform traditional fractional anisotropy-based methods by being more specific to individual's connectivity patterns [39] and less susceptible to the partial volume effect of crossing fibres and free water, as well as to provide better resolution in tractography [40].

2.5. Regions of Interest

To focus the analyses on the neural structures related to music therapy induced changes in TBI, the Automated Anatomical Labelling atlas 3 (AAL3) [41] was used to define the ROIs based on our previous studies [26,27]. Four regions were derived from the AAL3: right inferior frontal gyrus (pars operculum and triangularis), Rolandic operculum, and inferior parietal lobule.

2.6. Data Analysis

Diffusion MRI connectometry [28] analyses were carried out using DSI Studio (http://dsi-studio.labsolver.org, version 7 April 2021). Connectometry was used to derive the correlational tractography that has longitudinal QA changes correlated with Group. To do this, two nonparametric multiple regression models were used to identify local connectome (i.e., QA) changes across time (TP2 > TP1 and TP3 > TP2) between the groups (AB and BA). Local connectomes exceeding a *t*-statistic threshold of 2 were selected and tracked using a deterministic fibre tracking algorithm [40] to obtain correlational tractography. The tracks were filtered by topology-informed pruning [42] with 4 iterations, and a length threshold of 20 voxel distance was used to identify significant tracts. Bootstrap resampling with 10,000 randomized permutations was used to obtain the null distribution of the track length and estimate the false discovery rates (FDR).

To evaluate whether the intervention-induced longitudinal QA changes were associated with behavioural gains in executive function, the mean QA change in the network of significant connectometry results was extracted for each patient and exported to SPSS (IBM SPSS Statistics for Windows, v.27.0. IBM Corp.: Armonk, NY, USA). Then, nonparametric correlations (Spearman, two-tailed) were calculated over the whole sample between the longitudinal mean QA change in the significant connectometry results and the longitudinal FAB score change to determine the structural relationship with behavioural gains. To control for multiple comparisons, FDR-correction was applied.

3. Results

The demographic, clinical, and musical background information of the patients is presented in Table 1. There were no significant differences between the AB (n = 16) and BA (n = 9) groups.

Table 1. Demographic, clinical, and musical background information (n = 25).

	AB	BA	Difference between Groups (p)
Demographic information			
Age	42.1 (14.9)	40.8 (11.5)	0.814 (t)
Gender (female/male)	7/9	3/6	0.691 (X^2)
Education in years	14.3 (2.7)	14.9 (2.1)	0.535 (t)
Clinical information			
TBI severity (moderate/severe)	13/3	5/4	0.170 (X^2)
GCS (severe/moderate/minor) [a]	2/3/10	2/0/6	0.357 (X^2)
PTA classification (mild/moderate/severe) [b]	9/3/2	3/3/2	0.330 (X^2)
Cause of injury (traffic-related/fall/other)	6/9/1	2/3/4	0.072 (X^2)
Time since injury (months)	8.4 (6.0)	7.1 (6.1)	0.622 (t)
Lesion laterality [c] (left/right/both)	3/1/11	3/0/6	0.603 (t)
DAI [c] (yes/no)	6/9	6/3	0.400 (X^2)
Hemorrhages, bleeds or ischemic injury [c] (yes/no)	10/5	5/4	0.678 (X^2)
GOSE [d]	5.2 (1.5)	5.6 (1.1)	0.541 (t)
NOS-TBI [e]	2.0 (2.1)	1.8 (2.3)	0.812 (t)
Musical background			
Instrument playing (yes/no)	11/6	5/3	1.000 (X^2)
Years of playing	5.2 (11.3)	3.8 (5.8)	0.783 (t)
Singing (yes/no)	9/7	3/6	0.411 (X^2)
Years of singing	7.9 (13.7)	1.3 (3.0)	0.170 (t)
Dancing (yes/no)	9/7	4/5	0.688 (X^2)
Years of dancing	5.4 (10.9)	4.8 (9.8)	0.889 (t)

[a] 3–8 = severe, 9–12 = moderate, 13–15 = minor; [b] 1 = mild (<1 day), 2 = moderate (1–7 days), 3 = severe (>1 weeks); [c] Based on MRI findings; [d] Glasgow Outcome Scale Extended; [e] Neurological Outcome Scale for TBI.

The connectometry analyses comparing the QA changes from baseline (TP1) to 3-month (TP2) stage between the groups revealed that the group receiving the NMT (AB) showed greater QA increase (TP2 > TP1) compared to the group receiving only standard care (BA) in the right dorsal pathways (arcuate fasciculus, superior longitudinal fasciculus, frontal aslant tract) and in the right thalamic radiation and corticostriatal tract (FDR = 0.005; d = 0.97, Figure 2A). The mean increased QA in this network of results correlated with increased FAB score (r = 0.46, p = 0.021). No significant QA increases from TP1 to TP2 were observed in the BA group compared to the AB group.

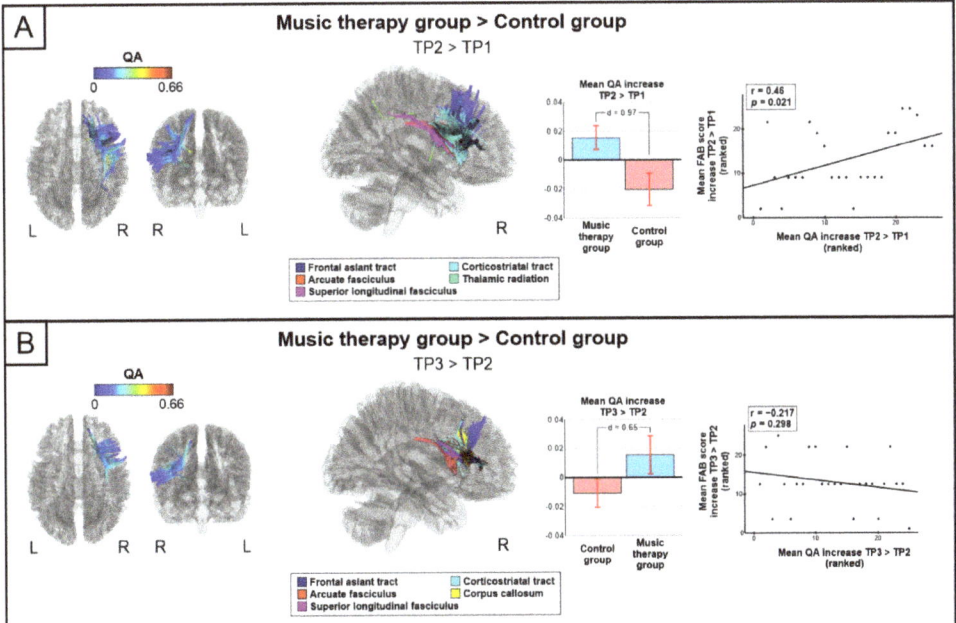

Figure 2. Music therapy induced structural white matter connectometry changes. Significant connectometry changes showing increased structural white matter connectivity between (**A**) music therapy and control group (TP2 > TP1) and (**B**) music therapy and control group (TP3 > TP2). Mean longitudinal QA change correlations (Spearman, two-tailed) to FAB score change are shown with scatter plots. Bar plots for mean QA in the significant connectivity results for both groups are shown: bar = mean, error-bar = standard error of mean, d = Cohen's d, L = left, QA = quantitative anisotropy, R = Right, TP = time point.

Similar findings were observed when comparing the groups between from the 3-month (TP2) to the 6-month (TP3) stage: the group receiving the NMT (BA) showed greater QA increase (TP3 > TP2) in the right dorsal pathways (arcuate fasciculus, superior longitudinal fasciculus, frontal aslant tract) and in the right corticostriatal tract as well as in the corpus callosum (FDR = 0.009; d = 0.65, Figure 2B) compared to the group receiving only standard care (AB). Significant correlations between the mean increased QA and increased FAB score were not observed. There were no significant QA increases from TP2 to TP3 in the AB group compared to the BA group.

4. Discussion

This structural white matter connectometry study set out to determine structural connectome changes induced by NMT and their relation to improved executive function in patients with TBI. Our novel findings were that compared to standard care, NMT enhanced structural connectivity in right frontal dorsal and projection pathways as well as in the corpus callosum. The enhanced structural connectivity was associated with improved executive function. To our best knowledge, this is the first study on patients to link treatment-induced white matter neuroplasticity changes with improved cognitive outcome in TBI. This study provides novel and crucial information about the neural mechanisms of music therapy induced brain recovery following TBI.

Executive dysfunction is considered to be the core clinical feature of TBI [20], particularly in moderate-to-severe cases, on which our study focused on, contributing significantly to both acute and chronic disability. Executive function is a broad term referring to higher order cognitive processes that enable individuals to regulate their thoughts and actions during goal-directed behaviour [43]. These processes are widely thought to include inhibition of prepotent responses, attentional control, task switching and working memory updating [44]. Neurally, executive function contributes to the coordination of these processes across a network of brain structures that need to work in concert. A large-scale quantitative meta-analysis of 193 functional neuroimaging studies has revealed that such executive control network comprises dorsolateral prefrontal, anterior cingulate, and parietal cortices [45]. To allow efficient communication, these spatially distributed brain regions are structurally connected via white matter pathways [46]. The three dominant structural components of this executive control network are (i) interhemispheric connections via the corpus callosum, (ii) fronto-parietal pathways, mainly the superior longitudinal fasciculus connecting dorsolateral prefrontal cortex and the parietal lobe, and (iii) the corticostriatal pathways between right dorsolateral prefrontal cortex and striatum [46–48].

The dependence on multiple white matter pathways working in concert makes executive function vulnerable to reduced communication efficiency following DAI in TBI. This was reflected in a recent meta-analysis evaluating the relationships between white matter fractional anisotropy values and executive dysfunction following TBI [49]. Executive dysfunction in TBI was associated with damage to various white matter pathways, but was most significantly correlated with decreased fractional anisotropy values in the superior longitudinal fasciculus, an association tract connecting the frontal, parietal and temporal lobes [49]. Together with commissural tracts, association tracts are most critical for cognition because they transfer information between lobes and hemispheres [50]. They are also most vulnerable to injury in TBI [12–14] and undergo long-term degeneration after the initial injury [15,16], giving rise to the functional and cognitive outcomes in TBI [16,17].

The white matter is a biologically active component of the brain, amenable to treatment-induced modifications that bring about beneficial behavioural change [24,51]. In TBI, two principles of white matter structure and function are pertinent to acknowledge in the rehabilitation. First, the severity and prognosis are related to the degree of initial axonal injury, that is, if the axonal scaffolding on which myelin can regain its integrity is preserved, the axonal recovery is plausible, and therefore the restoration of function [52]. Second, white matter structure possesses the capacity of plasticity, that is, modification of its structure by experience [53]. Since neurogenesis has no known clinically meaningful effect on (adult) brain recovery, restoration of function relies upon the ability of spared neurons to grow neurites and form new synapses to rebuild and remodel the injured networks [54,55]. This requires neuronal activity, that is, stimulation via rehabilitation [56] that provides a fertile ground for neuroplasticity and has been shown to produce plastic changes in the white matter including activity-dependent myelination [57] and enhanced oligodendrogenesis [58].

Our present results showing that NMT-induced white matter plasticity changes underpinning the improved executive function comprise the right (i) corpus callosum, (ii) frontoparietal connections, and (iii) the right corticostriatal tract parallel strongly with the previous evidence on the structural core of the executive control network [46–48,59] as well as with the evidence on critical white matter damage loci in TBI giving rise to executive dysfunction [49]. Our results are also well in line with previous DTI studies which have reported neuroplasticity changes in the arcuate fasciculus [60,61], superior longitudinal fasciculus [62,63], corpus callosum [63,64], and corticospinal tract [65] induced by musical training in healthy subjects and in the frontal aslant tract induced by music-based rehabilitation in stroke patients [24]. While previous evidence on treatment-related white matter plasticity in TBI is scarce, our results argue that structural connectivity can be enhanced via treatments in TBI and that the treatment-related white matter changes are associated with improved cognitive outcome.

The present study has some potential limitations that need to be considered when evaluating the findings. Due to the study design, it is impossible to infer whether some components of the intervention, for example active or passive engagement during music-making or movements while playing musical instruments, were more relevant to clinical improvement than others. Moreover, although the study is the largest RCT utilizing NMT in moderate-to-severe TBI to date, the sample size remains relatively modest ($n = 25$) and may preclude the detection of smaller neuroplasticity effect sizes due to lack of statistical power. The limited sample size also prevents us from making more fine-grained analyses of what are the differences and commonalities in the patterns of white matter changes and executive function recovery between different time points. Therefore, future longitudinal studies with a stratification of patients by time since injury as well as lesion site would be warranted to explicitly test the relationship of music therapy induced cognitive and neuroplasticity changes across the recovery spectrum.

5. Conclusions

In conclusion, the present results suggest that the positive effects of neurological music therapy on executive function recovery in TBI are underpinned by structural white matter reorganization within the structural executive function network. Clinically, together with our previous results [26,27,66], this evidence suggests that music therapy is a feasible tool to induce structural white matter neuroplasticity in the post-TBI brain that underpin improved executive function.

Author Contributions: Conceptualization, S.-T.S., S.L., J.P., S.K. and T.S.; Data curation, S.-T.S., N.M.-M. and L.K.; Formal analysis, A.J.S.; Funding acquisition, T.S.; Investigation, S.-T.S., N.M.-M., S.L., M.H., M.A. and L.K.; Methodology, A.J.S., S.-T.S., S.L., L.K. and J.P.; Project administration, S.-T.S. and T.S.; Resources, S.L. and T.S.; Software, A.J.S. and N.M.-M.; Supervision, N.M.-M., S.K. and T.S.; Visualization, A.J.S.; Writing—original draft, A.J.S. and T.S.; Writing—review & editing, A.J.S., S.-T.S., N.M.-M., S.L., M.H., M.A., L.K., J.P., S.K. and T.S. All authors have read and agreed to the published version of the manuscript.

Funding: Financial support was provided by the Academy of Finland, (grants 277693, 299044, 306625), European Research Council (grant 803466), University of Helsinki (grant 313/51/2013), Social Insurance Institution of Finland (grant no. 18/26/2013), Yrjö Johansson Foundation (grant no. 6464), Finnish Association of People with Physical Disabilities and Helsinki Uusimaa Hospital district (grants 461/13/01/00/2015, 154/13/01/2016), Finnish Cultural Foundation (grant 191230), Orion Research Foundation sr, Maire Taponen Foundation and Signe, and Ane Gyllenberg Foundation.

Institutional Review Board Statement: The study was conducted according to the guidelines of the Declaration of Helsinki, and approved by the Coordinating Ethics Committee of the Hospital District of Helsinki and Uusimaa (reference number 338/13/03/00/2012).

Informed Consent Statement: Informed consent was obtained from all subjects involved in the study.

Data Availability Statement: Anonymized data reported in this manuscript are available from the corresponding author upon reasonable request and subject to approval by the appropriate regulatory committees and officials. No custom codes were used in any of the analyses.

Acknowledgments: Open access funding provided by University of Helsinki. We would like to thank the multi-disciplinary team of experts who helped in the planning and implementation of the study: music therapists Päivi Jordan-Kilkki and Esa Ala-Ruona, Mari Tervaniemi, neurologists Anne Vehmas and Susanna Melkas, research nurse Veera Lotvonen, neuropsychologists Jaana Sarajuuri and Titta Ilvonen and the staff of Validia Rehabilitation Helsinki. Above all, we want to thank the patients with TBI and their family members who participated in the study.

Conflicts of Interest: The authors declare no conflict of interest.

References

1. Maas, A.I.R.; Menon, D.K.; David Adelson, P.D.; Andelic, N.; Bell, M.J.; Belli, A.; Bragge, P.; Brazinova, A.; Büki, A.; Chesnut, R.M.; et al. Traumatic brain injury: Integrated approaches to improve prevention, clinical care, and research. *Lancet Neurol.* **2017**, *16*, 987–1048. [CrossRef]
2. Colantonio, A.; Ratcliff, G.; Chase, S.; Kelsey, S.; Escobar, M.; Vernich, L. Long term outcomes after moderate to severe traumatic brain injury. *Disabil. Rehabil.* **2004**, *26*, 253–261. [CrossRef] [PubMed]
3. Strich, S.J. Diffuse degeneration of the cerebral white matter in severe dementia following head injury. *J. Neurol. Neurosurg. Psychiatry* **1956**, *19*, 163–185. [CrossRef] [PubMed]
4. Peerless, S.J.; Rewcastle, N.B. Shear injuries of the brain. *Can. Med. Assoc. J.* **1967**, *96*, 577–582.
5. Hoofien, D.; Gilboa, A.; Vakil, E.; Donovick, P.J. Traumatic brain injury (TBI) 10–20 years later: A comprehensive outcome study of psychiatric symptomatology, cognitive abilities and psychosocial functioning. *Brain Inj.* **2001**, *15*, 189–209. [CrossRef]
6. Langlois, J.A.; Rutland-Brown, W.; Wald, M.M. The epidemiology and impact of traumatic brain injury: A brief overview. *J. Head Trauma Rehabil.* **2006**, *21*, 375–378. [CrossRef]
7. Dikmen, S.S.; Corrigan, J.D.; Levin, H.S.; MacHamer, J.; Stiers, W.; Weisskopf, M.G. Cognitive outcome following traumatic brain injury. *J. Head Trauma Rehabil.* **2009**, *24*, 430–438. [CrossRef]
8. McDonald, B.C.; Flashman, L.A.; Saykin, A.J. Executive dysfunction following traumatic brain injury: Neural substrates and treatment strategies. *NeuroRehabilitation* **2002**, *17*, 333–344. [CrossRef]
9. Kinnunen, K.M.; Greenwood, R.; Powell, J.H.; Leech, R.; Hawkins, P.C.; Bonnelle, V.; Patel, M.C.; Counsell, S.J.; Sharp, D.J. White matter damage and cognitive impairment after traumatic brain injury. *Brain* **2011**, *134*, 449–463. [CrossRef]
10. Sharp, D.J.; Scott, G.; Leech, R. Network dysfunction after traumatic brain injury. *Nat. Rev. Neurol.* **2014**, *10*, 156–166. [CrossRef]
11. Scheid, R.; Walther, K.; Guthke, T.; Preul, C.; Von Cramon, D.Y. Cognitive sequelae of diffuse axonal injury. *Arch. Neurol.* **2006**, *63*, 418–424. [CrossRef] [PubMed]
12. Brandstack, N.; Kurki, T.; Tenovuo, O. Quantitative diffusion-tensor tractography of long association tracts in patients with traumatic brain injury without associated findings at routine MR imaging. *Radiology* **2013**, *267*, 231–239. [CrossRef] [PubMed]
13. Palacios, E.M.; Owen, J.P.; Yuh, E.L.; Wang, M.B.; Vassar, M.J.; Ferguson, A.R.; Diaz-Arrastia, R.; Giacino, J.T.; Okonkwo, D.O.; Robertson, C.S.; et al. The evolution of white matter microstructural changes after mild traumatic brain injury: A longitudinal DTI and NODDI study. *Sci. Adv.* **2020**, *6*, eaaz6892. [CrossRef]
14. Douglas, D.B.; Iv, M.; Douglas, P.K.; Anderson, A.; Vos, S.B.; Bammer, R.; Zeineh, M.; Wintermark, M. Diffusion tensor imaging of TBI: Potentials and challenges. *Top. Magn. Reson. Imaging* **2015**, *24*, 241–251. [CrossRef] [PubMed]
15. Johnson, V.E.; Stewart, J.E.; Begbie, F.D.; Trojanowski, J.Q.; Smith, D.H.; Stewart, W. Inflammation and white matter degeneration persist for years after a single traumatic brain injury. *Brain* **2013**, *136*, 28–42. [CrossRef]
16. Farbota, K.D.; Bendlin, B.B.; Alexander, A.L.; Rowley, H.A.; Dempsey, R.J.; Johnson, S.C. Longitudinal diffusion tensor imaging and neuropsychological correlates in traumatic brain injury patients. *Front. Hum. Neurosci.* **2012**, *6*, 160. [CrossRef]
17. Hellström, T.; Westlye, L.T.; Kaufmann, T.; Trung Doan, N.; Søberg, H.L.; Sigurdardottir, S.; Nordhøy, W.; Helseth, E.; Andreassen, O.A.; Andelic, N. White matter microstructure is associated with functional, cognitive and emotional symptoms 12 months after mild traumatic brain injury. *Sci. Rep.* **2017**, *7*, 1–14. [CrossRef]
18. Braeckman, K.; Descamps, B.; Caeyenberghs, K.; Vanhove, C. Longitudinal DTI changes following cognitive training therapy in a mild traumatic brain injury rat model. *Front. Neurosci.* **2018**, *12*. [CrossRef]
19. Cernich, A.N.; Kurtz, S.M.; Mordecai, K.L.; Ryan, P.B. Cognitive rehabilitation in traumatic brain injury. *Curr. Treat. Options Neurol.* **2010**, *12*, 412–423. [CrossRef]
20. Cicerone, K.; Levin, H.; Malec, J.; Stuss, D.; Whyte, J.; Edwards, E. Cognitive rehabilitation interventions for executive function: Moving from bench to bedside in patients with traumatic brain injury. *J. Cogn. Neurosci.* **2006**, *18*, 1212–1222. [CrossRef]
21. Sihvonen, A.J.; Särkämö, T.; Leo, V.; Tervaniemi, M.; Altenmüller, E.; Soinila, S. Music-based interventions in neurological rehabilitation. *Lancet Neurol.* **2017**, *16*, 648–660. [CrossRef]
22. Särkämö, T.; Tervaniemi, M.; Laitinen, S.; Forsblom, A.; Soinila, S.; Mikkonen, M.; Autti, T.; Silvennoinen, H.M.; Erkkilä, J.; Laine, M.; et al. Music listening enhances cognitive recovery and mood after middle cerebral artery stroke. *Brain* **2008**, *131*, 866–876. [CrossRef]
23. Sihvonen, A.J.; Leo, V.; Ripollés, P.; Lehtovaara, T.; Ylönen, A.; Rajanaro, P.; Laitinen, S.; Forsblom, A.; Saunavaara, J.; Autti, T.; et al. Vocal music enhances memory and language recovery after stroke: Pooled results from two RCTs. *Ann. Clin. Transl. Neurol.* **2020**, *7*, 2272–2287. [CrossRef] [PubMed]
24. Sihvonen, A.J.; Ripollés, P.; Leo, V.; Saunavaara, J.; Parkkola, R.; Rodriguez-Fornells, A.; Soinila, S.; Särkämö, T.; Rodríguez-Fornells, A.; Soinila, S.; et al. Vocal music listening enhances post-stroke language network reorganization. *eNeuro* **2021**, *8*, 34140351. [CrossRef] [PubMed]
25. Särkämö, T.; Ripollés, P.; Vepsäläinen, H.; Autti, T.; Silvennoinen, H.M.; Salli, E.; Laitinen, S.; Forsblom, A.; Soinila, S.; Rodríguez-Fornells, A. Structural changes induced by daily music listening in the recovering brain after middle cerebral artery stroke: A voxel-based morphometry study. *Front. Hum. Neurosci.* **2014**, *8*, 245. [CrossRef]
26. Siponkoski, S.T.; Martínez-Molina, N.; Kuusela, L.; Laitinen, S.; Holma, M.; Ahlfors, M.; Jordan-Kilkki, P.; Ala-Kauhaluoma, K.; Melkas, S.; Pekkola, J.; et al. Music Therapy Enhances Executive Functions and Prefrontal Structural Neuroplasticity after Traumatic Brain Injury: Evidence from a Randomized Controlled Trial. *J. Neurotrauma* **2020**, *37*, 618–634. [CrossRef]

27. Martínez-Molina, N.; Siponkoski, S.T.; Kuusela, L.; Laitinen, S.; Holma, M.; Ahlfors, M.; Jordan-Kilkki, P.; Ala-Kauhaluoma, K.; Melkas, S.; Pekkola, J.; et al. Resting-State Network Plasticity Induced by Music Therapy after Traumatic Brain Injury. *Neural Plast.* **2021**, *2021*, 6682471. [CrossRef]
28. Yeh, F.C.; Badre, D.; Verstynen, T. Connectometry: A statistical approach harnessing the analytical potential of the local connectome. *Neuroimage* **2016**, *125*, 162–171. [CrossRef]
29. Hula, W.D.; Panesar, S.; Gravier, M.L.; Yeh, F.C.; Dresang, H.C.; Dickey, M.W.; Fernandez-Miranda, J.C. Structural white matter connectometry of word production in aphasia: An observational study. *Brain* **2020**, *143*, 2532–2544. [CrossRef]
30. Dresang, H.C.; Hula, W.D.; Yeh, F.-C.; Warren, T.; Dickey, M.W. White-Matter Neuroanatomical Predictors of Aphasic Verb Retrieval. *Brain Connect.* **2021**, *11*, 319–330. [CrossRef]
31. Traumatic Brain Injury. Current Care Guidelines. Working group Set up by the Finnish Medical Society Duodecim, Finnish Neurological Society, Societas Medicinae Physicalis et Rehabilitationis Fenniae, Finnish Neurosurgical Society, Finnish Neuropsychological Society and Association of Finnish Insurance Medicine Doctors, Helsinki. Helsinki: The Finnish Medical Society Duodecim, 2021 (Referred 6.4.2022). Available online: www.kaypahoito.fi (accessed on 6 April 2022).
32. Wilson, J.T.L.; Pettigrew, L.E.L.; Teasdale, G.M. Structured interviews for the Glasgow Outcome Scale and the extended Glasgow Outcome Scale: Guidelines for their use. *J. Neurotrauma* **1998**, *15*, 573–580. [CrossRef] [PubMed]
33. Wilde, E.A.; McCauley, S.R.; Kelly, T.M.; Weyand, A.M.; Pedroza, C.; Levin, H.S.; Clifton, G.L.; Schnelle, K.P.; Shah, M.V.; Moretti, P. The neurological outcome scale for traumatic brain injury (NOS-TBI): I. Construct validity. *J. Neurotrauma* **2010**, *27*, 983–989. [CrossRef] [PubMed]
34. Dubois, B.; Slachevsky, A.; Litvan, I.; Pillon, B. The FAB: A frontal assessment battery at bedside. *Neurology* **2000**, *55*, 1621–1626. [CrossRef]
35. Yeh, F.C.; Tseng, W.Y.I. NTU-90: A high angular resolution brain atlas constructed by q-space diffeomorphic reconstruction. *Neuroimage* **2011**, *58*, 91–99. [CrossRef] [PubMed]
36. Yeh, F.C.; Wedeen, V.J.; Tseng, W.Y.I. Generalized q-sampling imaging. *IEEE Trans. Med. Imaging* **2010**, *29*, 1626–1635. [CrossRef]
37. Schilling, K.G.; Yeh, F.C.; Nath, V.; Hansen, C.; Williams, O.; Resnick, S.; Anderson, A.W.; Landman, B.A. A fiber coherence index for quality control of B-table orientation in diffusion MRI scans. *Magn. Reson. Imaging* **2019**, *58*, 82–89. [CrossRef]
38. Yeh, F.C.; Liu, L.; Hitchens, T.K.; Wu, Y.L. Mapping immune cell infiltration using restricted diffusion MRI. *Magn. Reson. Med.* **2017**, *77*, 603–612. [CrossRef]
39. Yeh, F.C.; Vettel, J.M.; Singh, A.; Poczos, B.; Grafton, S.T.; Erickson, K.I.; Tseng, W.Y.I.; Verstynen, T.D. Quantifying Differences and Similarities in Whole-Brain White Matter Architecture Using Local Connectome Fingerprints. *PLoS Comput. Biol.* **2016**, *12*, e1005203. [CrossRef]
40. Yeh, F.C.; Verstynen, T.D.; Wang, Y.; Fernández-Miranda, J.C.; Tseng, W.Y.I. Deterministic diffusion fiber tracking improved by quantitative anisotropy. *PLoS ONE* **2013**, *8*, e80713. [CrossRef]
41. Rolls, E.T.; Huang, C.C.; Lin, C.P.; Feng, J.; Joliot, M. Automated anatomical labelling atlas 3. *Neuroimage* **2020**, *206*, 116189. [CrossRef]
42. Yeh, F.C.; Panesar, S.; Barrios, J.; Fernandes, D.; Abhinav, K.; Meola, A.; Fernandez-Miranda, J.C. Automatic Removal of False Connections in Diffusion MRI Tractography Using Topology-Informed Pruning (TIP). *Neurotherapeutics* **2019**, *16*, 52–58. [CrossRef] [PubMed]
43. Friedman, N.P.; Miyake, A. Unity and diversity of executive functions: Individual differences as a window on cognitive structure. *Cortex* **2017**, *86*, 186–204. [CrossRef]
44. Miyake, A.; Friedman, N.P.; Emerson, M.J.; Witzki, A.H.; Howerter, A.; Wager, T.D. The Unity and Diversity of Executive Functions and Their Contributions to Complex "Frontal Lobe" Tasks: A Latent Variable Analysis. *Cogn. Psychol.* **2000**, *41*, 49–100. [CrossRef] [PubMed]
45. Niendam, T.A.; Laird, A.R.; Ray, K.L.; Dean, Y.M.; Glahn, D.C.; Carter, C.S. Meta-analytic evidence for a superordinate cognitive control network subserving diverse executive functions. *Cogn. Affect. Behav. Neurosci.* **2012**, *12*, 241–268. [CrossRef]
46. Shen, K.; Welton, T.; Lyon, M.; McCorkindale, A.N.; Sutherland, G.T.; Burnham, S.; Fripp, J.; Martins, R.; Grieve, S.M. Structural core of the executive control network: A high angular resolution diffusion MRI study. *Hum. Brain Mapp.* **2020**, *41*, 1226–1236. [CrossRef]
47. Sasson, E.; Doniger, G.M.; Pasternak, O.; Tarrasch, R.; Assaf, Y. White matter correlates of cognitive domains in normal aging with diffusion tensor imaging. *Front. Neurosci.* **2013**, *7*, 32. [CrossRef] [PubMed]
48. Gallen, C.L.; Turner, G.R.; Adnan, A.; D'Esposito, M. Reconfiguration of brain network architecture to support executive control in aging. *Neurobiol. Aging* **2016**, *44*, 42–52. [CrossRef]
49. Zhang, J.; Tian, L.; Zhang, L.; Cheng, R.; Wei, R.; He, F.; Li, J.; Luo, B.; Ye, X. Relationship between white matter integrity and post-traumatic cognitive deficits: A systematic review and meta-analysis. *J. Neurol. Neurosurg. Psychiatry* **2019**, *90*, 98–107. [CrossRef] [PubMed]
50. Filley, C.M. White matter: Organization and functional relevance. *Neuropsychol. Rev.* **2010**, *20*, 158–173. [CrossRef]
51. Filley, C.M.; Kelly, J.P. White Matter and Cognition in Traumatic Brain Injury. *J. Alzheimers. Dis.* **2018**, *65*, 345–362. [CrossRef]
52. Medana, I.M.; Esiri, M.M. Axonal damage: A key predictor of outcome in human CNS diseases. *Brain* **2003**, *126*, 515–530. [CrossRef] [PubMed]

53. Zatorre, R.J.; Fields, R.D.; Johansen-Berg, H. Plasticity in gray and white: Neuroimaging changes in brain structure during learning. *Nat. Neurosci.* **2012**, *15*, 528–536. [CrossRef] [PubMed]
54. Tomassini, V.; Matthews, P.M.; Thompson, A.J.; Fuglo, D.; Geurts, J.J.; Johansen-Berg, H.; Jones, D.K.; Rocca, M.A.; Wise, R.G.; Barkhof, F.; et al. Neuroplasticity and functional recovery in multiple sclerosis. *Nat. Rev. Neurol.* **2012**, *8*, 635–646. [CrossRef] [PubMed]
55. Cramer, S.C.; Sur, M.; Dobkin, B.H.; O'Brien, C.; Sanger, T.D.; Trojanowski, J.Q.; Rumsey, J.M.; Hicks, R.; Cameron, J.; Chen, D.; et al. Harnessing neuroplasticity for clinical applications. *Brain* **2011**, *134*, 1591–1609. [CrossRef]
56. Murphy, T.H.; Corbett, D. Plasticity during stroke recovery: From synapse to behaviour. *Nat. Rev. Neurosci.* **2009**, *10*, 861–872. [CrossRef]
57. Fields, R.D. A new mechanism of nervous system plasticity: Activity-dependent myelination. *Nat. Rev. Neurosci.* **2015**, *16*, 756–767. [CrossRef]
58. Gibson, E.M.; Purger, D.; Mount, C.W.; Goldstein, A.K.; Lin, G.L.; Wood, L.S.; Inema, I.; Miller, S.E.; Bieri, G.; Zuchero, J.B.; et al. Neuronal activity promotes oligodendrogenesis and adaptive myelination in the mammalian brain. *Science* **2014**, *344*, 1252304. [CrossRef]
59. Bettcher, B.M.; Mungas, D.; Patel, N.; Elofson, J.; Dutt, S.; Wynn, M.; Watson, C.L.; Stephens, M.; Walsh, C.M.; Kramer, J.H. Neuroanatomical substrates of executive functions: Beyond prefrontal structures. *Neuropsychologia* **2016**, *85*, 100–109. [CrossRef]
60. Vaquero, L.; Rousseau, P.N.; Vozian, D.; Klein, D.; Penhune, V. What you learn & when you learn it: Impact of early bilingual & music experience on the structural characteristics of auditory-motor pathways. *Neuroimage* **2020**, *213*, 116689. [CrossRef]
61. Halwani, G.F.; Loui, P.; Rüber, T.; Schlaug, G. Effects of practice and experience on the arcuate fasciculus: Comparing singers, instrumentalists, and non-musicians. *Front. Psychol.* **2011**, *2*, 156. [CrossRef]
62. Engel, A.; Hijmans, B.S.; Cerliani, L.; Bangert, M.; Nanetti, L.; Keller, P.E.; Keysers, C. Inter-individual differences in audio-motor learning of piano melodies and white matter fiber tract architecture. *Hum. Brain Mapp.* **2014**, *35*, 2483–2497. [CrossRef] [PubMed]
63. Loui, P.; Raine, L.B.; Chaddock-Heyman, L.; Kramer, A.F.; Hillman, C.H. Musical instrument practice predicts white matter microstructure and cognitive abilities in childhood. *Front. Psychol.* **2019**, *10*, 1198. [CrossRef] [PubMed]
64. Habibi, A.; Damasio, A.; Ilari, B.; Veiga, R.; Joshi, A.A.; Leahy, R.M.; Haldar, J.P.; Varadarajan, D.; Bhushan, C.; Damasio, H. Childhood music training induces change in micro and macroscopic brain structure: Results from a longitudinal study. *Cereb. Cortex* **2018**, *28*, 4336–4347. [CrossRef] [PubMed]
65. Bengtsson, S.L.; Nagy, Z.; Skare, S.; Forsman, L.; Forssberg, H.; Ullén, F. Extensive piano practicing has regionally specific effects on white matter development. *Nat. Neurosci.* **2005**, *8*, 1148–1150. [CrossRef]
66. Siponkoski, S.-T.; Koskinen, S.; Laitinen, S.; Holma, M.; Ahlfors, M.; Jordan-Kilkki, P.; Ala-Kauhaluoma, K.; Martínez-Molina, N.; Melkas, S.; Laine, M.; et al. Effects of neurological music therapy on behavioural and emotional recovery after traumatic brain injury: A randomized controlled cross-over trial. *Neuropsychol. Rehabil.* **2021**, 1–33. [CrossRef]

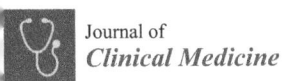

Article

Refined Analysis of Chronic White Matter Changes after Traumatic Brain Injury and Repeated Sports-Related Concussions: Of Use in Targeted Rehabilitative Approaches?

Francesco Latini [1,*,†], Markus Fahlström [2,†], Fredrik Vedung [1], Staffan Stensson [3], Elna-Marie Larsson [2], Mark Lubberink [4,5], Yelverton Tegner [6], Sven Haller [2,7], Jakob Johansson [8], Anders Wall [4,9], Gunnar Antoni [10] and Niklas Marklund [1,11]

1. Section of Neurosurgery, Department of Medical Sciences, Uppsala University, 75185 Uppsala, Sweden; fredrik.vedung@neuro.uu.se (F.V.); niklas.marklund@neuro.uu.se (N.M.)
2. Section of Radiology, Department of Surgical Sciences, Uppsala University, 75185 Uppsala, Sweden; markus.fahlstrom@radiol.uu.se (M.F.); elnamarielarsson@me.com (E.-M.L.); sven.haller@surgsci.uu.se (S.H.)
3. Rehabilitation and Pain Centre, Uppsala University Hospital, 75185 Uppsala, Sweden; staffan.stenson@akademiska.se
4. PET Centre, Uppsala University Hospital, 75185 Uppsala, Sweden; mark.lubberink@radiol.uu.se (M.L.); anders.wall@akademiska.se (A.W.)
5. Medical Physics, Uppsala University Hospital, 75185 Uppsala, Sweden
6. Division of Health, Medicine and Rehabilitation, Department of Health, Education and Technology, Luleå University of Technology, 97187 Luleå, Sweden; yelverton@tegner.com
7. Affidea CDRC Centre de Diagnostic Radiologique de Carouge SA, Clos de la Fonderie, 1227 Geneva, Switzerland
8. Section of Anesthesiology, Department of Surgical Sciences, Uppsala University, 75185 Uppsala, Sweden; jakob.johansson@surgsci.uu.se
9. Section of Nuclear Medicine and PET, Department of Surgical Sciences, Uppsala University, 75185 Uppsala, Sweden
10. Department of Medicinal Chemistry, Uppsala University, 75185 Uppsala, Sweden; gunnar.antoni@ilk.uu.se
11. Section of Neurosurgery, Department of Clinical Sciences Lund, Skåne University Hospital, Lund University, 22184 Lund, Sweden
* Correspondence: francesco.latini@neuro.uu.se; Tel.: +46-764244653
† These authors contributed equally to this work.

Abstract: Traumatic brain injury (TBI) or repeated sport-related concussions (rSRC) may lead to long-term memory impairment. Diffusion tensor imaging (DTI) is helpful to reveal global white matter damage but may underestimate focal abnormalities. We investigated the distribution of post-injury regional white matter changes after TBI and rSRC. Six patients with moderate/severe TBI, and 12 athletes with rSRC were included ≥6 months post-injury, and 10 (age-matched) healthy controls (HC) were analyzed. The Repeatable Battery for the Assessment of Neuropsychological Status was performed at the time of DTI. Major white matter pathways were tracked using q-space diffeomorphic reconstruction and analyzed for global and regional changes with a controlled false discovery rate. TBI patients displayed multiple classic white matter injuries compared with HC ($p < 0.01$). At the regional white matter analysis, the left frontal aslant tract, anterior thalamic radiation, and the genu of the corpus callosum displayed focal changes in both groups compared with HC but with different trends. Both TBI and rSRC displayed worse memory performance compared with HC ($p < 0.05$). While global analysis of DTI-based parameters did not reveal common abnormalities in TBI and rSRC, abnormalities to the fronto-thalamic network were observed in both groups using regional analysis of the white matter pathways. These results may be valuable to tailor individualized rehabilitative approaches for post-injury cognitive impairment in both TBI and rSRC patients.

Keywords: traumatic brain injury; sport related concussion; memory impairment; diffusion tensor imaging; white matter lesions; rehabilitative approaches

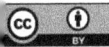

1. Introduction

Traumatic brain injury (TBI) affects more than 27 million people worldwide every year, often resulting in cognitive and functional deficits, the impairment of daily life functioning, and reduced quality of life [1–5].

Sport-related concussion (SRC), defined as a mild TBI, affects millions of athletes each year [6,7]. While most SRC-induced symptoms resolve within 2–3 weeks, headache, dizziness, confusion, and nausea may be long-lasting. Athletes with persisting symptoms beyond the first three months post-injury are often called the "miserable minority" reflecting a discrepancy into the debate concerning the psychological vs. organic origins of symptoms [8]. In fact, the treatment of these persisting cognitive deficits is challenging, in part since gross structural abnormalities on routine neuroimaging [e.g., structural magnetic resonance imaging (MRI), and computed tomography (CT)] are rare in repeated SRC (rSRC) compared with moderate and severe TBI [2,3,5,8]. Some of these athletes without traumatic damages visible at the routine morphological MRI sequences are not systematically considered for rehabilitation programs, and the possible long-term consequences of the brain injury are often neglected without a structural visible injury [9,10]. For these athletes, a diagnosis of a mild or major neurocognitive disorder caused by brain injury is commonly used [11], mostly based on the impaired cognitive function only [11,12]. Memory impairment has also often been linked to microstructural damage in the brain, and it affects patients both acutely and chronically after TBI [2,8,13,14].

The use of advanced MRI techniques, such as diffusion tensor imaging (DTI), can, in higher detail, reveal the presence of white matter injury that may cause injury-induced symptoms following TBI and SRC [8,15–17]. DTI can both qualitatively and quantitatively demonstrate pathology not detected by other modalities and is, therefore, an important tool not only in the research setting but in the clinical setting as well [18]. Altered DTI-based parameters in the subacute post-injury stage suggests different levels of white matter damage [19,20]. Robust evidence has shown a vulnerability of white matter bundles near the midline, such as the fornix and cingulum, to TBI-induced shearing forces [21–23]. Investigations of DTI-based parameters for specific regions such as the corpus callosum (CC), internal capsule (IC), and corona radiata (CR), indicates that baseline fractional anisotropy (FA) and mean diffusivity (MD) were associated with executive function and reaction time, respectively [24–26]. Other cognitive domains, including memory, may also depend on regional white matter integrity rather than generalized white matter injury [2,4,8,13,18,27–30]. Since there may be different subtypes of SRC, requiring specific rehabilitative therapies, refined white matter analysis is needed to understand the anatomical basis of the persisting symptoms [31].

Inter-subject differences in the mechanism of injury, as well as other biomechanical factors such as head and body composition, make it highly probable that, despite some commonalities, many areas of injury will differ among both patients and athletes [18,32]. The general interpretation of DTI-based-parameter alteration may therefore suffer these differences at group level, especially if the mean values of FA or MD are analyzed [18]. The further application of individualized assessments of regional brain injury are needed to realize the full potential of DTI as a research and clinical tool. These reasons may explain why, despite the general evidence, DTI is still not integrated in the clinical care of patients with TBI or SRC [9].

This work has two aims: first, to assess whether fiber tract analysis (local/regional) reveals alterations in DTI-based parameters not seen on whole tract analysis (global) nor morphological MRI in patients with TBI or rSRC athletes; second, to assess possible connections between local white matter alterations and long-term cognitive status in both groups.

2. Materials and Methods

2.1. Study Cohorts

Six patients were enrolled after a moderate (defined as Glasgow coma scale (GCS) score 9–13, loss of consciousness ≥5 min, and/or focal neurologic deficits [33]) to severe (GCS score ≤ 8) TBI and treated at the neuro-critical care unit ≥6 months at the department of neuro-surgery, Uppsala University hospital. Athletes of both sexes with rSRC and ≥6 months duration of post-concussion symptoms, according to the 4th edition of the Diagnostic and Statistical Manual of Mental Disorders, were recruited [34,35]. Ten age-matched HCs with no previous TBI, neurological condition, or current or previous active participation in any contact sport were recruited as a control group. The Regional Research Ethics Committee in Uppsala granted permission for the study (Dnr 2015/012). Written informed consent was obtained from all included patients/athletes and HCs. All research was conducted in accordance with the ethical standards given in the Helsinki Declaration of 1975, as revised in 2008.

2.2. Image Acquisition and Data Processing

High-resolution 3D-T1-weighted- (T1w), 3D-T2 fluid attenuated inversion recovery (T2-FLAIR), and susceptibility-weighted angiography (SWAN) images were acquired for morphological evaluation.

DTI was acquired with a single-shot echo-planar imaging sequence using the following imaging parameters: repetition time = 14,384 ms, echo-time = 78.6 ms, voxel size = $2 \times 2 \times 2$ mm^3, 73 slices, b-value = 1000 s/mm^2 with 32-directions on a 3.0 Tesla PET/MR-system (Signa PET/MR, GE Healthcare, Milwaukee, Waukesha, WI, USA). Motion and eddy current correction of acquired DTI data was performed in eddy, FSL (http://fsl.fmrib.ox.ac.uk/fsl/fslwiki; last accessed 11 October 2021) [36]. The diffusion data were reconstructed in MNI space using q-space diffeomorphic reconstruction (QSDR) in DSI studio with a diffusion sampling length ratio of 1.25. The output resolution was 2 mm. Briefly, QSDR is a white-matter-based nonlinear registration approach that directly reconstructs diffusion information in MNI space. As such, parametric images of FA, AD, and RD were calculated in MNI space. Detail information on QSDR can be found in Yeh et al. [37]. The QSDR function also provides a R^2-value between subject and MNI diffusion data. A value greater than 0.6 suggests a good registration result. A value greater than 0.6 was reported for all subjects. Major projection, commissural, and association white matter pathways (37 tracts in total) have previously been reconstructed within the HCP-1021 template following the anatomical criteria used for the Brain-Grid DTT reference atlas [38], which were applied to each subject.

Along-tract mapping was performed in DSI Studio. All included white matter pathways were stretched to correspond to straight lines. FA, AD, and RD were sampled along these lines and regressed using a kernel density estimator with default regression bandwidth at 1.0. Each point of these lines corresponds to one coordinate in the tract file generating indices for a given pathway. These were arranged from start to end with a corresponding DTI-based parameter for each given index for each subject.

2.3. Neuropsychology

The repeatable battery for the assessment of neuropsychological status (RBANS) [39], an objective test to measure neuro-cognitive functions including attention, verbal functions, visuospatial, immediate, and delayed memory, was performed by a trained neuropsychologist at the time of MRI investigation. Here, RBANS was used to estimate the neuro-cognitive burden in TBI and rSRC.

2.4. Data and Statistical Analysis

2.4.1. General White Matter Changes/Damages

The Shapiro–Wilks test was performed on the underlaying data for each analysis to test for normality; parametric or non-parametric statistical methods were chosen accordingly.

A Kruskal–Wallis test with Dunn's test to correct for multiple comparisons was used to test whole white matter pathway DTI-bases parameter differences between TBI, rSRC, and HCs for all white matter pathways, respectively. Furthermore, the median and interquartile range was calculated for TBI, rSRC, and HC and for all white matter pathways and DTI-based parameters, respectively. General changes were defined as a whole white matter pathway with significantly decreased total average FA and significantly increased total average AD or RD [19,20]. For all performed statistical analysis, derived p-values < 0.05 were considered significant. Statistical analysis and graphic plots were created using GraphPad Prism 9 (v 9.3.1., GraphPad Software, La Jolla, CA, USA).

2.4.2. Focal White Matter Changes/Damages

Focal along-tract analysis was performed using multiple unpaired t-tests comparing each white matter pathway index in TBI vs. HC and rSRC vs. HC for all DTI-based parameters and white matter pathways, respectively. The false discovery rate (FDR) was controlled using the Benjamini–Hochberg procedure with Q = 10%. In this regard, the number of false positives is kept below 10% of the number of significant indices. We chose a group of ten sequential significant indices to indicate a significant difference compared to HCs.

2.4.3. Neuropsychological Test

For descriptive analysis, the average and standard deviation (SD) of each subpart of the RBANS index was calculated. A group comparison on each subpart between TBI vs. HCs and rSRC vs. HCs were performed using an unpaired t-test for independent samples for comparison between groups.

3. Results

3.1. Participants

Six TBI patients (four males, two females, mean age 27 ± 7), 12 rSRC athletes (6 males, 6 females, mean age 26 ± 7) and 10 HCs (five males, five females, mean age 26 ± 5) were enrolled. No TBI patient had any known psychiatric or psychological disorder prior to the injury. Four TBI patients had cerebral contusions, and 2 had multiple cerebral microbleeds (CMB) suggesting diffuse axonal injury. Of the TBI patients, four had a good clinical recovery on the Glasgow outcome scale (GOS 5) and two a moderate disability (GOS 4). rSRC athletes had attained a median of 6 sports-related concussions (range 3–10). Concussion symptoms were assessed by the sport concussion assessment tool (SCAT)-3 [40], displaying high symptom severity. Non-specific white matter lesions were found in 2 rSRC athletes. Clinical and radiological data are summarized in Table 1.

Table 1. Summary of the clinical and radiological data of the three groups.

Clinical/Radiological Factors	Groups		
	TBI	SRC	HC
Number of patients	6	12	10
Age-mean (SD)	27 (7)	26 (7)	26 (5)
Gender-M/F	4/2	6/6	5/5
Concussions-no (range)	-	6 (3–10)	-
Contusions-no	4	-	-
DAI-no	2	-	-
Time since last TBI or SRC (months)	19 (8)	23 (6–132)	-
Length of Hospital stay (days)	17 (9)	-	-

Table 1. Cont.

Clinical/Radiological Factors		Groups		
		TBI	SRC	HC
Injury Mechanisms				
	Fall	3	-	-
	Motor vehicle accident	3	-	-
	Sports-related	-	12	-
Neurologic status				
	GCS at admission (range)	12 (5–14)	-	-
	GCS at discharge (range)	14 (8–15)	-	-
	GOS at the time of MRI (n of pts)	5 (4), 4(2)	-	-
Symptoms (SCAT)				
	SSS (range)	-	48.5 (3–91)	-
	NOS (range)	-	18 (2–22)	-

In athletes, concussion symptoms were assessed by the sport concussion assessment tool (SCAT). The symptom evaluation score lists 22 symptoms with a severity range of 0–6, and the symptom severity score (SSS) is the sum of all symptom scorings (range 0–132). The number of symptoms (NOS) is the sum of each symptom with a severity score between 1 and 6 (range 0–22). TBI: Traumatic brain injury, SRC: Sport-related concussions, and HI: healthy controls. DAI = diffuse axonal injury; GCS = Glasgow coma scale SCAT = sports concussion assessment tool; SSS = symptom severity score; NOS = number of symptoms; GOS: Glasgow outcome scale; non-parametric data (number of SRCs, time since last SRC, SSS, NOS, GCS) is presented as medians and range, and parametric data (age, time since TBI and length of hospital stay) is presented as means ± standard deviations (SD).

3.2. General White Matter Changes/Injuries

Differences in DTI-based parameters were observed in 29 white matter pathways in TBI patients compared to HCs (see Table 2). No rSRC athlete displayed significantly increased AD or RD or significantly decreased FA for any of the included white matter pathways (Table 2). On the other hand, six white matter pathways displayed significant difference in DTI parameters in rSRC compared with HC. The six structures displayed a completely different trend in DTI parameters with a higher FA and lower AD and RD compared with HC (Table 2). The median and interquartile range for all white matter pathways and DTI-based parameters are presented in electronic Supplementary Material Table S1 (ESM1).

Table 2. Analysis of global white matter damage.

White Matter Structure	AD		FA		RD		Injured	
	TBI vs. HC	SRC vs. HC	TBI vs. HC	SRC vs. HC	TBI vs. HC	SRC vs. HC	TBI	SRC
AC	<0.0001	<0.0001	<0.0001	<0.0001	<0.0001	<0.0001	Y	N
AF L	<0.0001	<0.0001	<0.0001	<0.0001	0.4062	<0.0001	N	N
AF R	0.0006	>0.9999	0.0603	0.6801	0.0002	0.3323	Y	N
Internal capsule Anterior L	<0.0001	0.8410	<0.0001	0.0226	<0.0001	0.5070	Y	N
Internal capsule Anterior R	<0.0001	0.2387	0.0416	<0.0001	<0.0001	>0.9999	Y	N
FAT L	0.0007	>0.9999	0.0125	>0.9999	<0.0001	>0.9999	Y	N
FAT R	0.0178	>0.9999	0.0149	0.6267	0.0006	0.2962	Y	N
ATR L	<0.0001	0.1121	<0.0001	0.0588	<0.0001	0.5310	Y	N
ATR R	<0.0001	>0.9999	<0.0001	0.6583	<0.0001	0.2591	Y	N
Ci L	0.1709	0.0003	<0.0001	0.2943	<0.0001	0.0295	N	N

Table 2. Cont.

White Matter Structure	AD		FA		RD		Injured	
	TBI vs. HC	SRC vs. HC	TBI vs. HC	SRC vs. HC	TBI vs. HC	SRC vs. HC	TBI	SRC
Ci R	<0.0001	<0.0001	0.0006	0.0026	<0.0001	0.0017	Y	N
CS L	<0.0001	0.1422	0.0006	>0.9999	<0.0001	>0.9999	Y	N
CS R	<0.0001	>0.9999	0.0322	0.8871	<0.0001	>0.9999	Y	N
External capsule L	<0.0001	0.8449	0.0374	0.0980	<0.0001	0.5370	Y	N
External capsule R	<0.0001	>0.9999	0.0410	>0.9999	<0.0001	0.6081	Y	N
FM	<0.0001	0.4771	0.0006	0.0028	<0.0001	<0.0001	Y	N
Fo L	<0.0001	<0.0001	<0.0001	0.0011	<0.0001	0.0001	Y	N
Fo R	<0.0001	<0.0001	<0.0001	<0.0001	<0.0001	<0.0001	Y	N
Genu CC	0.0019	>0.9999	<0.0001	0.3754	<0.0001	0.0060	Y	N
hSLF L	<0.0001	0.5733	0.0002	0.8185	<0.0001	0.8285	Y	N
hSLF R	<0.0001	>0.9999	0.0005	0.7111	<0.0001	>0.9999	Y	N
IFOF L	<0.0001	0.3086	0.0036	0.0009	<0.0001	0.1810	Y	N
IFOF R	<0.0001	>0.9999	0.2301	>0.9999	<0.0001	0.7752	Y	N
ILF L	0.0116	0.3316	0.0157	>0.9999	<0.0001	>0.9999	Y	N
ILF R	<0.0001	>0.9999	0.0140	>0.9999	<0.0001	0.6816	Y	N
MLF L	0.1890	0.0226	0.2841	0.0774	<0.0001	0.3796	N	N
MLF R	0.5220	>0.9999	0.0011	0.0105	<0.0001	<0.0001	N	N
OR L	<0.0001	0.6411	0.0207	0.5038	<0.0001	>0.9999	Y	N
OR R	<0.0001	>0.9999	>0.9999	>0.9999	<0.0001	0.8799	N	N
Internal capsule posterior L	<0.0001	0.0622	<0.0001	>0.9999	<0.0001	>0.9999	Y	N
Internal capsule posterior R	<0.0001	>0.9999	0.0144	0.8507	<0.0001	>0.9999	Y	N
UF L	<0.0001	0.3353	0.1033	0.0110	<0.0001	0.0007	Y	N
UF R	0.1262	0.4169	0.0729	0.7228	0.0022	0.0070	N	N
VO L	0.5318	>0.9999	0.0022	>0.9999	<0.0001	>0.9999	N	N
VO R	0.4149	0.1643	0.1207	0.0106	0.0240	0.3355	N	N
vSLF L	0.0027	0.0081	0.2355	>0.9999	0.0249	>0.9999	Y	N
vSLF R	<0.0001	0.0105	0.0012	0.5643	<0.0001	0.5110	Y	N

Adjusted *p*-values are presented for each comparison between traumatic brain injury (TBI), healthy controls (HC), and repeated sport-related concussions (rSRC) and HC including, all DTI-based metrics and white matter pathways. Values in red emphasize results wherein the axial diffusivity (AD) or radial diffusivity (RD) values are increased in comparison to HC, defining the criteria for white matter pathway injury. Values in green emphasize results wherein AD or RD decreases, which is contradictory to the theory presented. Y: yes (injured), N: not injured, L: left, R: right; AC: anterior commissure; AF: arcuate fasciculus; FAT: frontal aslant tract; ATR: anterior thalamic radiation; Ci: cingulum; CS: cortico-spinal tract; FM: forceps major; Fo: fornix; CC: corpus callosum; hSLF: horizontal component of superior longitudinal fasciculus; IFOF: inferior fronto-occipital fasciculus; ILF: inferior longitudinal fasciculus; MLF: middle longitudinal fasciculus; OR: optic radiation; UF: uncinate fasciculus; VO: vertical occipital fasciculus; vSLF: vertical component of superior longitudinal fasciculus.

3.3. Focal White Matter Changes/Injuries

Three white matter structures displayed regional differences in DTI-based parameters in both groups compared to HCs. The left frontal aslant tract (FAT) displayed lower FA and higher RD in the fronto-opercular region in TBI patients. The same pathway displayed higher FA and lower RD in the supplementary motor area region in rSRC patients. The right anterior thalamic radiation (ATR) displayed lower FA and higher AD and RD in TBI patients localized mostly at the thalamic level. The rSRC group displayed higher FA and lower AD and RD mostly at the thalamic level. The genu of the corpus callosum (CC) showed lower FA, higher AD and RD in the TBI group close to the midline. In the rSRC group, the focal analysis showed higher AD and lower RD close to the midline (Figure 1).

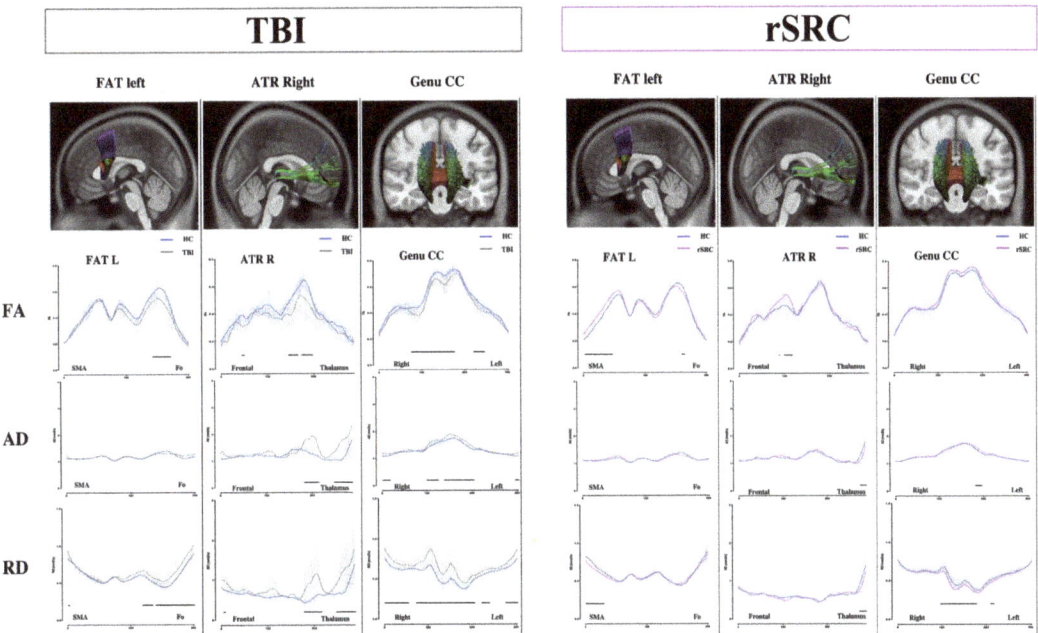

Figure 1. Focal analysis of three white matter pathways with white matter changes identified in both TBI patients and in rSRC patients compared with HC. False discovery rate (FDR) analysis was performed, as such significant differences are displayed as continuous lines on the x axis of each DTI-based parameter for each white matter pathway. The left frontal aslant tract (FAT) displayed lower FA and higher RD in the fronto-opercular region in TBI patients, while a higher FA and lower RD in the supplementary motor area region were found in the rSRC group. The right anterior thalamic radiation (ATR) displayed lower FA and higher AD and RD in the TBI group localized mostly at the thalamic level, while the rSRC group displayed higher FA and lower AD and RD mostly at the thalamic level. The genu of the corpus callosum (CC) showed lower FA and higher AD and RD in the TBI group close to the midline, while the rSRC group displayed a higher AD and lower RD close to the midline. TBI: traumatic brain injuries; rSRC: repeated sport related concussions; HC: healthy controls; AD: axial diffusivity; RD: radial diffusivity; FAT: frontal aslant tract; ATR: anterior thalamic radiation; CC: corpus callosum.

3.4. Neuropsychology

Both TBI patients and rSRC athletes were impaired on the RBANS global outcome analysis compared with HC (TBI: 75 ± 24; rSRC: 80 ± 17; HC: 105.5 ± 2; TBI to HC: $p = 0.03$ rSRC to HC: $p = 0.006$). RBANS Memory scores were lower in both TBI, and SRC when compared to HC ($p = 0.048$ and $p = 0.04$; respectively). The RBANS Verbal scores were lower in rSRC athletes compared to HC ($p = 0.048$) although not in TBI ($p = 0.07$). No significative difference was detected among the groups for the other RBANS functional domains (Figure 2).

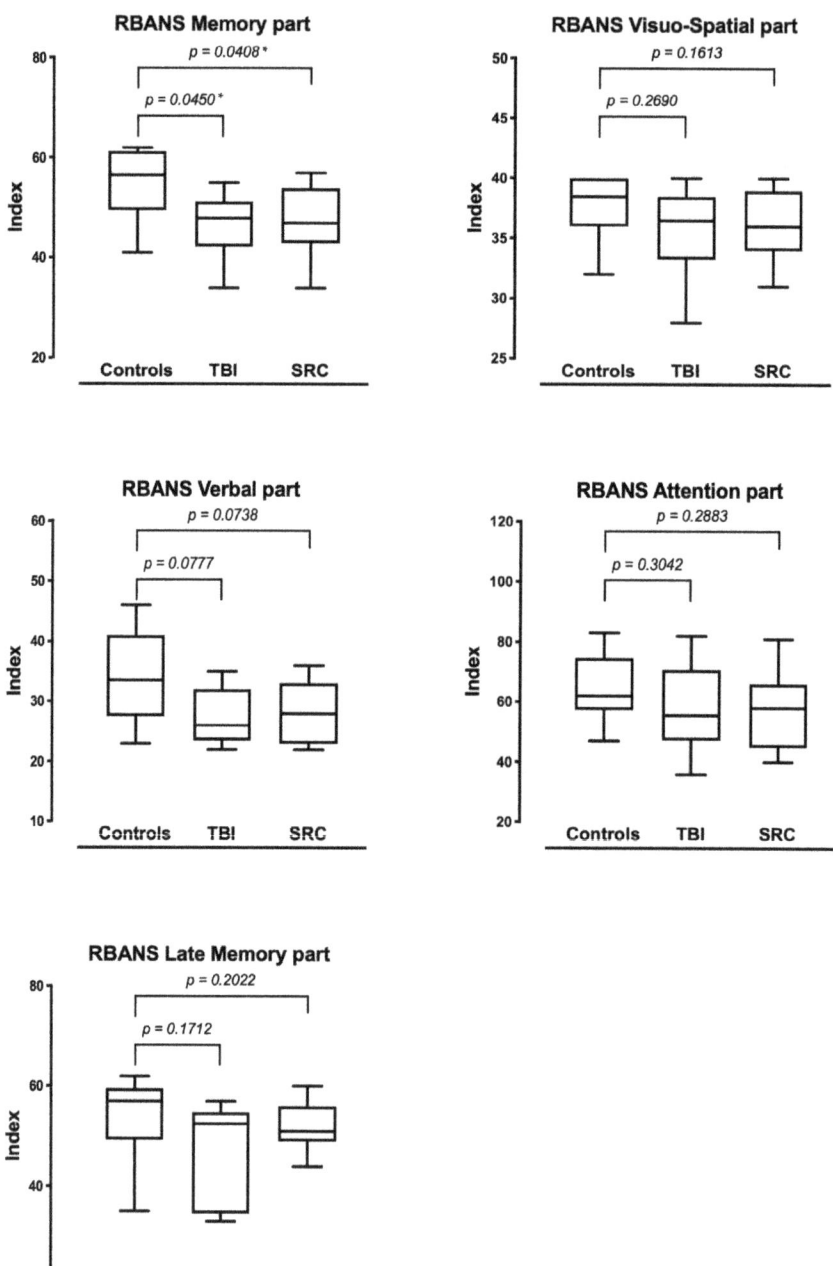

Figure 2. Each domain of RBANS is shown for TBI, rSRC, and HC. Significant differences in RBANS Memory score were detected between HC and TBI patients, as well as rSRC athletes. For the other domains of the RBANS, there were no significant differences among the groups. TBI: traumatic brain injuries; rSRC: repeated sport-related concussions; HC: healthy controls; RBANS: repeatable battery for the assessment of neuropsychological status. * Statistical significance with p value < 0.05.

4. Discussion

The most important finding in our study was that focal regional differences in white matter pathways were observed at the chronic stage post-injury in both TBI patients and rSRC athletes who had a similar impairment on memory testing in comparison to healthy, age-matched controls (HC). For the development of novel treatments, and for precision rehabilitation, an enhanced understanding of the structural basis of persistent symptoms is crucial [41].

White matter changes, demonstrated by differences in DTI-based parameters, have been previously identified in TBI patients [19,21,25,28,30]. Furthermore, differences in DTI-based parameters are also seen in patients with only minor cognitive impairment and in patients with normal conventional MRI, supporting the role of DTI in detecting subtle injuries missed by other modalities [8,20,25,30,42]. In our study, TBI patients displayed significant changes in DTI-based parameters compared with HC in 29 of the 37 analyzed white matter structures in the global white matter analysis. Using the same analysis interpreting the mean values for each single white matter in rSRC athletes, no white matter pathways displayed global axonal or myelin abnormalities compared with HC. However, a different trend in DTI parameters compared with HC was observed in six white matter pathways compared with HC. It is suggested that different injury mechanisms and levels of energy produced by trauma to cortical and subcortical structures may be explaining factors [15,26,28,30]. This variability leads to a lack of consensus on the interpretation of chronic DTI-based parameters after TBI or rSRC [16,21,23]. In fact, DTI has been demonstrated to be sensitive to a wide range of group differences, although no specific trends have been consistently identified [29,43]. For this reason, we performed post-hoc analyses to investigate specific and focal injuries to white matter pathways. A similar method was previously used to analyze regional white matter changes after radiation therapy in DTI-based parameters [44] and to investigate white matter anomalies in a patient with visual snow syndrome [45]. We found a different level of regional differences in the same white matter networks only partially revealed by the global analysis. Several white matter pathways displayed regionally decreased AD and RD in their midline segments in rSRC, in agreement with previous reports in chronic rSRC [16,46–48]. On the other hand, there are conflicting results showing increased AD and RD indicative of damage to axonal fibers or myelin, respectively [43,49]. Plausibly, focal and/or incomplete damage to myelin or axonal fibers may not affect the entire pathway in terms of DTI-based metrics at the chronic stage. Incomplete damage to both myelin and axons in rSRC may induce a myelin repair process with a change in the dominant cell type contributing to the signal, with axonal bundles being replaced by astrocytes and/or microglia [15]. Hence, significantly higher AD and RD and, potentially, lower FA in rSRC patients could be expected at the chronic stage [16,21,42,50]. Animal models showed that neuronal shrinkage can occur in the absence of cell death or perisomatic axotomy [16,51]. Decreased AD and RD post injury may be related to such shrinkage, leading to less surface area along axons for parallel diffusion [16,51].

These data suggest that the time course of physiological recovery extends longer than initially thought in rSRC athletes [17]. In addition, previous inconsistent results matching cognitive outcome and DTI may depend on the different DTI analysis methods used [22–24,43,51,52]. Changes in DTI-based parameters may be subtle and difficult to detect due to technical factors (such as the number of DTI directions, the algorithm used for the analysis, normalization process, the technique of tractography, the choice of global or focal indices' analysis among others) [52–55]. When the structural injury is focal and/or partially repaired, analysis of regional DTI-based metrics changes should be investigated to identify anatomical and possible links to functional information/dysfunction.

Both TBI patients and rSRC athletes performed significantly worse in the memory domain. This result agrees with other studies demonstrating impaired neuropsychological outcome in TBI patients and rSRC athletes during the subacute/chronic stage [2,4,5,7,20,23,39,56]. In patients with evidence of structural and functional abnormalities after TBI, effective cognitive rehabilitation interventions initiated post TBI enhance the recovery process and minimize the functional disability [57]. In rSRC patients, the persistence of symptoms long beyond the generally accepted time frame for recovery may reflect the development of post-concussion syndrome (PCS) [58,59]. There is, however, no consensus regarding the clinical neuroradiological criteria for PCS and, increasingly, the term persistent post-concussive symptoms (PPCS) is used [60]. Despite persisting symptoms, many of these athletes have normal MRI investigations [59]. The possible evidence of white matter alterations may represent an important factor to consider to plan early education [61], cognitive behavioral therapy [62], and/or aerobic exercise therapy [63], which have been shown to be effective in certain patients with post-concussion syndrome [59]. Moreover, since memory seems the common most affected domain in our two populations, the specific use of external memory aids and computer-assisted strategies may be indicated, since they have also been shown to improve attention, memory, and executive skills after TBI and therefore may be of help in SRC patients with memory impairment [10,64–66].

The indication for tailored cognitive rehabilitation based on the affected white matter networks and functional impairment would therefore be necessary to either restore or compensate for memory deficits or other functional impairments commonly debilitating to rSRC patients, as well as for TBI patients [67,68].

4.1. Functional Correlates of Regional White Matter Injuries

We found FAT, ATR, and CC to be among the abnormal white matter pathways due to significant variations in DTI-based parameters, at the regional analysis in both TBI and rSRC athletes. The two groups displayed similar functional outcome and a similar mid-line location for the DTI-based parameters changes at the regional analyses for the ATR and CC. FAT is a key component of a cortico-basal ganglia- thalamic-cerebellar circuit involved in action control [69,70]. In both hemispheres, the FAT plays a role in selecting among competing representations for actions that require the same motor resources (mainly the articulatory apparatus on the left hemisphere and the oculomotor and manual/limb action systems on the right hemisphere) [69,71,72]. Its damage has been related to impairment in speech and language functions, as well as executive functions, visual–motor activities, inhibitory control, working memory, and attention [69,71]. The damage/changes to segments of ATR can also be observed in the midline fluid percussion brain injury, a rodent model of diffuse TBI wherein memory deficits are observed [73]. Electrophysiological evidence suggests a crucial role for ATR connectivity in human memory formation, connecting the anterior and midline thalamic nuclear groups to the frontal lobe [74–79]. Commissural white matter pathways such as the genu and splenium of the CC are more vulnerable in their segment close to the midline due to a close relationship with fibrotic structures such as the falx cerebri [28,80,81]. Lesions or regional changes of the CC are known to disable the interhemispheric communication of multiple memory systems and disturb memory function [82–84], in particular in long-term verbal memory performance [85,86].

Taken together, these findings suggest that regional differences in the frontal and fronto-thalamic networks (FAT, ATR) may be key contributors to the poor memory performance observed in our study. The additional involvement of the genu of CC, may have resulted in a lack of interhemispheric modulation and resilience leading to a less compensable functional impairment [82–87]. Knowledge of the presence of such white matter changes is of importance to individualize treatment strategies [41].

4.2. Limitations

Our study has some limitations. The sample size of the three groups is small, especially the TBI group. Although the groups are thoroughly characterized and matched (age and gender) the injury mechanisms resulting in the TBI or rSRC were heterogeneous. Hence, our results should, therefore, be interpreted with caution. The limited sample size influenced our analysis and some of the variables such as age, gender, and hospitalization time were not included as confounding factors in this article. Since the TBI group is too small and other studies from our group did not identify significant differences among subgroups of rSRC athletes [88], we did not include the other variables in our analysis, which was beyond the aim of this article. We aimed to investigate differences in white matter changes with two different methods and to match the neuropsychological outcome with diffusion changes in the two groups. Further studies with larger cohorts are needed to clarify the role of the confounding factors in TBI and rSRC subjects at the chronic phase. We also believe that only longitudinal studies with repeated investigations would minimize the risk of hidden differences between the groups displaying trends for possible recovery. Another limitation is that we cannot exclude that possible comorbidities, such as post-traumatic stress disorder (PTSD), which has been described in TBI patients, might have contributed to the worse performance on memory domain by the TBI group [89]. On the other hand, the similar performance in rSRC athlete, the different background of the TBI patients included in this study and the absence of similar white matter alterations as previously reported may indicate a different reason for the results presented in this article.

To our knowledge, this is the first study applying focal injury analysis to white matter pathways in both TBI patients and rSRC athletes. Hence, another limitation may be linked to our methods with the creation of several small indices for each DTI-based parameter together with the intrinsic sensitivity to noise. We defined regional differences as a minimum of 10 consecutive indices reaching the pre-determined significant levels in comparison to controls at group level in both direction (increased or decreased when compared with healthy controls). We believe the FDR analysis may represent a reliable and solid way to discriminate the effects of confounds through the analysis of voxel's spatial neighborhood. Another limitation is the possible role of cerebral contusions and CMB on our DTI results. Post-traumatic lesions such as contusions and CMB can be associated with lasting changes in perilesional white matter properties, even remotely from the lesion, and midsagittal CMB have been associated with cognitive decline after TBI [90–92]. Since we did not anatomically normalize CMB, an effect on the DTI results cannot be excluded. However, at the time of DTI, neither acquisition nor an expansive effect of the contusions was present, nor was a significant deformation of anatomical structures detected. The quality of the normalization process was carefully assessed before the analysis. In view of the differences in acquisition period and the different trend in AD and RD between TBI and rSRC, a major role for CMB is unlikely. Further studies with more advanced models of white matter investigations are necessary to minimize the effects of confounds and to, in detail, assess network vulnerability in TBI and rSRC.

5. Conclusions

In our study, TBI patients and rSRC athletes displayed different morphological images and different DTI abnormalities at the first level analysis of white matter but shared a similarly impaired memory performance at the chronic stage after injury. DTI analysis detected white matter pathway changes especially in TBI patients but underestimated focal or incomplete abnormalities when the white matter pathway was considered as one entity. At the regional analysis, similar regions of the left FAT, the genu of the CC, and the right ATR displayed different focal changes in both rSRC and TBI patients, reflecting possible differences in trauma and recovery mechanisms. The concomitant presence of white matter findings and the functional impairment observed in both TBI patients and rSRC athletes may suggest a long-term chronic impairment in some subgroups of patients despite the normal standard MRI images. This information seems crucial to better interpret the functional outcome of athletes with rSRC and to tailor individualized rehabilitative plans.

Supplementary Materials: The following supporting information can be downloaded at: https://www.mdpi.com/article/10.3390/jcm11020358/s1, Table S1: Median with interquartile range for all white matter pathways and DTI-based parametric values.

Author Contributions: Author contributions included conception and study design, F.L., M.F. and N.M.; data collection or acquisition, F.V., S.S., E.-M.L., M.L., Y.T., J.J., A.W., G.A. and N.M.; statistical analysis, M.F.; interpretation of results, F.L., M.F., E.-M.L., S.H. and N.M.; drafting the manuscript work, F.L., M.F. and N.M.; and approval of the final version to be published and agreement to be accountable for the integrity and accuracy of all aspects of the work, All authors. All authors have read and agreed to the published version of the manuscript.

Funding: Swedish Brain Foundation FO2020-0147, FO2019-0190, FO2018-0166, Swedish Research Council (SRC) 2018-02500_VR, SRC under the framework of EU-ERA-NET NEURON CnsAFlame, Swedish Research Council for Sport Science P2019-0133, P2020-0116, P2021-0105, Bissen Brain Walk and Selander Foundation—all to N.M.

Institutional Review Board Statement: The study was conducted according to the guidelines of the Declaration of Helsinki and approved by the institutional ethics review board (2015/210/2).

Informed Consent Statement: Informed consent was obtained from all subjects involved in the study. Written informed consent has been obtained from the patients to publish this paper.

Data Availability Statement: The data that support the findings of this study are available on request from the corresponding author. The data are not publicly available due to privacy and ethical restrictions.

Conflicts of Interest: N.M. and Y.T. are scientific advisors for PolarCool Inc. The other authors have no competing/conflict of interests to declare.

References

1. GBD 2016 Traumatic Brain Injury and Spinal Cord Injury Collaborators. Global, Regional, and National Burden of Traumatic Brain Injury and Spinal Cord Injury, 1990–2016: A Systematic Analysis for the Global Burden of Disease Study 2016. *Lancet Neurol.* **2019**, *18*, 56–87. [CrossRef]
2. Dikmen, S.S.; Corrigan, J.D.; Levin, H.S.; Machamer, J.; Stiers, W.; Weisskopf, M.G. Cognitive Outcome Following Traumatic Brain Injury. *J. Head Trauma Rehabil.* **2009**, *24*, 430–438. [CrossRef] [PubMed]
3. Sariaslan, A.; Sharp, D.J.; D'Onofrio, B.M.; Larsson, H.; Fazel, S. Long-Term Outcomes Associated with Traumatic Brain Injury in Childhood and Adolescence: A Nationwide Swedish Cohort Study of a Wide Range of Medical and Social Outcomes. *PLoS Med.* **2016**, *13*, e1002103. [CrossRef]
4. Filley, C.M.; Kelly, J.P. White Matter and Cognition in Traumatic Brain Injury. *JAD* **2018**, *65*, 345–362. [CrossRef]
5. Marklund, N.; Bellander, B.-M.; Godbolt, A.K.; Levin, H.; McCrory, P.; Thelin, E.P. Treatments and Rehabilitation in the Acute and Chronic State of Traumatic Brain Injury. *J. Intern. Med.* **2019**, *285*, 608–623. [CrossRef] [PubMed]
6. Langlois, J.A.; Rutland-Brown, W.; Wald, M.M. The Epidemiology and Impact of Traumatic Brain Injury: A Brief Overview. *J. Head Trauma Rehabil.* **2006**, *21*, 375–378. [CrossRef]
7. McKeithan, L.; Hibshman, N.; Yengo-Kahn, A.M.; Solomon, G.S.; Zuckerman, S.L. Sport-Related Concussion: Evaluation, Treatment, and Future Directions. *Med. Sci.* **2019**, *7*, 44. [CrossRef]
8. Kraus, M.F.; Susmaras, T.; Caughlin, B.P.; Walker, C.J.; Sweeney, J.A.; Little, D.M. White Matter Integrity and Cognition in Chronic Traumatic Brain Injury: A Diffusion Tensor Imaging Study. *Brain* **2007**, *130*, 2508–2519. [CrossRef]
9. Pavlovic, D.; Pekic, S.; Stojanovic, M.; Popovic, V. Traumatic Brain Injury: Neuropathological, Neurocognitive and Neurobehavioral Sequelae. *Pituitary* **2019**, *22*, 270–282. [CrossRef]
10. Knight, S.; Takagi, M.; Fisher, E.; Anderson, V.; Lannin, N.A.; Tavender, E.; Scheinberg, A. A Systematic Critical Appraisal of Evidence-Based Clinical Practice Guidelines for the Rehabilitation of Children With Moderate or Severe Acquired Brain Injury. *Arch. Phys. Med. Rehabil.* **2019**, *100*, 711–723. [CrossRef] [PubMed]
11. Wortzel, H.S.; Arciniegas, D.B. The DSM-5 Approach to the Evaluation of Traumatic Brain Injury and Its Neuropsychiatric Sequelae. *NeuroRehabilitation* **2014**, *34*, 613–623. [CrossRef] [PubMed]
12. Dwyer, B.; Katz, D.I. Postconcussion Syndrome. *Handb. Clin. Neurol.* **2018**, *158*, 163–178. [CrossRef] [PubMed]
13. Arenth, P.M.; Russell, K.C.; Scanlon, J.M.; Kessler, L.J.; Ricker, J.H. Corpus Callosum Integrity and Neuropsychological Performance after Traumatic Brain Injury: A Diffusion Tensor Imaging Study. *J. Head Trauma Rehabil.* **2014**, *29*, E1–E10. [CrossRef] [PubMed]
14. Raskin, S.A.; Williams, J.; Aiken, E.M. A Review of Prospective Memory in Individuals with Acquired Brain Injury. *Clin. Neuropsychol.* **2018**, *32*, 891–921. [CrossRef] [PubMed]
15. Newcombe, V.; Chatfield, D.; Outtrim, J.; Vowler, S.; Manktelow, A.; Cross, J.; Scoffings, D.; Coleman, M.; Hutchinson, P.; Coles, J.; et al. Mapping Traumatic Axonal Injury Using Diffusion Tensor Imaging: Correlations with Functional Outcome. *PLoS ONE* **2011**, *6*, e19214. [CrossRef]
16. Lancaster, M.A.; Meier, T.B.; Olson, D.V.; McCrea, M.A.; Nelson, L.D.; Muftuler, L.T. Chronic Differences in White Matter Integrity Following Sport-Related Concussion as Measured by Diffusion MRI: 6-Month Follow-Up. *Hum. Brain Mapp.* **2018**, *39*, 4276–4289. [CrossRef]

17. Mohammadian, M.; Roine, T.; Hirvonen, J.; Kurki, T.; Posti, J.P.; Katila, A.J.; Takala, R.S.K.; Tallus, J.; Maanpää, H.-R.; Frantzén, J.; et al. Alterations in Microstructure and Local Fiber Orientation of White Matter Are Associated with Outcome after Mild Traumatic Brain Injury. *J. Neurotrauma* **2020**, *37*, 2616–2623. [CrossRef] [PubMed]
18. Hulkower, M.B.; Poliak, D.B.; Rosenbaum, S.B.; Zimmerman, M.E.; Lipton, M.L. A Decade of DTI in Traumatic Brain Injury: 10 Years and 100 Articles Later. *Am. J. Neuroradiol.* **2013**, *34*, 2064–2074. [CrossRef]
19. Shenton, M.E.; Hamoda, H.M.; Schneiderman, J.S.; Bouix, S.; Pasternak, O.; Rathi, Y.; Vu, M.-A.; Purohit, M.P.; Helmer, K.; Koerte, I.; et al. A Review of Magnetic Resonance Imaging and Diffusion Tensor Imaging Findings in Mild Traumatic Brain Injury. *Brain Imaging Behav.* **2012**, *6*, 137–192. [CrossRef]
20. Veeramuthu, V.; Narayanan, V.; Kuo, T.L.; Delano-Wood, L.; Chinna, K.; Bondi, M.W.; Waran, V.; Ganesan, D.; Ramli, N. Diffusion Tensor Imaging Parameters in Mild Traumatic Brain Injury and Its Correlation with Early Neuropsychological Impairment: A Longitudinal Study. *J. Neurotrauma* **2015**, *32*, 1497–1509. [CrossRef]
21. Aoki, Y.; Inokuchi, R.; Gunshin, M.; Yahagi, N.; Suwa, H. Diffusion Tensor Imaging Studies of Mild Traumatic Brain Injury: A Meta-Analysis. *J. Neurol. Neurosurg. Psychiatry* **2012**, *83*, 870–876. [CrossRef]
22. Zhang, J.; Wei, R.-L.; Peng, G.-P.; Zhou, J.-J.; Wu, M.; He, F.-P.; Pan, G.; Gao, J.; Luo, B.-Y. Correlations between Diffusion Tensor Imaging and Levels of Consciousness in Patients with Traumatic Brain Injury: A Systematic Review and Meta-Analysis. *Sci. Rep.* **2017**, *7*, 2793. [CrossRef] [PubMed]
23. Zhang, J.; Tian, L.; Zhang, L.; Cheng, R.; Wei, R.; He, F.; Li, J.; Luo, B.; Ye, X. Relationship between White Matter Integrity and Post-Traumatic Cognitive Deficits: A Systematic Review and Meta-Analysis. *J. Neurol. Neurosurg. Psychiatry* **2019**, *90*, 98–107. [CrossRef] [PubMed]
24. de la Plata, C.D.M.; Yang, F.G.; Wang, J.Y.; Krishnan, K.; Bakhadirov, K.; Paliotta, C.; Aslan, S.; Devous, M.D.; Moore, C.; Harper, C.; et al. Diffusion Tensor Imaging Biomarkers for Traumatic Axonal Injury: Analysis of Three Analytic Methods. *J. Int. Neuropsychol. Soc.* **2011**, *17*, 24–35. [CrossRef] [PubMed]
25. Moen, K.G.; Vik, A.; Olsen, A.; Skandsen, T.; Håberg, A.K.; Evensen, K.A.I.; Eikenes, L. Traumatic Axonal Injury: Relationships between Lesions in the Early Phase and Diffusion Tensor Imaging Parameters in the Chronic Phase of Traumatic Brain Injury: Traumatic Axonal Injury Lesions in Chronic TBI. *J. Neurosci. Res.* **2016**, *94*, 623–635. [CrossRef] [PubMed]
26. Hashim, E.; Caverzasi, E.; Papinutto, N.; Lewis, C.E.; Jing, R.; Charles, O.; Zhang, S.; Lin, A.; Graham, S.J.; Schweizer, T.A.; et al. Investigating Microstructural Abnormalities and Neurocognition in Sub-Acute and Chronic Traumatic Brain Injury Patients with Normal-Appearing White Matter: A Preliminary Diffusion Tensor Imaging Study. *Front. Neurol.* **2017**, *8*, 97. [CrossRef] [PubMed]
27. Maller, J.J.; Thomson, R.H.S.; Lewis, P.M.; Rose, S.E.; Pannek, K.; Fitzgerald, P.B. Traumatic Brain Injury, Major Depression, and Diffusion Tensor Imaging: Making Connections. *Brain Res. Rev.* **2010**, *64*, 213–240. [CrossRef] [PubMed]
28. Zappalà, G.; de Schotten, M.T.; Eslinger, P.J. Traumatic Brain Injury and the Frontal Lobes: What Can We Gain with Diffusion Tensor Imaging? *Cortex* **2012**, *48*, 156–165. [CrossRef] [PubMed]
29. Asken, B.M.; DeKosky, S.T.; Clugston, J.R.; Jaffee, M.S.; Bauer, R.M. Diffusion Tensor Imaging (DTI) Findings in Adult Civilian, Military, and Sport-Related Mild Traumatic Brain Injury (MTBI): A Systematic Critical Review. *Brain Imaging Behav.* **2018**, *12*, 585–612. [CrossRef]
30. Castaño Leon, A.M.; Cicuendez, M.; Navarro, B.; Munarriz, P.M.; Cepeda, S.; Paredes, I.; Hilario, A.; Ramos, A.; Gómez, P.A.; Lagares, A. What Can Be Learned from Diffusion Tensor Imaging from a Large Traumatic Brain Injury Cohort?: White Matter Integrity and Its Relationship with Outcome. *J. Neurotrauma* **2018**, *35*, 2365–2376. [CrossRef]
31. Makdissi, M.; Schneider, K.J.; Feddermann-Demont, N.; Guskiewicz, K.M.; Hinds, S.; Leddy, J.J.; McCrea, M.; Turner, M.; Johnston, K.M. Approach to Investigation and Treatment of Persistent Symptoms Following Sport-Related Concussion: A Systematic Review. *Br. J. Sports Med.* **2017**, *51*, 958–968. [CrossRef]
32. Ware, J.B.; Hart, T.; Whyte, J.; Rabinowitz, A.; Detre, J.A.; Kim, J. Inter-Subject Variability of Axonal Injury in Diffuse Traumatic Brain Injury. *J. Neurotrauma* **2017**, *34*, 2243–2253. [CrossRef]
33. Ingebrigtsen, T.; Romner, B.; Kock-Jensen, C. Scandinavian Guidelines for Initial Management of Minimal, Mild, and Moderate Head Injuries. The Scandinavian Neurotrauma Committee. *J. Trauma* **2000**, *48*, 760–766. [CrossRef] [PubMed]
34. Guze, S.B. Diagnostic and Statistical Manual of Mental Disorders, 4th Ed. (DSM-IV). *AJP* **1995**, *152*, 1228. [CrossRef]
35. McIntyre, M.; Amiri, M.; Kumbhare, D. Postconcussion Syndrome: A Diagnosis of Past Diagnostic and Statistical Manual of Mental Disorders. *Am. J. Phys. Med. Rehabil.* **2021**, *100*, 193–195. [CrossRef]
36. Andersson, J.L.R.; Sotiropoulos, S.N. An Integrated Approach to Correction for Off-Resonance Effects and Subject Movement in Diffusion MR Imaging. *Neuroimage* **2016**, *125*, 1063–1078. [CrossRef]
37. Yeh, F.-C.; Tseng, W.-Y.I. NTU-90: A High Angular Resolution Brain Atlas Constructed by q-Space Diffeomorphic Reconstruction. *Neuroimage* **2011**, *58*, 91–99. [CrossRef]
38. Latini, F.; Fahlström, M.; Berntsson, S.G.; Larsson, E.-M.; Smits, A.; Ryttlefors, M. A Novel Radiological Classification System for Cerebral Gliomas: The Brain-Grid. *PLoS ONE* **2019**, *14*, e0211243. [CrossRef]
39. McKay, C.; Casey, J.E.; Wertheimer, J.; Fichtenberg, N.L. Reliability and Validity of the RBANS in a Traumatic Brain Injured Sample. *Arch. Clin. Neuropsychol.* **2007**, *22*, 91–98. [CrossRef] [PubMed]
40. Yengo-Kahn, A.M.; Hale, A.T.; Zalneraitis, B.H.; Zuckerman, S.L.; Sills, A.K.; Solomon, G.S. The Sport Concussion Assessment Tool: A Systematic Review. *Neurosurg. Focus* **2016**, *40*, E6. [CrossRef] [PubMed]

41. Iverson, G.L. Network Analysis and Precision Rehabilitation for the Post-Concussion Syndrome. *Front. Neurol.* **2019**, *10*, 489. [CrossRef]
42. Bazarian, J.J.; Zhong, J.; Blyth, B.; Zhu, T.; Kavcic, V.; Peterson, D. Diffusion Tensor Imaging Detects Clinically Important Axonal Damage after Mild Traumatic Brain Injury: A Pilot Study. *J. Neurotrauma* **2007**, *24*, 1447–1459. [CrossRef]
43. Winklewski, P.J.; Sabisz, A.; Naumczyk, P.; Jodzio, K.; Szurowska, E.; Szarmach, A. Understanding the Physiopathology Behind Axial and Radial Diffusivity Changes—What Do We Know? *Front. Neurol.* **2018**, *9*, 92. [CrossRef]
44. Houri, J.; Karunamuni, R.; Connor, M.; Pettersson, N.; McDonald, C.; Farid, N.; White, N.; Dale, A.; Hattangadi-Gluth, J.A.; Moiseenko, V. Analyses of Regional Radiosensitivity of White Matter Structures along Tract Axes Using Novel White Matter Segmentation and Diffusion Imaging Biomarkers. *Phys. Imaging Radiat. Oncol.* **2018**, *6*, 39–46. [CrossRef]
45. Latini, F.; Fahlström, M.; Marklund, N.; Feresiadou, A. White Matter Abnormalities in a Patient with Visual Snow Syndrome: New Evidence from a Diffusion Tensor Imaging Study. *Eur. J. Neurol.* **2021**, *28*, 2789–2793. [CrossRef] [PubMed]
46. Chamard, E.; Lefebvre, G.; Lassonde, M.; Theoret, H. Long-Term Abnormalities in the Corpus Callosum of Female Concussed Athletes. *J. Neurotrauma* **2016**, *33*, 1220–1226. [CrossRef] [PubMed]
47. Henry, L.C.; Tremblay, J.; Tremblay, S.; Lee, A.; Brun, C.; Lepore, N.; Theoret, H.; Ellemberg, D.; Lassonde, M. Acute and Chronic Changes in Diffusivity Measures after Sports Concussion. *J. Neurotrauma* **2011**, *28*, 2049–2059. [CrossRef]
48. Meier, T.B.; Bergamino, M.; Bellgowan, P.S.F.; Teague, T.K.; Ling, J.M.; Jeromin, A.; Mayer, A.R. Longitudinal Assessment of White Matter Abnormalities Following Sports-Related Concussion. *Hum. Brain Mapp.* **2016**, *37*, 833–845. [CrossRef] [PubMed]
49. Wheeler-Kingshott, C.A.M.; Cercignani, M. About "Axial" and "Radial" Diffusivities. *Magn. Reson. Med.* **2009**, *61*, 1255–1260. [CrossRef]
50. Song, S.-K.; Yoshino, J.; Le, T.Q.; Lin, S.-J.; Sun, S.-W.; Cross, A.H.; Armstrong, R.C. Demyelination Increases Radial Diffusivity in Corpus Callosum of Mouse Brain. *Neuroimage* **2005**, *26*, 132–140. [CrossRef]
51. Singleton, R.H.; Zhu, J.; Stone, J.R.; Povlishock, J.T. Traumatically Induced Axotomy Adjacent to the Soma Does Not Result in Acute Neuronal Death. *J. Neurosci.* **2002**, *22*, 791–802. [CrossRef]
52. Farquharson, S.; Tournier, J.-D.; Calamante, F.; Fabinyi, G.; Schneider-Kolsky, M.; Jackson, G.D.; Connelly, A. White Matter Fiber Tractography: Why We Need to Move beyond DTI. *J. Neurosurg.* **2013**, *118*, 1367–1377. [CrossRef]
53. Vos, S.B.; Jones, D.K.; Viergever, M.A.; Leemans, A. Partial Volume Effect as a Hidden Covariate in DTI Analyses. *Neuroimage* **2011**, *55*, 1566–1576. [CrossRef] [PubMed]
54. Gardner, A.; Kay-Lambkin, F.; Stanwell, P.; Donnelly, J.; Williams, W.H.; Hiles, A.; Schofield, P.; Levi, C.; Jones, D.K. A Systematic Review of Diffusion Tensor Imaging Findings in Sports-Related Concussion. *J. Neurotrauma* **2012**, *29*, 2521–2538. [CrossRef]
55. Feigl, G.C.; Hiergeist, W.; Fellner, C.; Schebesch, K.-M.M.; Doenitz, C.; Finkenzeller, T.; Brawanski, A.; Schlaier, J. Magnetic Resonance Imaging Diffusion Tensor Tractography: Evaluation of Anatomic Accuracy of Different Fiber Tracking Software Packages. *World Neurosurg.* **2014**, *81*, 144–150. [CrossRef] [PubMed]
56. Manley, G.; Gardner, A.J.; Schneider, K.J.; Guskiewicz, K.M.; Bailes, J.; Cantu, R.C.; Castellani, R.J.; Turner, M.; Jordan, B.D.; Randolph, C.; et al. A Systematic Review of Potential Long-Term Effects of Sport-Related Concussion. *Br. J. Sports Med.* **2017**, *51*, 969–977. [CrossRef]
57. Rees, L.; Marshall, S.; Hartridge, C.; Mackie, D.; Weiser, M. Erabi Group Cognitive Interventions Post Acquired Brain Injury. *Brain Inj.* **2007**, *21*, 161–200. [CrossRef]
58. Willer, B.; Leddy, J.J. Management of Concussion and Post-Concussion Syndrome. *Curr. Treat Options Neurol.* **2006**, *8*, 415–426. [CrossRef]
59. Leddy, J.J.; Sandhu, H.; Sodhi, V.; Baker, J.G.; Willer, B. Rehabilitation of Concussion and Post-Concussion Syndrome. *Sports Health* **2012**, *4*, 147–154. [CrossRef] [PubMed]
60. Rickards, T.A.; Cranston, C.C.; McWhorter, J. Persistent Post-Concussive Symptoms: A Model of Predisposing, Precipitating, and Perpetuating Factors. *Appl. Neuropsychol. Adult* **2020**, 1–11. [CrossRef]
61. Mittenberg, W.; Canyock, E.M.; Condit, D.; Patton, C. Treatment of Post-Concussion Syndrome Following Mild Head Injury. *J. Clin. Exp. Neuropsychol.* **2001**, *23*, 829–836. [CrossRef]
62. Al Sayegh, A.; Sandford, D.; Carson, A.J. Psychological Approaches to Treatment of Postconcussion Syndrome: A Systematic Review. *J. Neurol. Neurosurg. Psychiatry* **2010**, *81*, 1128–1134. [CrossRef] [PubMed]
63. Leddy, J.J.; Kozlowski, K.; Donnelly, J.P.; Pendergast, D.R.; Epstein, L.H.; Willer, B. A Preliminary Study of Subsymptom Threshold Exercise Training for Refractory Post-Concussion Syndrome. *Clin. J. Sport Med.* **2010**, *20*, 21–27. [CrossRef] [PubMed]
64. Bergquist, T.; Gehl, C.; Mandrekar, J.; Lepore, S.; Hanna, S.; Osten, A.; Beaulieu, W. The Effect of Internet-Based Cognitive Rehabilitation in Persons with Memory Impairments after Severe Traumatic Brain Injury. *Brain Inj.* **2009**, *23*, 790–799. [CrossRef] [PubMed]
65. Chen, S.H.; Thomas, J.D.; Glueckauf, R.L.; Bracy, O.L. The Effectiveness of Computer-Assisted Cognitive Rehabilitation for Persons with Traumatic Brain Injury. *Brain Inj.* **1997**, *11*, 197–209. [CrossRef]
66. Tam, S.-F.; Man, W.-K. Evaluating Computer-Assisted Memory Retraining Programmes for People with Post-Head Injury Amnesia. *Brain Inj.* **2004**, *18*, 461–470. [CrossRef] [PubMed]
67. Iaccarino, M.A.; Bhatnagar, S.; Zafonte, R. Rehabilitation after Traumatic Brain Injury. *Handb. Clin. Neurol.* **2015**, *127*, 411–422. [CrossRef] [PubMed]

68. Barman, A.; Chatterjee, A.; Bhide, R. Cognitive Impairment and Rehabilitation Strategies After Traumatic Brain Injury. *Indian J. Psychol. Med.* **2016**, *38*, 172–181. [CrossRef]
69. Dick, A.S.; Garic, D.; Graziano, P.; Tremblay, P. The Frontal Aslant Tract (FAT) and Its Role in Speech, Language and Executive Function. *Cortex* **2019**, *111*, 148–163. [CrossRef]
70. Vergani, F.; Lacerda, L.; Martino, J.; Attems, J.; Morris, C.; Mitchell, P.; de Schotten, M.T.; Dell'Acqua, F. White Matter Connections of the Supplementary Motor Area in Humans. *J. Neurol. Neurosurg. Psychiatry* **2014**, *85*, 1377–1385. [CrossRef]
71. La Corte, E.; Eldahaby, D.; Greco, E.; Aquino, D.; Bertolini, G.; Levi, V.; Ottenhausen, M.; Demichelis, G.; Romito, L.M.; Acerbi, F.; et al. The Frontal Aslant Tract: A Systematic Review for Neurosurgical Applications. *Front. Neurol.* **2021**, *12*, 51. [CrossRef]
72. Baker, C.M.; Burks, J.D.; Briggs, R.G.; Smitherman, A.D.; Glenn, C.A.; Conner, A.K.; Wu, D.H.; Sughrue, M.E. The Crossed Frontal Aslant Tract: A Possible Pathway Involved in the Recovery of Supplementary Motor Area Syndrome. *Brain Behav.* **2018**, *8*, e00926. [CrossRef] [PubMed]
73. Lifshitz, J.; Rowe, R.K.; Griffiths, D.R.; Evilsizor, M.N.; Thomas, T.C.; Adelson, P.D.; McIntosh, T.K. Clinical Relevance of Midline Fluid Percussion Brain Injury: Acute Deficits, Chronic Morbidities, and the Utility of Biomarkers. *Brain Inj.* **2016**, *30*, 1293–1301. [CrossRef]
74. Aggleton, J.P.; Brown, M.W. Episodic Memory, Amnesia, and the Hippocampal-Anterior Thalamic Axis. *Behav. Brain Sci.* **1999**, *22*, 425–444; discussion 444–489. [CrossRef]
75. Sweeney-Reed, C.M.; Zaehle, T.; Voges, J.; Schmitt, F.C.; Buentjen, L.; Kopitzki, K.; Esslinger, C.; Hinrichs, H.; Heinze, H.-J.; Knight, R.T.; et al. Corticothalamic Phase Synchrony and Cross-Frequency Coupling Predict Human Memory Formation. *Elife* **2014**, *3*, e05352. [CrossRef]
76. Sweeney-Reed, C.M.; Zaehle, T.; Voges, J.; Schmitt, F.C.; Buentjen, L.; Kopitzki, K.; Hinrichs, H.; Heinze, H.-J.; Rugg, M.D.; Knight, R.T.; et al. Thalamic Theta Phase Alignment Predicts Human Memory Formation and Anterior Thalamic Cross-Frequency Coupling. *Elife* **2015**, *4*, e07578. [CrossRef] [PubMed]
77. de Bourbon-Teles, J.; Bentley, P.; Koshino, S.; Shah, K.; Dutta, A.; Malhotra, P.; Egner, T.; Husain, M.; Soto, D. Thalamic Control of Human Attention Driven by Memory and Learning. *Curr. Biol.* **2014**, *24*, 993–999. [CrossRef]
78. Carrera, E.; Bogousslavsky, J. The Thalamus and Behavior: Effects of Anatomically Distinct Strokes. *Neurology* **2006**, *66*, 1817–1823. [CrossRef] [PubMed]
79. Nishio, Y.; Hashimoto, M.; Ishii, K.; Ito, D.; Mugikura, S.; Takahashi, S.; Mori, E. Multiple Thalamo-Cortical Disconnections in Anterior Thalamic Infarction: Implications for Thalamic Mechanisms of Memory and Language. *Neuropsychologia* **2014**, *53*, 264–273. [CrossRef]
80. Bigler, E.D. The Lesion(s) in Traumatic Brain Injury: Implications for Clinical Neuropsychology. *Arch. Clin. Neuropsychol.* **2001**, *16*, 95–131. [CrossRef]
81. Ok, B.S.; Lyong, K.O.; Ho, K.S.; Soo, K.M.; Min, S.S.; Woo, C.Y.; Mok, B.W.; Ho, J.S. Relation between Cingulum Injury and Cognition in Chronic Patients with Traumatic Brain Injury; Diffusion Tensor Tractography Study. *NeuroRehabilitation* **2013**, *33*, 465–471. [CrossRef]
82. Gazzaniga, M.S. Cerebral Specialization and Interhemispheric CommunicationDoes the Corpus Callosum Enable the Human Condition? *Brain* **2000**, *123*, 1293–1326. [CrossRef] [PubMed]
83. Glickstein, M.; Berlucchi, G. Classical Disconnection Studies of the Corpus Callosum. *Cortex* **2008**, *44*, 914–927. [CrossRef] [PubMed]
84. Schulte, T.; Müller-Oehring, E.M. Contribution of Callosal Connections to the Interhemispheric Integration of Visuomotor and Cognitive Processes. *Neuropsychol. Rev.* **2010**, *20*, 174–190. [CrossRef]
85. Yaldizli, Ö.; Penner, I.-K.; Frontzek, K.; Naegelin, Y.; Amann, M.; Papadopoulou, A.; Sprenger, T.; Kuhle, J.; Calabrese, P.; Radü, E.W.; et al. The Relationship between Total and Regional Corpus Callosum Atrophy, Cognitive Impairment and Fatigue in Multiple Sclerosis Patients. *Mult. Scler.* **2014**, *20*, 356–364. [CrossRef] [PubMed]
86. McDonald, S.; Rushby, J.A.; Dalton, K.I.; Allen, S.K.; Parks, N. The Role of Abnormalities in the Corpus Callosum in Social Cognition Deficits after Traumatic Brain Injury. *Soc. Neurosci.* **2018**, *13*, 471–479. [CrossRef]
87. van der Knaap, L.J.; van der Ham, I.J.M. How Does the Corpus Callosum Mediate Interhemispheric Transfer? A Review. *Behav. Brain Res.* **2011**, *223*, 211–221. [CrossRef]
88. Marklund, N.; Vedung, F.; Lubberink, M.; Tegner, Y.; Johansson, J.; Blennow, K.; Zetterberg, H.; Fahlström, M.; Haller, S.; Stenson, S.; et al. Tau Aggregation and Increased Neuroinflammation in Athletes after Sports-Related Concussions and in Traumatic Brain Injury Patients—A PET/MR Study. *Neuroimage Clin.* **2021**, *30*, 102665. [CrossRef]
89. Mohamed, A.Z.; Cumming, P.; Nasrallah, F.A. White Matter Alterations Are Associated With Cognitive Dysfunction Decades After Moderate-to-Severe Traumatic Brain Injury and/or Posttraumatic Stress Disorder. *Biol. Psychiatry Cogn. Neurosci. Neuroimaging* **2021**, *6*, 1100–1109. [CrossRef]
90. Andreasen, S.; Andersen, K.; Conde, V.; Dyrby, T.; Puonti, O.; Kammersgaard, L.; Madsen, C.; Madsen, K.; Poulsen, I.; Siebner, H. Limited Colocalization of Microbleeds and Microstructural Changes After Severe Traumatic Brain Injury. Available online: https://pubmed.ncbi.nlm.nih.gov/31588844/?from_single_result=limited+colocalization%2C+Andreasen+S&expanded_search_query=limited+colocalization%2C+Andreasen+S (accessed on 23 May 2020).

91. Haller, S.; Vernooij, M.W.; Kuijer, J.P.A.; Larsson, E.-M.; Jäger, H.R.; Barkhof, F. Cerebral Microbleeds: Imaging and Clinical Significance. *Radiology* **2018**, *287*, 11–28. [CrossRef] [PubMed]
92. Rostowsky, K.A.; Maher, A.S.; Irimia, A. Macroscale White Matter Alterations Due to Traumatic Cerebral Microhemorrhages Are Revealed by Diffusion Tensor Imaging. *Front. Neurol.* **2018**, *9*, 948. [CrossRef] [PubMed]

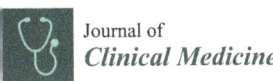

Article

Abnormal Dorsal Caudate Activation Mediated Impaired Cognitive Flexibility in Mild Traumatic Brain Injury

Hui Xu [1,2,*], Xiuping Zhang [3] and Guanghui Bai [1,4,*]

1. Department of Radiology, The Second Affiliated Hospital and Yuying Children's Hospital of Wenzhou Medical University, Wenzhou 325027, China
2. Research Center, Institut Universitaire de Gériatrie de Montréal, Montreal, QC H3W 1W5, Canada
3. School of Psychology, Beijing Language and Culture University, Beijing 100083, China; zhangxp@blcu.edu.cn
4. Wenzhou Key Laboratory of Basic Science and Translational Research of Radiation Oncology, Wenzhou 325027, China
* Correspondence: huixujx@gmail.com (H.X.); bghu79@126.com (G.B.)

Abstract: Background: Mild traumatic brain injury (mTBI) is an important but less recognized public health concern. Previous studies have demonstrated that patients with mTBI have impaired executive function, which disrupts the performance of daily activities. Few studies have investigated neural mechanisms of cognitive flexibility in mTBI patients using objective tools such as the psychological experiment paradigm. Here, we aimed to examine neural correlates of cognitive flexibility in mTBI. Methods: Sixteen mTBI patients and seventeen matched healthy controls (HCs) underwent functional MRI during a rule-based task-switching experimental paradigm. Linear models were used to obtain within-group activation maps and areas of differential activation between the groups. In addition, we conducted mediation analyses to evaluate the indirect effect of abnormal dorsal caudate activation on the association between information processing speed and cognitive flexibility in mTBI. Results: mTBI patients exhibited significantly longer reaction time in the task switching (TS) condition compared to HCs, reflecting impaired cognitive flexibility. In addition, the patients showed reduced activation in the dorsal caudate (dCau), anterior cingulate cortex, and other frontal regions during the TS condition. Mediation analysis revealed that the reduced dCau activation had a significant effect on the relationship between information processing speed and cognitive flexibility in mTBI. Conclusions: Abnormal dorsal caudate activation in mTBI mediates impaired cognitive flexibility, which indicated dorsal caudate might be playing a vital role in the cognitive flexibility of mTBI patients. These findings highlight an alternative target for clinical interventions for the improvement of cognitive functions in mTBI.

Keywords: mild traumatic brain injury; functional MRI; cognitive flexibility; task switching; dorsal caudate

1. Introduction

Mild traumatic brain injury (mTBI) is an important but less recognized public health concern [1], which accounts for nearly 80% of all traumatic brain injuries [2,3]. Patients with mTBI have impaired executive function, which disrupts the normal performance of daily activities [4]. Executive function is a high-level cognitive function in human beings [5]. As a core component of the executive function, cognitive flexibility defines the ability of individuals to constantly adjust their behavioral responses according to the changing external environment [6,7]. Many studies have demonstrated executive dysfunction in patients with various diseases and the patients exhibit impaired cognitive flexibility [8–12].

Previous studies conducting magnetic resonance imaging (MRI) found that patients with traumatic brain injury have executive dysfunction, and showed impaired cognitive flexibility and altered information processing speed on the behavior level [13]. A previous study that employed graph theory analysis showed that patients exhibited reduced centrality of characteristic vectors of caudate and cingulate cortex, which could accurately predict executive dysfunction in traumatic brain injury [13]. Another study that conducted a word-based working memory task in patients with severe traumatic brain injury showed that the abnormal activation response of caudate was negatively correlated with the patient's cognitive fatigue under complex conditions, but was positively associated with cognitive fatigue under simple conditions [14]. In addition, one task-switching study showed that patients with local caudate atrophy had abnormal cognitive flexibility, and needed sufficient cognitive load during task switching, but exhibited a significantly increased error rate [15].

Besides, other studies demonstrated that patients with traumatic brain injury had widespread altered white matter microstructure, and the damage to the upper radiation crown from the caudate to the anterior auxiliary motor zone was significantly associated with the switching cost required for patients to achieve task switching, which could predict impaired cognitive flexibility in the patients [16]. Therefore, patients with traumatic brain injury exhibited impaired cognitive flexibility with altered behavioral responses as well as structural and functional abnormalities in the hub region caudate. However, these studies mainly focused on the cognitive dysfunction in patients with moderate to severe traumatic brain injury.

Moreover, previous studies mostly employed specific neuropsychological measurement tools such as the Wisconsin Card Sorting Test to assess cognitive function [17], but were limited by subjective judgments and the expectation effect; it has been proved that when individuals with mild head injury are informed of this, they may experience cognitive difficulties and perform worse on neuropsychological tests compared to the individuals who are uninformed [18,19]. In addition, other studies conducted different psychological experimental tasks to measure cognitive functions in patients with traumatic brain injury, such as working memory tasks [20–22] and the go/no-go task [23,24], which were performed mainly to measure working memory and inhibitory control ability, respectively. Furthermore, few studies have investigated cognitive flexibility in mTBI patients and its associated neural mechanisms using objective tools such as the psychological experiment paradigm.

To explore underlying neural mechanisms of cognitive flexibility in mTBI patients, we performed a rule-based cognitive control experimental paradigm with functional MRI. Here, we first investigated specific behavioral patterns of cognitive impairment in the mTBI patients, and then explored abnormal brain activation in task conditions. Thereafter, we assessed the relationship between altered brain activation, information processing speed and cognitive flexibility. We aimed to identify neural correlates of impaired cognitive flexibility in mTBI.

2. Materials and Methods

2.1. Participants

Sixteen mTBI patients (6 females, mean age 25.8 ± 2.8 years) were recruited from the local emergency department. Diagnosis of the mTBI was assessed by two experienced neurologists following the World Health Organization's Collaborating Centre for Neurotrauma Task Force [4]. To be included in this study, all mTBI patients had to have met the following inclusion criteria: (1) a Glasgow Coma Scale score of 13–15; (2) one or more of loss of consciousness (if present) <30 min, post-traumatic amnesia (if present) <24 h, and/or other transient neurological abnormalities such as focal signs, seizure, and intracranial lesion not necessitating surgery. We excluded patients with a history of neurological disease, long-standing psychiatric condition, head injury, substance or alcohol abuse, clinical symptoms of depression and anxiety, intubation and/or presence of a skull fracture as well as administration of sedatives on arrival in the emergency department, spinal cord injury. Patients with a manifestation of mTBI due to medications by other injuries (e.g., systemic injuries, facial injuries, or intubation) or other sources such as psychological trauma, language barrier, or coexisting medical conditions as well as those caused by penetrating craniocerebral injury were also excluded from this study. In addition, 17 age- and sex-matched healthy controls (HCs) were also enrolled (5 females, mean age 27.8 ± 3.3 years).

2.2. Neuropsychological Tests

Several neuropsychological performance tests were performed. The tests included Trail-Making Test Part-A (TMT-A) for rote memory assessment, Forward Digit Span (FDS) and Backward Digit Span (BDS) test of Wechsler Adult Intelligence Scale-III for working memory assessment and Digit Symbol Coding (DSC) task for cognitive function assessment and information processing speed. On the other hand, we employed self-reported symptomatology assessments such as Insomnia, which was evaluated using the Insomnia Severity Index (ISI) for sleep quality and short-form Headache Impact Test (HIT) for severity of headaches. All the neuropsychological tests were performed by an experienced clinical psychologist blinded to this study.

2.3. Experimental Design and Procedures

We employed a modified version of the rule-based task-switching experimental paradigm [25–27], where participants responded to the target digital stimuli based on the cues presented initially. It is a highly time-efficient event-related fMRI paradigm, which has been designed to specifically probe for cognitive flexibility and stability. Participants were instructed to perform one of three task conditions on numerical stimuli based on a cue presented simultaneously during each trial (Figure 1). The task was generated and presented using PsychToolBox and appeared on a uniform black background [28,29]. At each trial, participants were cued explicitly (using a square or diamond cue) as to which condition should be performed during the digit stimuli between 1 and 9 (excluding number 5). Three conditions were set in the experiment: ongoing (OG), distractor inhibition (DI) and task switch (TS). For the ongoing (OG) condition, a diamond cue was presented at the center of a screen with a digit stimulus on the left side, and participants were asked to indicate whether the digit was larger or smaller than five. On the other hand, for the distractor inhibition (DI) condition, a diamond cue was presented at the center of a screen with two-digit stimuli on each side, and participants were asked to indicate whether the left digit was larger or smaller than five, and had to inhibit their response to the right digit (assessing cognitive stability). For the task switch (TS) condition, a square cue was presented at the center of a screen with two-digit stimuli at each side, and the participants were asked to switch from the left digit to the right digit and then decide whether the right digit was odd or even (assessing cognitive flexibility). At each trial, the condition cue and digit stimuli were simultaneously presented for 2000 ms, followed by a variable inter-trial interval of 2000, 4000, or 6000 ms. Participants were required to accurately respond as quickly as possible within the limit of 2000 ms.

All participants received out-of-scanner practice with trial-to-trial feedback and were instructed to provide accurate and quick responses until they attained 95% accuracy. The task was split into two functional scanning runs of 84 trials each. Each run started and ended with two dummy scans (5 s) for scanner signal stabilization, while the participants looked at a fixation cross at the center of the screen.

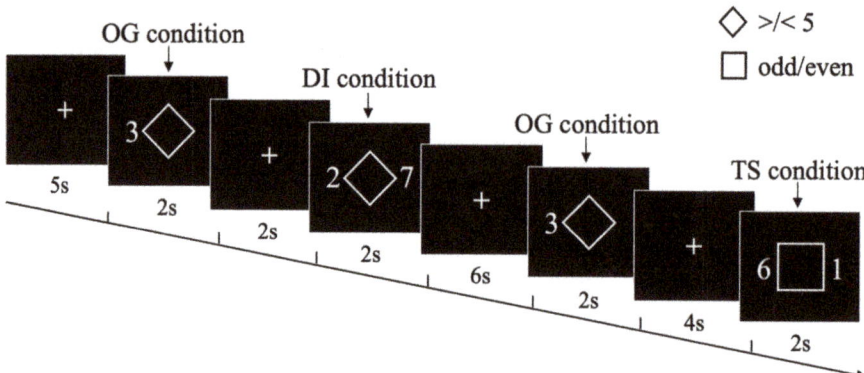

Figure 1. Schematic illustration of the rule-based task-switching experimental paradigm. During three task conditions [ongoing (OG) condition, distractor inhibition (DI) condition, task switch (TS) condition], depending on task cues (square vs. diamond), participants performed one of the different tasks on visually presented number stimuli (smaller/larger than 5 vs. odd/even).

2.4. fMRI Data Acquisition

Functional MRI images were acquired on a 3.0 Tesla MRI scanner (GE 750 Medical Systems), equipped with a single-shot, gradient-recalled echo planar imaging (EPI) sequence and a 32-channel head coil.

A total of 340 functional volumes were acquired in two runs, using a T2*-weighted BOLD-sensitive gradient-recalled, EPI sequence with 54 slices covering the whole brain [repetition time (TR) = 2500 ms, echo time (TE) = 30 ms, slice thickness = 3 mm, flip angle (FA) = 90°, field of view (FOV) = 216 mm × 216 mm, matrix size = 64 × 64, voxel size = 3 mm × 3 mm × 3 mm]. The first and last two volumes of each run were discarded to allow for stable magnetization.

Before performing functional MRI scan, a high-resolution T1-weighted magnetization prepared-rapid gradient echo scan was acquired with the following parameters: TR = 2300 ms, TE = 3.17 ms, FA = 9°, slice thickness = 1 mm, FOV = 256 mm × 256 mm, matrix size = 256 × 256.

We also captured multiple neuroimaging data (including T1-flair, T2-flair, T2, susceptibility-weighted imaging (SWI)) for all the mTBI patients. These data were used to assess the presence of focal lesions and cerebral microbleeds. Visible contusion lesions were not detected in any of the patients.

2.5. Statistical Analysis of Behavioral Data

All trials with a response time (RT) < 150 ms were eliminated. The RT analyses were limited to proper trials. Both RT and error rate (ER) data for the task behavioral performance were analyzed using ANOVAs, with "task condition" (OG, DI, TS) and "group" (mTBI patients, HCs) factors. The significant main effects and interactions were further explored by post hoc t tests using Bonferroni's correction. A $p < 0.05$ was used as statistically significant for all the behavior analyses.

2.6. fMRI Data Preprocessing and Statistical Analysis

Using FEAT in FSL v5.0, we analyzed whole-brain voxel-wise activation on the fMRI scans of the rule-based task-switching experimental paradigm [30]. We performed preprocessing of all individual fMRI runs using the following procedures: both the first and last 2 volumes were deleted, underwent motion correction (MCFLIRT) [31], brain extraction, spatial smoothing (6-mm full-width at half maximum kernel), and high-pass temporal filtering (0.01-Hz cutoff). In addition, linear registration (FLIRT) was performed in T1, fMRI, and MNI152 standard space. The degree of head motion from all participants was quantified, and according to the head motion criteria (translational or rotational motion parameters less than 2.0 mm or 2.0°), none of the participants were excluded (the mean translation was 0.08 ± 0.02 mm, and rotation was 0.04 ± 0.01°).

First-level (within-run) general linear model analyses in native fMRI space were conducted with FILM prewhitening, with 3 separate regressors (the onset of all stimuli for OG condition, DI condition and TS condition). Each one of them convolved with a double-gamma hemodynamic response function with the application of temporal filtering [32]. First-level contrast was set up to create voxel-wise contrast of parameter estimate maps of activation in different task conditions. The maps were then used for second-level (within-subject) analysis in the 2 runs. The maps were converted to MNI152 space and fixed effects analyses were performed with 3 contrasts to identify OG, DI or TS conditions. The resultant maps for each contrast were then used for third-level (group-level) FLAME 1 + 2 mixed-effects analyses which proved to have high statistic values at a small proportion of voxels in a relatively small sample size (threshold: cluster-based $p < 0.05$; whole-brain family-wise-error corrected $Z > 2.3$) [33], with 3 contrasts: OG, DI or TS activation. We employed Student's t test to analyze the effect of the group on brain activation of different task conditions using mTBI patients and HCs as factors.

2.7. Relationship between Abnormal Activation, Behavioral and Neuropsychological Measures in mTBI

To examine whether abnormal activation during different task conditions correlates with behavioral features and neuropsychological measures in mTBI, Spearman correlation analyses between abnormal activation, task behavioral performance and clinical parameters were performed in patients. The $p < 0.05$ was taken as a significant threshold with FDR (false discovery rate) corrected for multiple comparisons.

2.8. Mediation Analysis between Abnormal Dorsal Caudate Activation and Cognitive Flexibility in mTBI

To examine the indirect effect of abnormal dorsal caudate activation on the association between information processing speed and cognitive flexibility in mTBI patients, we conducted mediation analysis using SPSS PROCESS v3.4, with a 5000 bias-correction bootstrapping approach [34,35]. Here, the information processing speed (indexed by the scores of DSC task) was considered as the independent variable, abnormal dorsal caudate activation in the TS condition was considered as the mediator while cognitive flexibility (indexed by the RT of TS condition) was considered as the dependent variable. Age and education level were used as covariates in the mediation analysis. The estimation of indirect effects was considered significant when zero was not included in the bootstrapped 95% confidence interval (CI) (5000 iterations).

3. Results

3.1. Demographics and Neuropsychological Assessment

Our analysis showed that there were no significant differences in age ($t_{31} = -0.952$, $p > 0.05$), education level ($t_{31} = -1.297$, $p > 0.05$) or sex ($\chi^2_1 = 0.243$, $p > 0.05$) between groups. The mTBI patients presented significantly worse insomnia severity and headache compared to HCs (all $p < 0.01$). In addition, patients exhibited impaired information processing speed (reflected by the DSC task) compared with HCs ($p < 0.001$, Table 1). All mTBI patients exhibited the same injury severity with a Glasgow Coma Score of 15, loss of consciousness < 30 min, and post-traumatic amnesia < 24 h. The most common cause of injuries was acceleration/deceleration caused by traffic accidents (6/16, 37.5%), followed by falls (5/16, 31.2%), assaults (3/16, 18.8%), and others (2/16, 12.5%).

Table 1. Demographic characteristics and neuropsychological measures in mTBI patients and HCs.

	mTBI Patients (n = 16)	HCs (n = 17)	t/χ² Test	p-Value
Demographic characteristics				
Age (years)	25.8 ± 2.8	27.8 ± 3.3	−1.897	0.067
Sex (F/M)	6/10	5/12	0.243	0.622
Handedness (L/R)	0/16	0/17		
Education level (years)	13.9 ± 1.3	13.6 ± 1.6	0.316	0.754
Time post injury (days)	2.7 ± 1.3	-	-	-
Injury severity (n(%))				
GCS = 15	16(100%)	-	-	-
loss of conscious < 30 min	16(100%)	-	-	-
post-traumatic amnesia < 24 h	16(100%)	-	-	-
Injury causes (n(%))				
Traffic accident	6(37.5%)	-	-	-
Fall	5(31.2%)	-	-	-
Assault	3(18.8%)	-	-	-
Others	2(12.5%)	-	-	-
Information processing speed				
TMA-A score	50.0 ± 8.8	48.6 ± 8.1	0.461	0.648
DSC score	32.2 ± 5.1	45.7 ± 5.5	−7.343	$p < 0.001$
Working memory				
FDS score	8.5 ± 0.8	7.9 ± 1.1	1.874	0.07
BDS score	4.3 ± 0.8	3.8 ± 0.8	2.036	0.051
Self-reported symptom				
ISI score	7.1 ± 2.1	2.1 ± 1.1	8.704	$p < 0.01$
HIT score	48.1 ± 4.3	38.6 ± 6.1	5.091	$p < 0.01$

Values presented as Mean ± SD unless otherwise stated. mTBI, mild traumatic brain injury; HCs, healthy controls; GCS, Glasgow Coma Score; TMT-A, Trail-Making Test Part-A; FDS, Forward Digit Span; BDS, Backward Digit Span; DSC, Digit Symbol Coding; ISI, the Insomnia Severity Index; HIT, the short-form Headache Impact Test.

3.2. fMRI Behavioral Performance

Compared with HCs, patients with mTBI exhibited significantly longer RT in the TS condition [$F_{(1,31)} = 4.247, p = 0.048$], reflecting impaired cognitive flexibility on a behavioral level (Figure 2A). Furthermore, mTBI patients were significantly less accurate than HCs across all conditions ($p < 0.05$, Figure 2B). The detailed information about fMRI behavioral performance is described in the Supplementary Materials.

3.3. fMRI Brain Imaging Results

Compared with HCs, mTBI patients showed significantly reduced activation in widespread frontal regions across OG conditions (Table S1), which were mainly distributed in the medial superior frontal gyrus (mSFG), dorsolateral superior frontal gyrus (dlSFG), medial orbital gyrus (mOG), ventrolateral middle frontal gyrus (vlMFG) and rostrodorsal supramarginal gyrus (rdSG).

During the DI condition, mTBI patients exhibited significantly reduced activation in a broad cingulate-frontal network compared to HCs (Table S2), which included the posterior cingulate cortex (PCC), posterior insula (pIns) and other frontal regions.

In addition, for the TS condition, the mTBI patients showed significantly reduced activation in the dorsal caudate (dCau), anterior cingulate cortex (ACC), and other frontal regions (Figure 3, Table 2) compared with HCs.

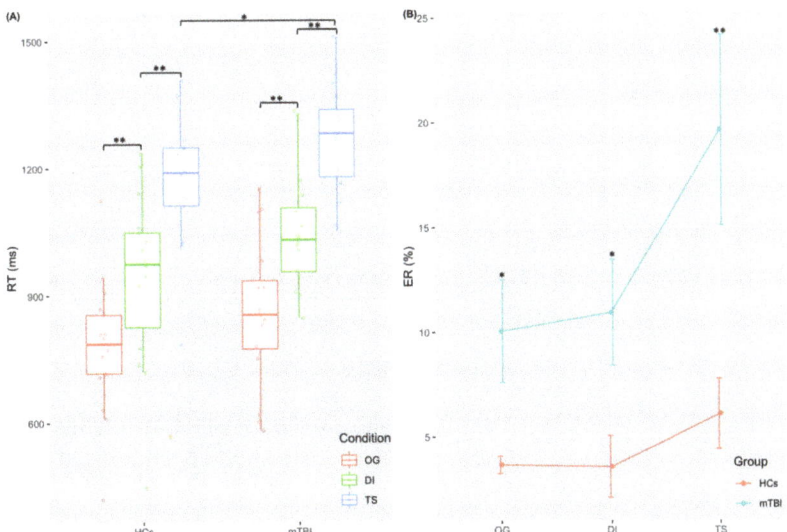

Figure 2. Behavioral results of fMRI task performance. (**A**) Mean response time (RT) during three conditions [ongoing (OG) condition, distractor inhibition (DI) condition, task switch (TS) condition] in mTBI patients and HCs; (**B**) Error rate (ER) during three conditions in mTBI patients and HCs. Error bars represent standard deviation. *: $p < 0.05$; **: $p < 0.01$. mTBI, mild traumatic brain injury; HCs, healthy controls.

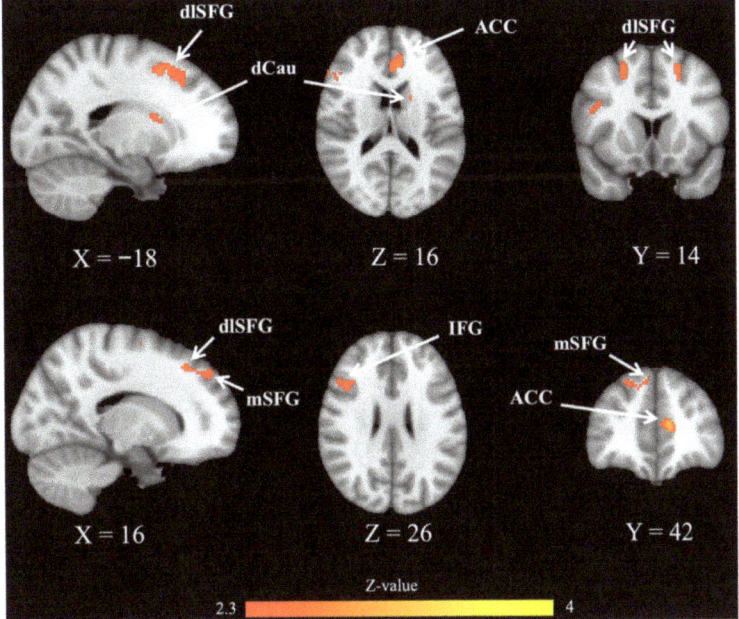

Figure 3. Brain activation results from the BOLD-fMRI analysis of the contrast mTBI < HC in task switching (TS) condition (FEW corrected). Compared with HCs, mTBI patients showed significantly reduced activation in the dorsal caudate (dCau), anterior cingulate cortex (ACC), medial superior frontal gyrus (mSFG), dorsolateral superior frontal gyrus (dlSFG).

Table 2. Results from the BOLD-fMRI analysis of the contrast mTBI < HCs in TS condition (FWE corrected).

Brain Regions	Hemisphere	BA	Peak MNI Coordinates			Z-Value	Size (Voxels)
			x	y	z		
dCau	L	NA	−18	8	14	2.638	112
dlSFG	L	8	−18	10	50	3.005	177
	R	6, 8	20	−6	64	3.295	421
mSFG	R	91	8	46	42	3.201	154
IFG	R	44, 45	44	10	20	3.109	268
ACC	L	32	−10	40	12	3.549	210

mTBI, mild traumatic brain injury; HCs, healthy controls; FWE, family wise error; TS, task switching; MNI, Montreal Neurological Institute; L, left; R, right; dCau, dorsal caudate; dlSFG, dorsolateral Superior Frontal Gyrus; mSFG, medial Superior Frontal Gyrus; IFG, inferior frontal gyrus; ACC, anterior cingulate cortex.

3.4. Relationship between Abnormal Activation, Behavioral and Neuropsychological Measures in mTBI

The reduced dCau activation of the TS condition in mTBI patients was positively correlated with information processing speed (indexed by DSC) ($p < 0.001$, FDR corrected), but negatively correlated with RT for TS condition ($p < 0.001$, FDR corrected). In addition, the RT for TS condition was negatively correlated with information processing speed in mTBI patients ($p < 0.001$, FDR corrected).

3.5. Abnormal Dorsal Caudate Activation Mediates the Relationship between Information Processing Speed and Cognitive Flexibility in mTBI

Mediation modeling was performed to test whether the magnitude of information about processing speed's effect on cognitive flexibility was dependent on reduced dCau activation. We found that reduced dCau activation had a significant mediating effect on the relationship between information processing speed and cognitive flexibility in mTBI patients (a ×b = −18.836, 95%CI: [−42.183, −5.347], $p < 0.05$, Figure 4).

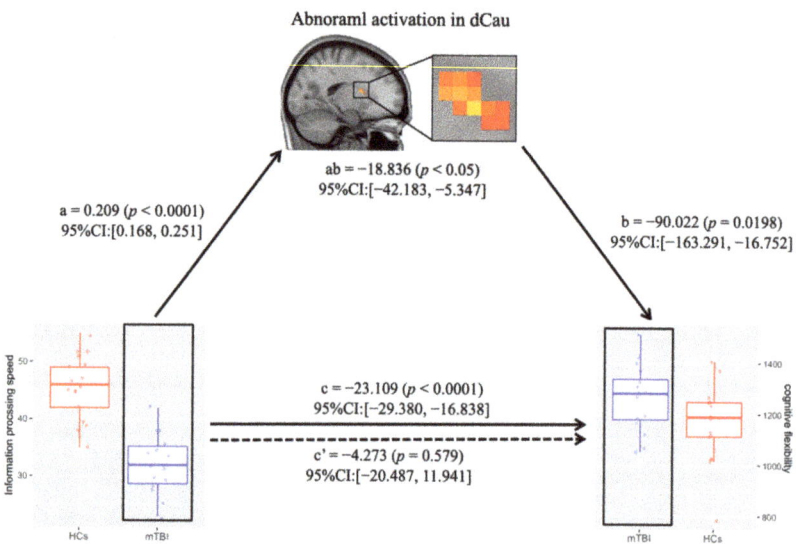

Figure 4. Abnormal dCau activation mediates the association between information processing speed and cognitive flexibility in mTBI patients. The illustration demonstrates that within mTBI patients, information processing speed affected cognitive flexibility through the abnormal dCau activation. mTBI, mild traumatic brain injury; HCs, healthy controls; dCau, dorsal caudate; CI, confidence interval.

4. Discussion

To the best of our knowledge, this is the first study to investigate the underlying mechanisms of cognitive flexibility in mTBI patients using a rule-based task-switching experimental paradigm. The mTBI patients exhibited a longer RT than HCs on the TS condition, accompanied by a significantly reduced activation in the dorsal caudate, anterior cingulate cortex and other frontal regions. Furthermore, the abnormal dorsal caudate activation mediated the relationship between information processing speed and cognitive flexibility in patients. Together, these results suggested that dorsal caudate might play a vital role in the cognitive flexibility of mTBI, thus providing an alternative clinical target for impaired cognitive functions in patients.

During the task behavioral performance, mTBI patients only showed significantly longer RT on TS condition compared to HCs, indicating that mTBI patients had impaired cognitive flexibility on the behavior level. These data were in sync with data from previous studies [15,16]. These studies used local-global task-switching tasks and showed that, compared with HCs, patients with traumatic brain injury had significantly longer RT and increased ER under TS condition. Although the studies performed different experimental paradigms, the findings demonstrated specific cognitive behavioral patterns in patients with traumatic brain injuries. Previous research found that patients with several neurocognitive disorders exhibited poor cognitive outcomes [36,37]. We speculated that the mTBI patients had specific behavioral response patterns on impaired cognitive flexibility, which could help in understanding cognitive dysfunction in mTBI.

By comparing the brain activation response of mTBI patients and HCs under different task conditions, we showed that during the OG condition, mTBI patients exhibited significantly weaker activation in widespread frontal brain regions. Plenty of MRI studies revealed that the frontal cortex is involved in different neural circuits with a subcortical nucleus, which plays a vital role in various kinds of cognitive functions [38–41]. Many clinical studies have demonstrated that mTBI patients often present significantly reduced activation in the frontal cortex during simple tasks [42,43]. On the other hand, the observed abnormal frontal activation in mTBI indicated that the patients had cognitive dysfunction. In addition, during the DI condition, mTBI patients showed significantly reduced activation in the PCC, pIns and other frontal regions. As a key hub in the default mode network, PCC is involved in the regulation of attention and self-referential processing [44–46]. It has been hypothesized that reduced PCC activation in mTBI reduces the ability of other stimuli to direct patients' attention away from the distract stimulus, as patients showed significantly longer RT for the DI condition compared with the OG condition.

In the TS condition, our analyses showed that patients had significantly longer RT and higher ER compared to HCs, thus reflecting impaired cognitive flexibility in mTBI. Furthermore, compared with HCs, mTBI patients exhibited reduced activation in dCau, ACC and other frontal regions. Previous studies showed that the ACC, a hub region in the salience network [47], plays an important role in cognitive control [23], and has a close projection loop with the caudate nucleus [48,49]. Several studies performed the Stroop task, and showed that conflicts between potential behaviors elicit a significant abnormal activation during conflict monitoring and action selection [50–53]. In addition, the interconnection of the caudate nucleus and ACC is involved in evaluating the consequences of behavior and adjusting behavioral response [53–55]. Previous studies have shown that the caudate nucleus is a susceptible hub region in mTBI [56], and its dysfunction was significantly associated with impaired cognitive function in patients [57]. In addition, the impaired white matter fiber from the caudate nucleus to the cerebral cortex could predict impairment of cognitive flexibility in mTBI patients [16]. In our study, mTBI patients might have altered white matter connections in the dorsal caudate, which resulted in reduced activation in the patients. Another study showed that the abnormal caudate activation in patients with traumatic brain injuries was significantly associated with cognitive fatigue [14]. Our results suggested that mTBI patients might need more cognitive load to perform cognitive flexibility responses, which would further cause cognitive fatigue, and finally lead to the abnormal activation of dorsal caudate [58].

Interestingly, we demonstrated that the abnormal activation of dorsal caudate played a significant mediating role between information processing speed and cognitive flexibility in mTBI patients. Many previous studies on traumatic brain injury have shown that structural and functional abnormalities of the caudate nucleus were significantly related to executive dysfunction in patients [14,57]. Besides, we showed that information processing speed was significantly related to cognitive flexibility in mTBI patients. This was consistent with the findings from previous studies, which showed that an individual's information processing speed ability is significantly associated with cognitive flexibility [59,60]. However, whether the impaired information processing speed or the abnormal dorsal caudate activation affects cognitive flexibility in mTBI patients remains unknown. Investigating the relationship between the information processing speed, abnormal dorsal caudate activation, and cognitive flexibility would help to understand the neural mechanisms of cognitive flexibility deficit in mTBI patients. Our mediation model showed that the abnormal dorsal caudate activation was a significant mediator between the patient's information processing speed and impaired cognitive flexibility.

There are some limitations that should be noticed. Firstly, it is still unclear whether the observed abnormal activation changes could be related to structural and resting-state functional alterations in mTBI patients. Future studies can combine multimodal MRI imaging to investigate the neural mechanism underlying cognitive flexibility in mTBI. Secondly, the difficulty level of the experimental task in this study was relatively high for patients. Thus, future studies can apply cognitive tasks with a moderately difficult level to investigate cognitive function in mTBI. Finally, the sample size of both groups was relatively small. Future studies with larger samples are needed to improve the reliability of the results and investigate the effect of different brain injury types on results.

5. Conclusions

In summary, we performed a rule-based task-switching paradigm to investigate the neural mechanism of impaired cognitive flexibility in mTBI. The mTBI patients showed reduced activation in the dorsal caudate, anterior cingulate cortex, and other frontal regions during the TS condition. Further mediation analysis revealed that impaired cognitive flexibility was mediated by abnormal dorsal caudate activation in mTBI. These findings may underscore the importance of dorsal caudate in impaired cognitive flexibility in mTBI, and abnormal dorsal caudate activation reflected in altered cognitive flexibility behavior in patients. Furthermore, our findings would provide an alternative target for clinical interventions for cognitive function improvement in mTBI. In future research, cognitive intervention together with transcranial magnetic stimulation targeted caudate or caudate-involved functional networks will be a great treatment intervention for cognitive impairment in mTBI patients.

Supplementary Materials: The following supporting information can be downloaded at: https://www.mdpi.com/article/10.3390/jcm11092484/s1, Table S1: Results from the BOLD-fMRI analysis of the contrast mTBI < HC in OG condition (FEW corrected); Table S2: Results from the BOLD-fMRI analysis of the contrast mTBI < HC in DI condition (FWE corrected).

Author Contributions: H.X. and G.B. conceived the study, designed the trial. X.Z. and H.X. supervised the conduct of the trial and data collection. H.X. and X.Z. provided statistical advice on study design and analyzed the data; H.X. drafted the manuscript, and all authors contributed substantially to its revision. H.X. and G.B. took responsibility for the paper as a whole. All authors have read and agreed to the published version of the manuscript.

Funding: This study was funded by the Natural Science Foundation of Zhejiang Province (No. LY19H180003, LY15H090016), Wenzhou Science and Technology Bureau in China (No. Y20180112, Y20140577), and Beijing New Health Industry Development Foundation (No. XM2020-02-002).

Institutional Review Board Statement: The study was conducted in accordance with the Declaration of Helsinki, and approved by the Institutional Review Board of of the Second Affiliated Hospital and Yuying Children's Hospital of Wenzhou Medical University (protocol code NCT05108909 and 2016).

Informed Consent Statement: Not applicable.

Data Availability Statement: The data that support the findings of this study are available on request from the corresponding author.

Conflicts of Interest: The authors declare that they have no conflict of interest.

References

1. Xu, H.; Tao, Y.; Zhu, P.; Li, D.; Zhang, M.; Bai, G.; Yin, B. Restoration of aberrant shape of caudate sub-regions associated with cognitive function improvement in mild traumatic brain injury. *J. Neurotrauma* **2022**, *39*, 348–357. [CrossRef] [PubMed]
2. Bruns, J., Jr.; Hauser, W.A. The epidemiology of traumatic brain injury: A review. *Epilepsia* **2003**, *44*, 2–10. [CrossRef] [PubMed]
3. Capizzi, A.; Woo, J.; Verduzco-Gutierrez, M. Traumatic Brain Injury: An Overview of Epidemiology, Pathophysiology, and Medical Management. *Med. Clin. N. Am.* **2020**, *104*, 213–238. [CrossRef] [PubMed]
4. Holm, L.; Cassidy, J.D.; Carroll, L.J.; Borg, J. Neurotrauma Task Force on Mild Traumatic Brain Injury of the WHO Collaborating Centre. Summary of the WHO Collaborating Centre for Neurotrauma Task Force on Mild Traumatic Brain Injury. *J. Rehabil. Med.* **2005**, *37*, 137–141. [CrossRef]
5. Gilbert, S.J.; Burgess, P.W. Executive function. *Curr. Biol.* **2008**, *18*, R110–R114. [CrossRef]
6. Friedman, N.P.; Robbins, T.W. The role of prefrontal cortex in cognitive control and executive function. *Neuropsychopharmacology* **2022**, *47*, 72–89. [CrossRef]
7. Ridderinkhof, K.R.; Ullsperger, M.; Crone, E.A.; Nieuwenhuis, S. The role of the medial frontal cortex in cognitive control. *Science* **2004**, *306*, 443–447. [CrossRef]
8. Chamberlain, S.R.; Fineberg, N.A.; Blackwell, A.D.; Robbins, T.W.; Sahakian, B.J. Motor inhibition and cognitive flexibility in obsessive-compulsive disorder and trichotillomania. *Am. J. Psychiatry* **2006**, *163*, 1282–1284. [CrossRef]
9. Chamberlain, S.R.; Fineberg, N.A.; Menzies, L.A.; Blackwell, A.D.; Bullmore, E.T.; Robbins, T.W.; Sahakian, B.J. Impaired cognitive flexibility and motor inhibition in unaffected first-degree relatives of patients with obsessive-compulsive disorder. *Am. J. Psychiatry* **2007**, *164*, 335–338. [CrossRef]
10. Ersche, K.D.; Barnes, A.; Jones, P.S.; Morein-Zamir, S.; Robbins, T.W.; Bullmore, E.T. Abnormal structure of frontostriatal brain systems is associated with aspects of impulsivity and compulsivity in cocaine dependence. *Brain* **2011**, *134*, 2013–2024. [CrossRef]
11. Moreno-Lopez, L.; Catena, A.; Fernandez-Serrano, M.J.; Delgado-Rico, E.; Stamatakis, E.A.; Perez-Garcia, M.; Verdejo-Garcia, A. Trait impulsivity and prefrontal gray matter reductions in cocaine dependent individuals. *Drug Alcohol Depend.* **2012**, *125*, 208–214. [CrossRef]
12. Vaghi, M.M.; Vertes, P.E.; Kitzbichler, M.G.; Apergis-Schoute, A.M.; van der Flier, F.E.; Fineberg, N.A.; Sule, A.; Zaman, R.; Voon, V.; Kundu, P.; et al. Specific Frontostriatal Circuits for Impaired Cognitive Flexibility and Goal-Directed Planning in Obsessive-Compulsive Disorder: Evidence From Resting-State Functional Connectivity. *Biol. Psychiatry* **2017**, *81*, 708–717. [CrossRef]
13. Fagerholm, E.D.; Hellyer, P.J.; Scott, G.; Leech, R.; Sharp, D.J. Disconnection of network hubs and cognitive impairment after traumatic brain injury. *Brain* **2015**, *138*, 1696–1709. [CrossRef]
14. Wylie, G.R.; Dobryakova, E.; DeLuca, J.; Chiaravalloti, N.; Essad, K.; Genova, H. Cognitive fatigue in individuals with traumatic brain injury is associated with caudate activation. *Sci. Rep.* **2017**, *7*, 8973. [CrossRef]
15. Leunissen, I.; Coxon, J.P.; Caeyenberghs, K.; Michiels, K.; Sunaert, S.; Swinnen, S.P. Subcortical volume analysis in traumatic brain injury: The importance of the fronto-striato-thalamic circuit in task switching. *Cortex* **2014**, *51*, 67–81. [CrossRef]
16. Leunissen, I.; Coxon, J.P.; Caeyenberghs, K.; Michiels, K.; Sunaert, S.; Swinnen, S.P. Task switching in traumatic brain injury relates to cortico-subcortical integrity. *Hum. Brain Mapp.* **2014**, *35*, 2459–2469. [CrossRef]
17. Grant, D.A.; Berg, E.A. A behavioral analysis of degree of reinforcement and ease of shifting to new responses in a Weigl-type card-sorting problem. *J. Exp. Psychol.* **1948**, *38*, 404–411. [CrossRef]
18. Ozen, L.J.; Fernandes, M.A. Effects of "diagnosis threat" on cognitive and affective functioning long after mild head injury. *J. Int. Neuropsychol. Soc.* **2011**, *17*, 219–229. [CrossRef]
19. Suhr, J.A.; Gunstad, J. "Diagnosis Threat": The effect of negative expectations on cognitive performance in head injury. *J. Clin. Exp. Neuropsychol.* **2002**, *24*, 448–457. [CrossRef]
20. Dobryakova, E.; Boukrina, O.; Wylie, G.R. Investigation of Information Flow During a Novel Working Memory Task in Individuals with Traumatic Brain Injury. *Brain Connect.* **2015**, *5*, 433–441. [CrossRef]
21. Fischer-Baum, S.; Miozzo, M.; Laiacona, M.; Capitani, E. Perseveration during verbal fluency in traumatic brain injury reflects impairments in working memory. *Neuropsychology* **2016**, *30*, 791–799. [CrossRef] [PubMed]
22. Sandry, J.; DeLuca, J.; Chiaravalloti, N. Working memory capacity links cognitive reserve with long-term memory in moderate to severe TBI: A translational approach. *J. Neurol.* **2015**, *262*, 59–64. [CrossRef] [PubMed]

23. Bonnelle, V.; Ham, T.E.; Leech, R.; Kinnunen, K.M.; Mehta, M.A.; Greenwood, R.J.; Sharp, D.J. Salience network integrity predicts default mode network function after traumatic brain injury. *Proc. Natl. Acad. Sci. USA* **2012**, *109*, 4690–4695. [CrossRef] [PubMed]
24. Sharp, D.J.; Beckmann, C.F.; Greenwood, R.; Kinnunen, K.M.; Bonnelle, V.; De Boissezon, X.; Powell, J.H.; Counsell, S.J.; Patel, M.C.; Leech, R. Default mode network functional and structural connectivity after traumatic brain injury. *Brain* **2011**, *134*, 2233–2247. [CrossRef] [PubMed]
25. Armbruster, D.J.; Ueltzhoffer, K.; Basten, U.; Fiebach, C.J. Prefrontal cortical mechanisms underlying individual differences in cognitive flexibility and stability. *J. Cogn. Neurosci.* **2012**, *24*, 2385–2399. [CrossRef]
26. Armbruster-Genc, D.J.; Ueltzhoffer, K.; Fiebach, C.J. Brain Signal Variability Differentially Affects Cognitive Flexibility and Cognitive Stability. *J. Neurosci.* **2016**, *36*, 3978–3987. [CrossRef]
27. Sekutowicz, M.; Schmack, K.; Steimke, R.; Paschke, L.; Sterzer, P.; Walter, H.; Stelzel, C. Striatal activation as a neural link between cognitive and perceptual flexibility. *Neuroimage* **2016**, *141*, 393–398. [CrossRef]
28. Hartmann, T.; Weisz, N. An Introduction to the Objective Psychophysics Toolbox. *Front. Psychol.* **2020**, *11*, 585437. [CrossRef]
29. Brainard, D.H. The Psychophysics Toolbox. *Spat. Vis.* **1997**, *10*, 433–436. [CrossRef]
30. Woolrich, M.W.; Ripley, B.D.; Brady, M.; Smith, S.M. Temporal autocorrelation in univariate linear modeling of FMRI data. *NeuroImage* **2001**, *14*, 1370–1386. [CrossRef]
31. Xu, H.; Chen, Y.; Tao, Y.; Zhang, Y.; Zhao, T.; Wang, M.; Fan, L.; Zheng, Y.; Guo, C. Modulation effect of acupuncture treatment on chronic neck and shoulder pain in female patients: Evidence from periaqueductal gray-based functional connectivity. *CNS Neurosci. Ther.* **2022**, *28*, 714–723. [CrossRef]
32. Woolrich, M.W.; Behrens, T.E.; Beckmann, C.F.; Jenkinson, M.; Smith, S.M. Multilevel linear modelling for FMRI group analysis using Bayesian inference. *NeuroImage* **2004**, *21*, 1732–1747. [CrossRef]
33. Chen, G.; Saad, Z.S.; Nath, A.R.; Beauchamp, M.S.; Cox, R.W. FMRI group analysis combining effect estimates and their variances. *NeuroImage* **2012**, *60*, 747–765. [CrossRef]
34. Hayes, A.F.; Preacher, K.J. Statistical mediation analysis with a multicategorical independent variable. *Br. J. Math. Stat. Psychol.* **2014**, *67*, 451–470. [CrossRef]
35. Preacher, K.J.; Rucker, D.D.; Hayes, A.F. Addressing Moderated Mediation Hypotheses: Theory, Methods, and Prescriptions. *Multivar. Behav. Res.* **2007**, *42*, 185–227. [CrossRef]
36. Esechie, A.; Bhardwaj, A.; Masel, T.; Raji, M. Neurocognitive sequela of burn injury in the elderly. *J. Clin. Neurosci.* **2019**, *59*, 1–5. [CrossRef]
37. Pollicina, I.; Maniaci, A.; Lechien, J.R.; Iannella, G.; Vicini, C.; Cammaroto, G.; Cannavicci, A.; Magliulo, G.; Pace, A.; Cocuzza, S.; et al. Neurocognitive Performance Improvement after Obstructive Sleep Apnea Treatment: State of the Art. *Behav. Sci.* **2021**, *11*, 180. [CrossRef]
38. Alvarez, J.A.; Emory, E. Executive function and the frontal lobes: A meta-analytic review. *Neuropsychol. Rev.* **2006**, *16*, 17–42. [CrossRef]
39. Cummings, J.L. Frontal-subcortical circuits and human behavior. *J. Psychosom. Res.* **1998**, *44*, 627–628. [CrossRef]
40. Mega, M.S.; Cummings, J.L. Frontal-subcortical circuits and neuropsychiatric disorders. *J. Neuropsychiatry Clin. Neurosci.* **1994**, *6*, 358–370. [CrossRef]
41. Wager, T.D.; Davidson, M.L.; Hughes, B.L.; Lindquist, M.A.; Ochsner, K.N. Prefrontal-subcortical pathways mediating successful emotion regulation. *Neuron* **2008**, *59*, 1037–1050. [CrossRef] [PubMed]
42. Reverberi, C.; Toraldo, A.; D'Agostini, S.; Skrap, M. Better without (lateral) frontal cortex? Insight problems solved by frontal patients. *Brain* **2005**, *128*, 2882–2890. [CrossRef] [PubMed]
43. Shimamura, A.P.; Janowsky, J.S.; Squire, L.R. Memory for the temporal order of events in patients with frontal lobe lesions and amnesic patients. *Neuropsychologia* **1990**, *28*, 803–813. [CrossRef]
44. Hahn, B.; Ross, T.J.; Stein, E.A. Cingulate activation increases dynamically with response speed under stimulus unpredictability. *Cereb. Cortex* **2007**, *17*, 1664–1671. [CrossRef]
45. Kaiser, R.H.; Andrews-Hanna, J.R.; Wager, T.D.; Pizzagalli, D.A. Large-Scale Network Dysfunction in Major Depressive Disorder: A Meta-analysis of Resting-State Functional Connectivity. *JAMA Psychiatry* **2015**, *72*, 603–611. [CrossRef]
46. Small, D.M.; Gitelman, D.R.; Gregory, M.D.; Nobre, A.C.; Parrish, T.B.; Mesulam, M.M. The posterior cingulate and medial prefrontal cortex mediate the anticipatory allocation of spatial attention. *NeuroImage* **2003**, *18*, 633–641. [CrossRef]
47. Xu, H.; Seminowicz, D.A.; Krimmel, S.R.; Zhang, M.; Gao, L.; Wang, Y. Altered Structural and Functional Connectivity of Salience Network in Patients with Classic Trigeminal Neuralgia. *J. Pain* **2022**, in press. [CrossRef]
48. Kemp, J.M.; Powell, T.P. The cortico-striate projection in the monkey. *Brain* **1970**, *93*, 525–546. [CrossRef]
49. Yeterian, E.H.; Van Hoesen, G.W. Cortico-striate projections in the rhesus monkey: The organization of certain cortico-caudate connections. *Brain Res.* **1978**, *139*, 43–63. [CrossRef]
50. Ham, T.E.; de Boissezon, X.; Leff, A.; Beckmann, C.; Hughes, E.; Kinnunen, K.M.; Leech, R.; Sharp, D.J. Distinct frontal networks are involved in adapting to internally and externally signaled errors. *Cereb. Cortex* **2013**, *23*, 703–713. [CrossRef]
51. Heyder, K.; Suchan, B.; Daum, I. Cortico-subcortical contributions to executive control. *Acta Psychol.* **2004**, *115*, 271–289. [CrossRef]
52. Kerns, J.G.; Cohen, J.D.; MacDonald, A.W., 3rd; Cho, R.Y.; Stenger, V.A.; Carter, C.S. Anterior cingulate conflict monitoring and adjustments in control. *Science* **2004**, *303*, 1023–1026. [CrossRef]

53. Shenhav, A.; Botvinick, M.M.; Cohen, J.D. The expected value of control: An integrative theory of anterior cingulate cortex function. *Neuron* **2013**, *79*, 217–240. [CrossRef]
54. O'Reilly, R.C.; Frank, M.J. Making working memory work: A computational model of learning in the prefrontal cortex and basal ganglia. *Neural. Comput.* **2006**, *18*, 283–328. [CrossRef]
55. Wiecki, T.V.; Frank, M.J. A computational model of inhibitory control in frontal cortex and basal ganglia. *Psychol. Rev.* **2013**, *120*, 329–355. [CrossRef]
56. Xu, H.; Wang, X.; Chen, Z.; Bai, G.; Yin, B.; Wang, S.; Sun, C.; Gan, S.; Wang, Z.; Cao, J.; et al. Longitudinal Changes of Caudate-Based Resting State Functional Connectivity in Mild Traumatic Brain Injury. *Front. Neurol.* **2018**, *9*, 467. [CrossRef]
57. De Simoni, S.; Jenkins, P.O.; Bourke, N.J.; Fleminger, J.J.; Hellyer, P.J.; Jolly, A.E.; Patel, M.C.; Cole, J.H.; Leech, R.; Sharp, D.J. Altered caudate connectivity is associated with executive dysfunction after traumatic brain injury. *Brain* **2018**, *141*, 148–164. [CrossRef]
58. Wylie, G.R.; Flashman, L.A. Understanding the interplay between mild traumatic brain injury and cognitive fatigue: Models and treatments. *Concussion* **2017**, *2*, CNC50. [CrossRef]
59. Dajani, D.R.; Uddin, L.Q. Demystifying cognitive flexibility: Implications for clinical and developmental neuroscience. *Trends Neurosci.* **2015**, *38*, 571–578. [CrossRef]
60. McCabe, D.P.; Roediger, H.L.; McDaniel, M.A.; Balota, D.A.; Hambrick, D.Z. The relationship between working memory capacity and executive functioning: Evidence for a common executive attention construct. *Neuropsychology* **2010**, *24*, 222–243. [CrossRef]

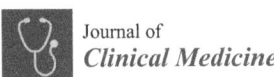

Article

Cortical and Subcortical Alterations and Clinical Correlates after Traumatic Brain Injury

Qiang Xue [1,†], Linbo Wang [2,†], Yuanyu Zhao [3], Wusong Tong [4], Jiancun Wang [1], Gaoyi Li [5], Wei Cheng [2], Liang Gao [6,*] and Yan Dong [6,*]

1. Department of Neurosurgery, Eastern Hepatobiliary Surgery Hospital, Navy Medical University, Shanghai 200433, China; smmuxq@foxmail.com (Q.X.); wc_jiancun@yeah.net (J.W.)
2. Institute of Science and Technology for Brain-inspired Intelligence, Fudan University, Shanghai 210023, China; linbowang@fudan.edu.cn (L.W.); wcheng.fdu@gmail.com (W.C.)
3. Department of Organ Transplantation, Changzheng Hospital, Navy Medical University, Shanghai 200070, China; zhaoyuanyu0617@163.com
4. Department of Neurosurgery, Shanghai Pudong New Area People's Hospital, Shanghai 201299, China; tongws0599@163.com
5. Department of Neurosurgery, People's Hospital of Putuo District, Tongji University School of Medicine, Shanghai 200061, China; ligaoyitongji@126.com
6. Department of Neurosurgery, Shanghai Tenth People's Hospital, Tongji University School of Medicine, Shanghai 200072, China
* Correspondence: lianggaoh@126.com (L.G.); smmudongyan@163.com (Y.D.)
† These authors contributed equally to this study.

Abstract: Background: Traumatic brain injury (TBI) often results in persistent cognitive impairment and psychiatric symptoms, while lesion location and severity are not consistent with its clinical complaints. Previous studies found cognitive deficits and psychiatric disorders following TBI are considered to be associated with prefrontal and medial temporal lobe lesions, however, the location and extent of contusions often cannot fully explain the patient's impairments. Thus, we try to find the structural changes of gray matter (GM) and white matter (WM), clarify their correlation with psychiatric symptoms and memory following TBI, and determine the brain regions that primary correlate with clinical measurements. **Methods**: Overall, 32 TBI individuals and 23 healthy controls were recruited in the study. Cognitive impairment and psychiatric symptoms were examined by Mini-Mental State Examination (MMSE), Hospital Anxiety and Depression Scale (HADS), and Wechsler Memory Scale-Chinese Revision (WMS-CR). All MRI data were scanned using a Siemens Prisma 3.0 Tesla MRI system. T1 MRI data and diffusion tensor imaging (DTI) data were processed to analyze GM volume and WM microstructure separately. **Results**: In the present study, TBI patients underwent widespread decrease of GM volume in both cortical and subcortical regions. Among these regions, four brain areas including the left inferior temporal gyrus and medial temporal lobe, supplementary motor area, thalamus, and anterior cingulate cortex (ACC) were highly implicated in the post-traumatic cognitive impairment and psychiatric complaints. TBI patients also underwent changes of WM microstructure, involving decreased fractional anisotropy (FA) value in widespread WM tracts and increased mean diffusivity (MD) value in the forceps minor. The changes of WM microstructure were significantly correlated with the decrease of GM volume. **Conclusions**: TBI causes widespread cortical and subcortical alterations including a reduction in GM volume and change in WM microstructure related to clinical manifestation. Lesions in temporal lobe may lead to more serious cognitive and emotional dysfunction, which should attract our high clinical attention.

Keywords: traumatic brain injury; gray matter volume; white matter track; prognosis

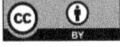

1. Introduction

Traumatic brain injury (TBI) is the leading cause of death and disability in individuals below age 45, which typically caused by motor vehicle crashes, falls, contact sports, or assaults. TBI often results in persistent cognitive impairment and psychiatric symptoms, including memory deficit, anxiety, and depression, which exert a negative impact on quality of life and rehabilitation process [1–3]. Due to the significant heterogeneity in the clinical presentation and neuropathological across TBI patients, it is challenging to predict the risk of comorbid psychiatric disorders and cognitive impairment [4]. Previous studies found that TBI severity is not correlated with neuropsychiatric outcome [5,6]. Meanwhile, previous findings for the correlation between lesion location and cognitive function and psychiatric complaints were inconsistent [7].

Although TBI is heterogeneous in the cause and intensity of impact, it still exhibits a featured pattern of anatomical injuries. The impact typically results in contusions involving the basal and polar regions of the frontal and temporal lobes [8,9]. Besides focal brain injuries, diffuse axonal injuries (DAI) occur after TBI, which frequently affect the frontal and temporal WM, corpus callosum, and brainstem [10]. Traditionally, cognitive deficits and psychiatric disorders following TBI are considered to be associated with prefrontal and medial temporal lobe lesions, however the location and extent of these contusions often cannot fully explain the patient's impairments [11–14]. During the acute and subacute stages of TBI, secondary damages including inflammation, apoptosis, excitotoxicity, and prolonged hypo-perfusion result in progressive and widespread white matter (WM) atrophy and gray matter (GM) volume loss across large areas of the brain spanning most of the cortex and subcortical areas over time [14–16]. These abnormalities in the parietal and occipital lobes and subcortical regions including basal ganglions and thalamus are closely related to post-traumatic cognitive functions and psychiatric symptoms [14,17,18]. Due to the heterogeneity inherent to study design and various pipelines of data pre-processing, parcellation, and analysis among the previous studies, the topographical distribution of morphometric changes and their clinical associations related to post-traumatic psychiatric symptoms and memory function remains inconsistent.

In the present study, we assessed the cortical and subcortical GM and WM damage and its relation to post-traumatic neuropsychological measurements of anxiety and depressive symptoms and memory function. We then investigated the relationships between disruption of WM microstructure and the decrease in GM volume. We aimed to obtain a comprehensive understanding of the relationship between the structural alterations and psychiatric symptoms and memory following TBI and determine the brain regions correlated with clinical measurements.

2. Materials and Methods

2.1. Participants

Overall, 32 patients with TBI were recruited from the Shanghai Pudong New Area People's Hospital. These patients were older than 18 years and with first-ever TBI and positive finding on cranial CT scans on admission. They were excluded from the study if suffering neurological or psychiatric disorders prior to TBI. The initial evaluation of severity of TBI took place within the first 24 h after injury during hospitalization based on Glasgow Coma Scale (GCS), which classifies TBI into three categories as mild (GCS 13–15), moderate (GCS 9–12), and severe (GCS 3–8). Twenty-three healthy participants without history of TBI, neurological, and psychiatric disorders were matched for age, gender, and education. The ethics committee of the Pudong New Area People's Hospital approved the study. Informed written consent for study participation was obtained from all patients and healthy controls.

2.2. Cognitive Functional Assessment and Neuropsychological Assessment

The global cognition was assessed with the Mini-Mental State Examination (MMSE), which includes items measuring orientation, attention, memory, language, and visual/spatial skills. MMSE scores range from 0 to 30, with a higher score indicating better cognitive performance. The Hospital Anxiety and Depression Scale (HADS), which is a brief self-assessment questionnaire measuring severity of emotional disorder and has been validated in TBI populations, was employed to evaluate the anxiety and depressive symptoms. The anxiety and depression subscales have seven items respectively. Wechsler Memory Scale-Chinese Revision (WMS-CR) picture, recognition, associative learning, comprehension memory, and digit span were administered to evaluate multiple categories of memory capacity. The sum of five subscales was calculated to reflect general memory function.

2.3. Image Acquisition

All MRI data were collected using a Siemens Prisma 3.0 Tesla MRI system (Prisma, Siemens, Erlangen, Germany) equipped with a 20-channel head coil. Participants assumed a supine position in the MRI scanner with cushions to restrict the mobility of their heads, thus minimizing the head motion. During rs-fMRI scanning, participants were guided to stay awake with their eyes closed without thinking about anything in particular. Structural images were acquired using a high-resolution T1-weighted MPRAGE sequence with 192 sagittal slices, TR/TE = 2530/2.98 ms, flip angle = 7°, FOV = 256 × 256 mm, matrix size = 256 × 256, voxel size = 1 × 1 × 1 mm^3, which facilitated the localization and co-registration of functional data. In addition, transverse turbo-spin-echo T2-weighted images for lesion localization were obtained with 30 axial slices, slice thickness = 5 mm, TR/TE = 6000/95 ms, flip angle = 120°, FOV = 220 × 220 mm, matrix size = 320 × 320, voxel size = 0.34 × 0.34 × 5 mm^3. Diffusion tensor images (DTI) were acquired using an echo planar imaging (EPI) sequence (30 gradient directions, 1 baseline (b = 0) image, b = 1000 s/mm^2, TR = 10,100 ms, TE = 92 ms, FOV = 256 × 256 mm, 75 axial slices, voxel size = 2.0 × 2.0 × 2.0 mm^3.

2.4. T1 MRI Data Processing and Analysis

The T1-weighted MRI images were preprocessed by using the CAT12 (Computational Anatomy Toolbox; http://dbm.neuro.uni-jena.de/cat12/; accessed on 1 June 2021) for grey matter extraction, which is an extension of SPM12 (Statistical Parametric Mapping) to provide computational anatomy. Images were segmented into GM, WM, and cerebrospinal fluid (CSF), and normalized to a standard template (Montreal Neurological Institute). Raw images of lower quality (CAT image quality rating <75%) were excluded. Cortical maps were smoothed using an 8-mm full width at half maximum kernel, prior to building the statistical model. After preprocessing, the Brainnetome Atlas was used to extract regional grey matter volume by averaging voxel GM within each regions of interest (ROI). Based on the Brainnetome Atlas, GM was segmented into 246 ROI.

2.5. Diffusion Tensor Imaging(DTI) Data Preprocessing and Analysis

The DTI data were preprocessed by using the FMRIB Diffusion Toolbox (FSL, FMRIB, Oxford, UK). Briefly, after correcting for the eddy-current effect and brain tissue extraction, the diffusion tensor model was fit to extract DTI measures. The output yielded voxel-wise maps of fractional anisotropy (FA), mean diffusivity (MD), radial diffusivity (RD), and axial diffusivity (AD). Next, DTI data from each participant were registered to a standard space (Montreal Neurological Institute, NMI, ICBM-152). To obtain a comprehensive WM segmentation, WM tracts were defined using JHU_ICBM_tracts_maxprob_thr25 atlas [19]. Finally, mean FA, MD, RD, and AD values were computed in each WM ROI in standard space for each participant.

2.6. Correlation Analysis and Statistical Analyses

Statistical analyses were conducted using Matlab 2018b. Continuous variables were described using means and standard deviations, and categorical variables were summarized using frequencies. The normality distribution of continuous data was verified with a one-sample Kolmogorov-Smirnov Test. Pearson correlation was used to investigate the relationship between the structural measures and clinical scores. Age, gender, and educational level were regressed out before correlation analysis. The independent *t*-test were applied to perform the group comparisons for continuous demographic and clinical variables. The categorical demographic was computed using a Chi-square test. Statistical significance was set at $p < 0.05$ (false discovery rate [FDR] corrected). Missing data were not included in all analysis.

3. Results

3.1. Demographic and Clinical Characteristics

Thirty-two TBI patients and 23 healthy controls were included in the present study, with the demographic and clinical parameters shown in Table 1. Overall, 31.25% of patients had moderate–severe and 68.75% mild TBI. Average time since injury was 8.47 months. There were no significant differences between the TBI group and healthy controls in terms of gender ($p = 0.949$), age ($p = 0.422$) or education years ($p = 0.756$). Relative to healthy controls, TBI patients had lower level of MMSE scores. Moreover, they performed worse on memory function tests and presented more anxiety and depressive symptoms.

Table 1. The demographic and clinical characteristics in TBI patients and healthy controls.

	TBI (n = 32)	Healthy Controls (n = 23)	p Value
Age, mean (SD), y	35.59 (10.64)	33.35 (9.42)	0.422
Male, No. (%)	22 (68.35%)	16 (69.57%)	0.949
Educational lever, mean (SD), y	9.22 (4.16)	9.57 (3.89)	0.756
Time since injury, mean (SD), m	8.41 (7.02)	NA	NA
GCS, No. (%)			
13–15	22 (68.75%)	NA	NA
9–12	6 (12.89%)	NA	NA
3–8	4 (12.50%)	NA	NA
MMSE, mean (SD)	27.281 (2.57)	29.26 (0.92)	0.001
HADS anxiety, mean (SD)	8.63 (4.65)	4.22 (2.43)	<0.001
HADS depression, mean (SD)	7.97 (5.96)	3.09 (2.25)	<0.001
Memory, mean (SD)	40.31 (13.54)	52.04 (7.10)	<0.001

TBI: traumatic brain injury; GCS: Glasgow coma scale; MMSE: mini mental state examination; HADS: hospital anxiety and depression scale; NA: not applicable.

3.2. Reduced GM Volumes in Patients with Traumatic Brain Injury

As shown in Figure 1A, focal lesions were mainly present in bilateral orbitofrontal and temporal cortical regions. Compared to healthy controls, TBI patients underwent widespread decrease of GM volume in the bilateral frontal and temporal gyrus, left cingulate gyrus, and right insular lobe, particularly in the right orbitofrontal, left inferior, and middle temporal lobe, and subgenual anterior cingulate cortex (Figure 1B, Table 2). In subcortical regions, decreased GM volumes were observed in the bilateral amygdala, right hippocampus, left nucleus accumbens, and bilateral rostral temporal thalamus.

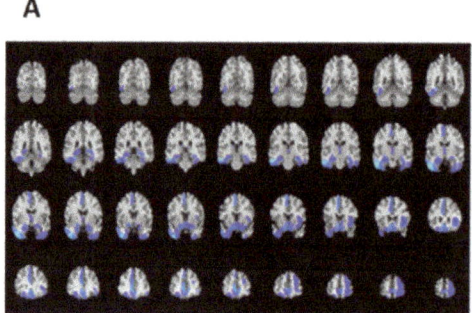
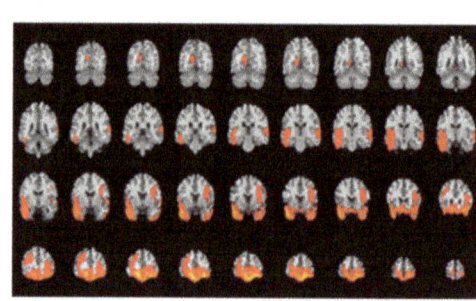

Figure 1. Lesion map following TBI (**A**) and differences in GM volumes between TBI participants and healthy controls (**B**).

Table 2. Brain regions with statistical difference between TBI patients and healthy controls.

Regions [#]	TBI (n = 32) Mean (±SD), mm^3	HC (n = 23) Mean (±SD), mm^3	% of Volumetric Decreases	p Value
SFG_L_7_1	679.38 ± 95.23	763.34 ± 80.17	11.00%	0.019
SFG_L_7_5	688.43 ± 90.55	762.78 ± 79.24	9.75%	0.033
SFG_L_7_6	617.15 ± 104.01	704.67 ± 91.78	12.42%	0.033
MFG_R_7_3	770.74 ± 175.19	914.94 ± 132.80	15.76%	0.041
MFG_R_7_7	724.51 ± 155.40	851.19 ± 112.29	14.88%	0.045
IFG_R_6_5	522.33 ± 75.282	601.15 ± 101.43	13.11%	0.034
OrG_L_6_1	415.58 ± 88.91	487.35 ± 65.21	14.73%	0.048
OrG_R_6_1	549.00 ± 129.35	677.97 ± 98.88	19.02%	0.017
OrG_L_6_3	760.58 ± 144.75	886.59 ± 110.28	14.21%	0.034
OrG_L_6_5	907.44 ± 148.74	1056.28 ± 137.44	14.09%	0.017
OrG_R_6_5	755.51 ± 134.16	879.01 ± 112.78	14.05%	0.033
OrG_R_6_6	412.28 ± 67.12	472.76 ± 56.05	12.79%	0.034
STG_L_6_1	632.45 ± 129.23	727.36 ± 90.08	13.05%	0.048
MTG_L_4_2	692.60 ± 151.93	835.50 ± 126.73	17.10%	0.017
ITG_L_7_1	252.28 ± 45.31	300.55 ± 45.66	16.06%	0.017
ITG_L_7_3	461.55 ± 84.69	568.62 ± 81.82	18.83%	0.005
ITG_R_7_3	410.09 ± 73.29	474.31 ± 55.33	13.54%	0.034
ITG_L_7_4	431.60 ± 89.55	551.51 ± 82.59	21.74%	<0.001
ITG_R_7_4	480.15 ± 80.21	553.43 ± 82.71	13.24%	0.035
ITG_L_7_7	497.54 ± 89.74	586.11 ± 92.01	15.11%	0.017
FuG_L_3_1	997.68 ± 149.18	1154.11 ± 146.99	13.55%	0.017
FuG_R_3_1	1111.18 ± 164.05	1244.75 ± 145.85	10.73%	0.047
FuG_L_3_3	948.99 ± 136.76	1061.95 ± 148.23	10.64%	0.050
PhG_L_6_5	115.27 ± 17.03	130.30 ± 18.02	11.53%	0.039
INS_R_6_2	246.82 ± 31.88	276.64 ± 37.96	10.78%	0.035
INS_R_6_3	285.86 ± 41.35	323.85 ± 54.10	11.73%	0.050
CG_L_7_3	470.88 ± 88.78	554.36 ± 66.22	15.06%	0.017
CG_L_7_7	633.52 ± 147.04	794.16 ± 118.78	20.23%	0.006
Amyg_L_2_1	185.75 ± 21.72	207.61 ± 26.65	10.53%	0.034
Amyg_R_2_1	267.19 ± 32.58	297.09 ± 38.82	10.07%	0.049
Amyg_L_2_2	93.16 ± 10.40	103.25 ± 12.28	9.77%	0.033
Amyg_R_2_2	140.75 ± 15.64	156.67 ± 18.30	10.16%	0.028
Hipp_L_2_1	666.67 ± 80.30	737.97 ± 80.84	9.66%	0.034
Hipp_L_2_2	485.14 ± 67.36	541.11 ± 64.92	10.34%	0.050
Hipp_R_2_2	566.44 ± 75.22	633.31 ± 60.04	10.56%	0.034
BG_L_6_3	368.88 ± 49.71	411.61 ± 48.00	10.38%	0.033
BG_R_6_3	456.63 ± 64.02	507.36 ± 57.34	10.00%	0.050
Tha_L_8_4	174.26 ± 30.13	198.40 ± 24.08	12.17%	0.034
Tha_R_8_4	185.47 ± 33.66	213.33 ± 28.92	13.06%	0.034

[#] Brainnetome atlas; TBI: traumatic brain injury; HC: healthy controls.

3.3. Correlations between GM Volume and Clinical Parameters in Patients with Traumatic Brain Injury

Although extensive atrophy was observed in the cortical and subcortical structures, only a small set of brain regions correlate with the clinical parameters, as shown in Table 3. There were significant correlations ($p < 0.05$ uncorrected) between MMSE scores and GM volumes in the left inferior temporal gyrus extending to the left fusiform gyrus and middle temporal gyrus, bilateral hippocampus, left anterior cingulate cortex (ACC), and left thalamus. Specifically, the total memory scores were associated with the GM volume of the left thalamus, right middle frontal gyrus, and insular lobe. Analysis of the anxiety and depressive symptoms showed that the GM volume of the supplementary motor area was correlated to anxiety and depressive symptoms. In addition, the anxiety symptoms were also significantly associated with the decreased GM volume of the left hippocampus. In brief, four brain areas–the left inferior temporal gyrus and medial temporal lobe, supplementary motor area, thalamus, and ACC–were highly implicated in the post-traumatic cognitive impairment and psychiatric complaints.

Table 3. Significant correlations between the GM volumes and clinical parameters in TBI patients.

Regions [#]	MMSE		Memory		HADS-A		HADS-D	
	r_Value	p_Value	r_Value	p_Value	r_Value	p_Value	r_Value	p_Value
SFG_L_7_1	NS	NS	NS	NS	NS	NS	0.36	0.04
SFG_L_7_5	NS	NS	NS	NS	0.37	0.03	NS	NS
MFG_R_7_3	NS	NS	−0.34	0.05	NS	NS	NS	NS
MTG_L_4_2	0.45	0.01	NS	NS	NS	NS	NS	NS
ITG_L_7_1	0.37	0.03	NS	NS	NS	NS	NS	NS
ITG_L_7_4	0.49	<0.01	NS	NS	NS	NS	NS	NS
ITG_L_7_7	0.36	0.04	NS	NS	NS	NS	NS	NS
FuG_L_3_1	0.45	0.01	NS	NS	NS	NS	NS	NS
FuG_L_3_3	0.58	<0.01	NS	NS	NS	NS	NS	NS
INS_R_6_2	NS	NS	−0.45	0.01	NS	NS	NS	NS
CG_L_7_3	0.40	0.02	NS	NS	NS	NS	NS	NS
Hipp_L_2_2	0.55	<0.01	NS	NS	0.38	0.03	NS	NS
Hipp_R_2_2	0.44	0.01	NS	NS	NS	NS	NS	NS
Tha_L_8_4	0.49	<0.01	0.51	<0.01	NS	NS	NS	NS

[#] Brainnetome atlas; NS: not significant MMSE: mini mental state examination; HADS-A: hospital anxiety and depression scale: anxiety; HADS-D: hospital anxiety and depression scale: depression.

3.4. WM Microstructure Alterations in Patients with Traumatic Brain Injury

Compared with the healthy controls, TBI patients showed a significantly decreased FA value in widespread WM tracts, including the left inferior fronto-occipital fasciculus (IFOF), left superior longitudinal fasciculus (SLF), bilateral uncinate fasciculus (UF), forceps major, and forceps minor (Figure 2, Table 4). Mean diffusivity of WM regions showed significant difference in the forceps minor.

Table 4. Significant outcome of WM integrity between TBI patients and healthy controls.

Regions [#]	Fractional Anisotropy			Mean Diffusivity		
	TBI (n = 32) Mean (±SD)	HC (n = 23) Mean (±SD)	p-Value	TBI (n = 32) Mean (±SD)	HC (n = 23) Mean (±SD)	p-Value
Forceps.major	0.68 ± 0.02	0.70 ± 0.02	0.03	NS	NS	NS
Forceps.minor	0.53 ± 0.03	0.56 ± 0.03	0.01	0.00077 ± 0.000036	0.00073 ± 0.000043	0.04
Inferior.fronto-occipital.fasciculus.L	0.51 ± 0.03	0.53 ± 0.03	0.04	NS	NS	NS
Superior.longitudinal.fasciculus.L	0.48 ± 0.03	0.49 ± 0.03	0.04	NS	NS	NS
Uncinate.fasciculus.L	0.48 ± 0.05	0.52 ± 0.03	0.03	NS	NS	NS
Uncinate.fasciculus.R	0.52 ± 0.05	0.55 ± 0.03	0.04	NS	NS	NS

[#] JHU White-Matter Tractography Atlas; NS: not significant; TBI: traumatic brain injury; HC: healthy controls.

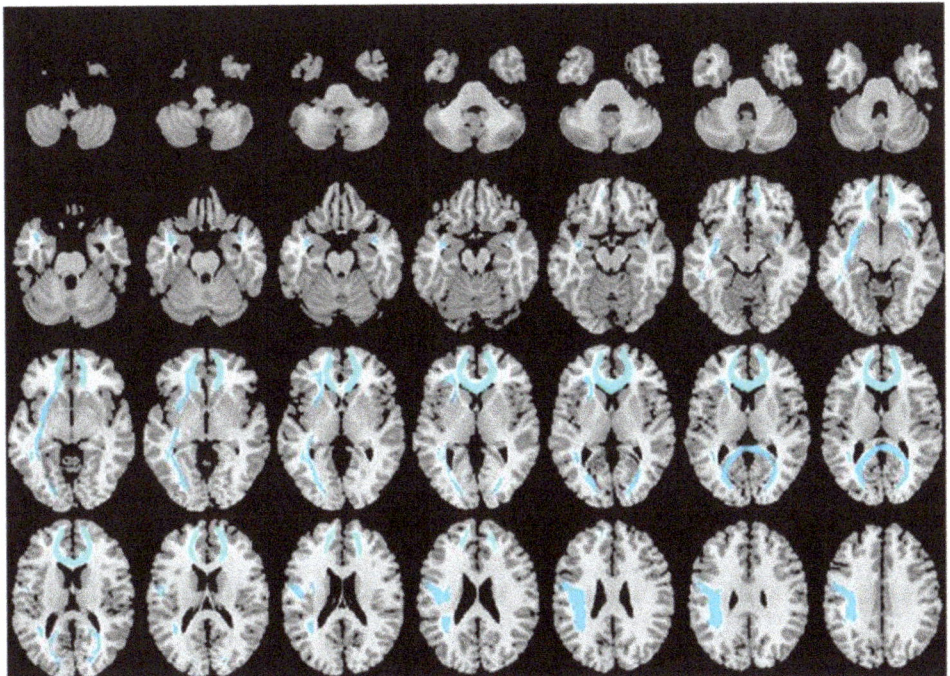

Figure 2. Voxel-wise Tract-Based Spatial Statistics differences in FA metrics between group.

As UF and IFOF traverse the temporal lobe, which is closely related to the post-traumatic cognitive function and psychiatric symptoms, we further explored the relationship between these two fiber tracks and the GM structures of the temporal gyrus and medial temporal lobe. GM volumes were significantly related to the FA of left UF and left IFOF in multiple regions of left temporal gyrus and left hippocampus (Table 5). No statistically significant association was found between SLF and the GM volumes of the supplementary motor area.

Table 5. The relationship between fractional anisotropy and GM volume in the temporal gyrus and medial temporal lobe of TBI Subjects.

	Left Uncinate Fasciculus		Left Inferior Fronto-Occipital Fasciculus	
Regions [#]	r	p	r	p
STG_L_6_1	0.358	0.041	NS	NS
STG_L_6_2	−0.439	0.011	−0.399	0.021
STG_L_6_5	0.435	0.011	NS	NS
STG_L_6_6	0.347	0.048	NS	NS
MTG_L_4_1	0.391	0.025	NS	NS
MTG_L_4_2	0.555	<0.001	NS	NS
MTG_L_4_3	0.491	0.004	0.427	0.013
ITG_L_7_1	0.504	0.003	0.573	<0.001
ITG_L_7_3	0.398	0.022	NS	NS
ITG_L_7_4	0.397	0.022	NS	NS

Table 5. Cont.

Regions [#]	Left Uncinate Fasciculus		Left Inferior Fronto-Occipital Fasciculus	
	r	p	r	p
ITG_L_7_5	0.403	0.020	NS	NS
ITG_L_7_6	0.542	0.001	0.530	0.002
FuG_L_3_1	0.471	0.006	NS	NS
FuG_L_3_3	NS	NS	0.379	0.029
PhG_L_6_1	0.422	0.014	NS	NS
PhG_L_6_2	NS	NS	0.387	0.026
PhG_L_6_4	0.464	0.007	0.359	0.040
PhG_L_6_5	0.598	<0.001	NS	NS
Hipp_L_2_1	0.559	<0.001	NS	NS
Hipp_L_2_1	0.512	0.002	NS	NS

[#] Brainnetome atlas; NS: not significant.

4. Discussion

In this work, we systemically investigated differences in whole-brain GM and WM between participants with TBI and healthy controls and explored their relationships with clinical measurements. We first demonstrated TBI patients underwent widespread decrease of GM volume in both cortical regions and subcortical regions. Among these regions, four brain areas including left inferior temporal gyrus and medial temporal lobe, supplementary motor area, thalamus, and ACC were highly implicated in the post-traumatic cognitive impairment and psychiatric complaints. We then found WM microstructure was disrupted in TBI patients, involving a decreased FA value in widespread WM tracts including the left IFOF, left SLF, bilateral UF, forceps major, and forceps minor, with an increased MD value in the forceps minor. Finally, we explored the consistency of structural damage in gray and WM, showing GM volumes were significantly related to the FA of left UF and left IFOF in multiple regions of left temporal gyrus and left hippocampus.

About 1.7 million people in the United States develop TBI each year, and more than 50,000 people have severe cognitive impairment [20]. In China, TBI occupies second place in the incidence of systemic trauma and first place in the fatality and disability rate [21]. Most TBI patients are young and middle-aged patients, and may suffer from long-time loss of living and working ability. The primary injury of TBI may not be serious, but due to changes in the local pathological environment after trauma, it is easy to induce diffuse axonal injury, which indicates damage to axons and surrounding fibers [22]. Patients gradually develop affective and cognitive dysfunction. Therefore, it is of great clinical significance to study the changes of brain microstructure after TBI and its relationship with cognitive–emotional function.

In accordance with previous reports, TBI patients presented common abnormalities of brain morphology despite heterogeneity in injury severity and mechanisms, extent of focal insults, and time since injury [23–25]. Despite widespread atrophy across the cortical and subcortical regions, only a relatively small subset of this pattern of damage–mainly in the left inferior temporal gyrus and medial temporal lobe, supplementary motor area, thalamus, and ACC–were highly implicated in the post-traumatic cognitive impairment and psychiatric complaints. Among 32 TBI patients, those with temporal lobe injury had more severe symptoms than those with frontal lobe injury, especially those with lesions on the inferior temporal gyrus. Moreover, TBI causes extensive changes in the WM microstructure, including the left IFOF, left SLF, bilateral UF, forceps major, and forceps minor. GM volumes in multiple subregions of left temporal lobe and left hippocampus were significantly related to the FA of left UF and left IFOF. This provides some inspiration for our clinical work.

Although the frontal lobe and temporal lobe are most likely to be injured in TBI, differences exist in their clinical manifestation and outcome [26,27]. Injury of the temporal lobe should be paid more attention; due to its anatomical position in the brain, the temporal lobe contains a large number of association fibers and commissural fibers. It has a complex integration effect on the frontal lobe, occipital lobe, and the sensory motor areas of parietal lobe, and plays a coordinating role between the anterior–posterior and left–right brain. The completion of brain function depends on the multi-synaptic information transmission of nerve fibers, and damage to the temporal lobe interrupts or affects the transmission of this information, resulting in cognitive and emotional dysfunction. Therefore, even small lesions in the temporal lobe should attract our high clinical attention. Early clinical monitoring of cognitive and emotional functions in patients with craniocerebral injury, and timely, comprehensive cognitive rehabilitation intervention is of great significance to prevent further functional decline and improve the quality of life of patients.

In our research, we demonstrated a widespread GM volume reduction in both cortical regions and subcortical regions. In addition to the reduction in GM volume at the immediate injury lesion, some deep structural GM volumes were also reduced and correlated with the patient's clinical presentation. Changes in the local metabolic environment and the occurrence of DAI may be responsible for this [28–30]. Eventually, patients have axonal and fiber damage, and gradually develop cognitive impairment and altered affective function. We also calculated the FA and MD values of the WM fiber tracts, and found a significantly decreased FA value in widespread WM tracts including the left IFOF, left SLF, bilateral UF, forceps major, and forceps minor, with a significantly increased MD value in the forceps minor. Among these fiber tracks, the forceps minor and forceps major are the interhemispheric fibers of the frontal cortex and occipital cortex, respectively, and the UF, IFOF, and SLF are intrahemispheric association fibers. The UF and IFOF connect the temporal lobe with orbital and polar frontal cortex, and the SLF links the frontal lobe with parietal lobe. This means that although the damage mostly occurs in the cerebral cortex in TBI patients, irreversible structural damage to WM fiber tracts still occurs, and both intrahemispheric associative fibers and interhemispheric fibers will break, leading to the appearance of symptoms in patients.

The human brain has an overall leftward posterior and rightward anterior asymmetry, which may help to provide cognitive advantages and solve spatial constraints [31,32]. Existing studies have confirmed that there is brain asymmetry in normal aging or neuropsychiatric and neurodegenerative diseases [33,34]. Under pathological conditions, the left hemisphere may be mainly affected [35]; we found such leftward lateralization in our research. Damage to the integrity of the left IFOF and left SLF is significantly stronger than that of the right side, which is also consistent with the reduction of GM volume of left temporal gyrus and left hippocampus. This can be explained as TBI promotes the degradation of WM in the non-dominant hemisphere or leads to the transformation of structure to the dominant hemisphere. However, any inference about the change direction of symmetry after TBI is complex and needs further exploration.

Early parcellation efforts aimed at defining regional boundaries using limited samples, including the widely used Brodmann atlas and automated anatomical labeling (AAL) atlas [36,37]. The Brainnetome Atlas is a connectivity-based parcellation of the brain, which establishes a priori, biologically valid brain parcellation scheme of the entire cortical and subcortical GM into sub-regions showing a coherent pattern of anatomical connections and provides a new framework for human brain research and in particular connectome analysis [38–41]. Thus, in this research we used The Brainnetome Atlas to more accurately describe the locations of the activation or connectivity in the brain.

We also analyzed the limitations of our research for further improvement. First, the population enrolled in this study was relatively small and consisted of Chinese only. With the different brain injured regions of patients, the degree of injury is not consistent, which may lead to high heterogeneity among patients and an impact on the results. Secondly, patients are often accompanied with cognitive impairment and emotional dysfunction;

these confounding factors will add to the difficulty of analysis of drawing conclusions on the correlation between changes in gray and WM structure and cognitive and affective dysfunction. Thirdly, the HADS scale for emotional dysfunction is a self-reported questionnaire. It is possible that TBI patients with cognitive impairment tend to overestimate or underestimate their mood problems, which may reduce the credibility of the conclusion. Finally, as a retrospective cross-sectional study, it is prone to produce selection bias and recall bias, which affects the precision of the outcome.

In conclusion, we shed light on differences in whole-brain GM and WM maps and explored their clinical significance. Briefly, four brain regions, including the left inferior temporal gyrus and medial temporal lobe, supplementary motor area, thalamus, and ACC, correlated to cognitive performance and psychiatric complaints following TBI, and injury of the temporal lobe should be paid more attention.

Author Contributions: Conceptualization, Y.D.; Data curation, Q.X. and J.W.; Formal analysis, L.W. and G.L.; Funding acquisition, L.G. and Y.D.; Investigation, Q.X., Y.Z., G.L. and Y.D.; Methodology, L.W., W.T. and W.C.; Project administration, L.G.; Resources, W.T. and L.G.; Software, J.W.; Supervision, W.C.; Writing—original draft, Q.X., Y.Z. and W.C.; Writing—review & editing, Y.D. All authors have read and agreed to the published version of the manuscript.

Funding: This research was funded by the National Natural Science Foundation of China (grant number 81671227). And The APC was funded by the same funding.

Informed Consent Statement: Informed consent was obtained from all subjects involved in the study.

Acknowledgments: We are grateful to the participating patients and the healthy controls. Without you, this study would not have been possible.

Conflicts of Interest: The authors declare no conflict of interest.

References

1. Bombardier, C.H.; Fann, J.R.; Temkin, N.R.; Esselman, P.C.; Barber, J.; Dikmen, S.S. Rates of major depressive disorder and clinical outcomes following traumatic brain injury. *JAMA* **2010**, *303*, 1938–1945. [CrossRef] [PubMed]
2. Ponsford, J.; Alway, Y.; Gould, K.R. Epidemiology and Natural History of Psychiatric Disorders After TBI. *J. Neuropsychiatry Clin. Neurosci.* **2018**, *30*, 262–270. [CrossRef] [PubMed]
3. Graham, N.S.; Sharp, D.J. Understanding neurodegeneration after traumatic brain injury: From mechanisms to clinical trials in dementia. *J. Neurol. Neurosurg. Psychiatry* **2019**, *90*, 1221–1233. [CrossRef] [PubMed]
4. Fazel, S.; Wolf, A.; Pillas, D.; Lichtenstein, P.; Långström, N. Suicide, fatal injuries, and other causes of premature mortality in patients with traumatic brain injury: A 41-year Swedish population study. *JAMA Psychiatry* **2014**, *71*, 326–333. [CrossRef]
5. Alway, Y.; Gould, K.R.; Johnston, L.; McKenzie, D.; Ponsford, J. A prospective examination of Axis I psychiatric disorders in the first 5 years following moderate to severe traumatic brain injury. *Psychol. Med.* **2016**, *46*, 1331–1341. [CrossRef]
6. Singh, R.; Mason, S.; Lecky, F.; Dawson, J. Comparison of early and late depression after TBI; (the SHEFBIT study). *Brain Inj.* **2019**, *33*, 584–591. [CrossRef]
7. Khellaf, A.; Khan, D.Z.; Helmy, A. Recent advances in traumatic brain injury. *J. Neurol.* **2019**, *266*, 2878–2889. [CrossRef]
8. Gentry, L.R.; Godersky, J.C.; Thompson, B. MR imaging of head trauma: Review of the distribution and radiopathologic features of traumatic lesions. *AJR Am. J. Roentgenol.* **1988**, *150*, 663–672. [CrossRef]
9. McAllister, T.W. Neurobiological consequences of traumatic brain injury. *Dialogues Clin. Neurosci.* **2011**, *13*, 287–300. [CrossRef]
10. Mesfin, F.B.; Gupta, N.; Hays Shapshak, A.; Taylor, R.S. Diffuse axonal injury. In *StatPearls*; StatPearls Publishing: Treasure Island, FL, USA, 2021.
11. Stuss, D.T. Traumatic brain injury: Relation to executive dysfunction and the frontal lobes. *Curr. Opin. Neurol.* **2011**, *24*, 584–589. [CrossRef]
12. Bigler, E.D. Distinguished Neuropsychologist Award Lecture 1999. The lesion(s) in traumatic brain injury: Implications for clinical neuropsychology. *Arch. Clin. Neuropsychol.* **2001**, *16*, 95–131. [CrossRef] [PubMed]
13. Misquitta, K.; Dadar, M.; Tarazi, A.; Hussain, M.W.; Alatwi, M.K.; Ebraheem, A.; Multani, N.; Khodadadi, M.; Goswami, R.; Wennberg, R.; et al. The relationship between brain atrophy and cognitive-behavioural symptoms in retired Canadian football players with multiple concussions. *Neuroimage Clin.* **2018**, *19*, 551–558. [CrossRef] [PubMed]
14. Lutkenhoff, E.S.; Wright, M.J.; Shrestha, V.; Real, C.; McArthur, D.L.; Buitrago-Blanco, M.; Vespa, P.M.; Monti, M.M. The subcortical basis of outcome and cognitive impairment in TBI: A longitudinal cohort study. *Neurology* **2020**, *95*, e2398–e2408. [CrossRef]
15. Johnson, V.E.; Stewart, J.E.; Begbie, F.D.; Trojanowski, J.Q.; Smith, D.H.; Stewart, W. Inflammation and WM degeneration persist for years after a single traumatic brain injury. *Brain* **2013**, *136 Pt 1*, 28–42. [CrossRef] [PubMed]

16. Xiong, Y.; Mahmood, A.; Chopp, M. Current understanding of neuroinflammation after traumatic brain injury and cell-based therapeutic opportunities. *Chin. J. Traumatol.* **2018**, *21*, 137–151. [CrossRef] [PubMed]
17. Lauer, J.; Moreno-López, L.; Manktelow, A.; Carroll, E.L.; Outtrim, J.G.; Coles, J.P.; Newcombe, V.F.; Sahakian, B.J.; Menon, D.K.; Stamatakis, E.A. Neural correlates of visual memory in patients with diffuse axonal injury. *Brain Inj.* **2017**, *31*, 1513–1520. [CrossRef]
18. Spitz, G.; Bigler, E.D.; Abildskov, T.; Maller, J.J.; O'Sullivan, R.; Ponsford, J.L. Regional cortical volume and cognitive functioning following traumatic brain injury. *Brain Cogn.* **2013**, *83*, 34–44. [CrossRef]
19. Mori, S.; Oishi, K.; Jiang, H.; Jiang, L.; Li, X.; Akhter, K.; Hua, K.; Faria, A.V.; Mahmood, A.; Woods, R. Stereotaxic WM atlas based on diffusion tensor imaging in an ICBM template. *Neuroimage* **2008**, *40*, 570–582. [CrossRef]
20. Marin, J.R.; Weaver, M.D.; Yealy, D.M.; Mannix, R.C. Trends in visits for traumatic brain injury to emergency departments in the United States. *JAMA* **2014**, *311*, 1917–1919. [CrossRef]
21. Lu, L.; Li, F.; Ma, Y.; Chen, H.; Wang, P.; Peng, M.; Chen, Y.C.; Yin, X. Functional connectivity disruption of the substantia nigra associated with cognitive impairment in acute mild traumatic brain injury. *Eur. J. Radiol.* **2019**, *114*, 69–75. [CrossRef]
22. Kanthimathinathan, H.K.; Mehta, H.; Scholefield, B.R.; Morris, K.P. Traumatic Brain Injury Practice Guidelines: Variability in U.K. PICUs. *Pediatr. Crit. Care Med.* **2021**, *22*, e270–e274. [CrossRef] [PubMed]
23. Gutierre, M.U.; Telles, J.P.M.; Welling, L.C.; Rabelo, N.N.; Teixeira, M.J.; Figueiredo, E.G. Biomarkers for traumatic brain injury: A short review. *Neurosurg. Rev.* **2021**, *44*, 2091–2097. [CrossRef] [PubMed]
24. Bourgeois-Tardif, S.; de Beaumont, L.; Rivera, J.C.; Chemtob, S.; Weil, A.G. Role of innate inflammation in traumatic brain injury. *Neurol. Sci.* **2021**, *42*, 1287–1299. [CrossRef] [PubMed]
25. Livny, A.; Biegon, A.; Kushnir, T.; Harnof, S.; Hoffmann, C.; Fruchter, E.; Weiser, M. Cognitive Deficits Post-Traumatic Brain Injury and Their Association with Injury Severity and GM Volumes. *J. Neurotrauma* **2017**, *34*, 1466–1472. [CrossRef]
26. Wallace, E.J.; Mathias, J.L.; Ward, L. The relationship between diffusion tensor imaging findings and cognitive outcomes following adult traumatic brain injury: A meta-analysis. *Neurosci. Biobehav. Rev.* **2018**, *92*, 93–103. [CrossRef]
27. Grassi, D.C.; Conceição, D.M.D.; Leite, C.D.C.; Andrade, C.S. Current contribution of diffusion tensor imaging in the evaluation of diffuse axonal injury. *Arq. Neuropsiquiatr.* **2018**, *76*, 189–199. [CrossRef]
28. Wallace, E.J.; Mathias, J.L.; Ward, L. Diffusion tensor imaging changes following mild, moderate and severe adult traumatic brain injury: A meta-analysis. *Brain Imaging Behav.* **2018**, *12*, 1607–1621. [CrossRef]
29. D'Souza, M.M.; Kumar, M.; Choudhary, A.; Kaur, P.; Kumar, P.; Rana, P.; Trivedi, R.; Sekhri, T.; Singh, A.K. Alterations of connectivity patterns in functional brain networks in patients with mild traumatic brain injury: A longitudinal resting-state functional magnetic resonance imaging study. *Neuroradiol. J.* **2020**, *33*, 186–197. [CrossRef]
30. Sporns, O. Graph theory methods: Applications in brain networks. *Dialogues Clin. Neurosci.* **2018**, *20*, 111–121. [CrossRef]
31. Duboc, V.; Dufourcq, P.; Blader, P.; Roussigné, M. Asymmetry of the Brain: Development and Implications. *Annu. Rev. Genet.* **2015**, *49*, 647–672. [CrossRef]
32. Minkova, L.; Habich, A.; Peter, J.; Kaller, C.P.; Eickhoff, S.B.; Klöppel, S. GM asymmetries in aging and neurodegeneration: A review and meta-analysis. *Hum. Brain Mapp.* **2017**, *38*, 5890–5904. [CrossRef] [PubMed]
33. Kalia, L.V.; Lang, A.E. Parkinson's disease. *Lancet* **2015**, *386*, 896–912. [CrossRef]
34. Zhong, Z.; Merkitch, D.; Karaman, M.M.; Zhang, J.; Sui, Y.; Goldman, J.G.; Zhou, X.J. High-Spatial-Resolution Diffusion MRI in Parkinson Disease: Lateral Asymmetry of the Substantia Nigra. *Radiology* **2019**, *291*, 149–157. [CrossRef] [PubMed]
35. He, Y.; Evans, A. Graph theoretical modeling of brain connectivity. *Curr. Opin. Neurol.* **2010**, *23*, 341–350. [CrossRef] [PubMed]
36. Manley, G.T.; Mac Donald, C.L.; Markowitz, A.J.; Stephenson, D.; Robbins, A.; Gardner, R.C.; Winkler, E.; Bodien, Y.G.; Taylor, S.R.; Yue, J.K.; et al. The Traumatic Brain Injury Endpoints Development (TED) Initiative: Progress on a Public-Private Regulatory Collaboration to Accelerate Diagnosis and Treatment of Traumatic Brain Injury. *J. Neurotrauma* **2017**, *34*, 2721–2730. [CrossRef] [PubMed]
37. Kwak, E.H.; Wi, S.; Kim, M.; Pyo, S.; Shin, Y.K.; Oh, K.J.; Han, K.; Kim, Y.W.; Cho, S.R. Factors affecting cognition and emotion in patients with traumatic brain injury. *NeuroRehabilitation* **2020**, *46*, 369–379. [CrossRef]
38. Pandit, A.S.; Expert, P.; Lambiotte, R.; Bonnelle, V.; Leech, R.; Turkheimer, F.E.; Sharp, D.J. Traumatic brain injury impairs small-world topology. *Neurology* **2013**, *80*, 1826–1833. [CrossRef]
39. Fagerholm, E.D.; Hellyer, P.J.; Scott, G.; Leech, R.; Sharp, D.J. Disconnection of network hubs and cognitive impairment after traumatic brain injury. *Brain* **2015**, *138 Pt 6*, 1696–1709. [CrossRef]
40. Raichle, M.E. The brain's default mode network. *Annu. Rev. Neurosci.* **2015**, *38*, 433–447. [CrossRef]
41. Palacios, E.M.; Owen, J.P.; Yuh, E.L.; Wang, M.B.; Vassar, M.J.; Ferguson, A.R.; Diaz-Arrastia, R.; Giacino, J.T.; Okonkwo, D.O.; Robertson, C.S.; et al. TRACK-TBI Investigators. The evolution of WM microstructural changes after mild traumatic brain injury: A longitudinal DTI and NODDI study. *Sci. Adv.* **2020**, *6*, eaaz6892. [CrossRef]

MDPI
St. Alban-Anlage 66
4052 Basel
Switzerland
Tel. +41 61 683 77 34
Fax +41 61 302 89 18
www.mdpi.com

Journal of Clinical Medicine Editorial Office
E-mail: jcm@mdpi.com
www.mdpi.com/journal/jcm

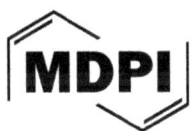

www.ingramcontent.com/pod-product-compliance
Lightning Source LLC
LaVergne TN
LVHW070400100526
838202LV00014B/1359